Multiple Pregnancy and Delivery

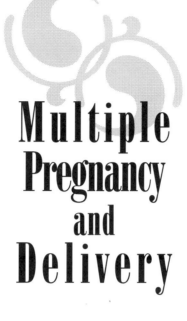

Multiple Pregnancy and Delivery

Stanley A. Gall, M.D.

Donald E. Baxter Professor and Chairman
Department of Obstetrics and Gynecology
University of Louisville School of Medicine
Louisville, Kentucky

with 68 illustrations

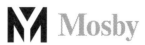

Mosby

St. Louis Baltimore Boston Carlsbad Chicago Naples New York Philadelphia Portland
London Madrid Mexico City Singapore Sydney Tokyo Toronto Wiesbaden

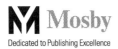
Mosby
Dedicated to Publishing Excellence

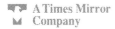
A Times Mirror
Company

Vice President and Publisher: Anne S. Patterson
Editor: Susie Baxter
Developmental Editor: Ellen Baker Geisel
Project Manager: Deborah L. Vogel
Production Editor: Karen L. Allman
Designer: Pati Pye
Manufacturing Supervisor: Linda M. Ierardi

Printed in the United States of America
Composition by Clarinda Company
Printing/binding by Courier

Mosby-Year Book, Inc.
11830 Westline Industrial Drive
St. Louis, Missouri 64146

International Standard Book Number 0-8151-3406-1

96 97 98 99 00 / 9 8 7 6 5 4 3 2 1

Contributors

William E. Ackerman III, M.D.
The Pain Care Center
Little Rock, Arkansas

Richard L. Berkowitz, M.D.
Professor and Chairman,
Department of Obstetrics, Gynecology, and Reproductive Science,
Mt. Sinai University School of Medicine;
Chief of Service,
Department of Obstetrics, Gynecology, and Reproductive Science,
Mount Sinai Medical Center,
New York, New York

Suneet P. Chauhan, M.D.
Assistant Professor,
Department of Obstetrics and Gynecology,
Medical College of Georgia
Augusta, Georgia

Frank A. Chervenak, M.D.
Professor, Department of Obstetrics and Gynecology,
Cornell University School of Medicine;
Director, Maternal-Fetal Medicine,
Department of Obstetrics and Gynecology,
The New York Hospital,
New York, New York

Arie Drugan, M.D.
Director, Division of Reproductive Genetics,
Department of Obstetrics and Gynecology,
Rambam Medical Center,
Haifa, Israel

Mark I. Evans, M.D., Ph.D.
Professor of Ob/Gyn, Microbiology and Genetics, and Pathology,
Wayne State University School of Medicine;
Professor and Vice-Chief of Obstetrics and Gynecology,
Director, Division of Reproductive Genetics and Center for Fetal Diagnosis and Therapy,
Department of Obstetrics and Gynecology,
Hutzel Hospital,
Detroit, Michigan

Stanley A. Gall, M.D.
Donald E. Baxter Professor and Chairman,
Department of Obstetrics and Gynecology,
University of Louisville School of Medicine;
Louisville, Kentucky

Michael O. Gardner, M.D., MPH
Assistant Professor,
Maternal Fetal Medicine,
University of New Mexico
Albuquerque, New Mexico

Alexandra Gerassimides, M.D.
Assistant Professor,
Department of Pathology,
University of Louisville School of Medicine;
Director, Division of Perinatal Pathology,
Department of Pathology,
University of Louisville Hospital,
Louisville, Kentucky

Larry C. Gilstrap III, M.D.
Professor of Obstetrics and Gynecology;
Director, Maternal-Fetal Medicine Fellowship Program,
Department of Obstetrics and Gynecology,
University of Texas Southwest Health Science Center,
Dallas, Texas

Mark P. Johnson, M.D.
Assistant Professor of Ob/Gyn, Molecular Biology and Genetics, and Pathology,
Wayne State University School of Medicine;
Associate Director,
Division of Reproductive Genetics,
Department of Obstetrics and Gynecology,
Hutzel Hospital,
Detroit, Michigan

Eric L. Krivchenia, M.S.
Genetic Counselor and Coordinator,
Department of Obstetrics and Gynecology,
Division of Reproductive Genetics,
Hutzel Hospital,
Detroit, Michigan

Dennis M. O'Connor, M.D.
Associate Professor of Obstetrics and Gynecology and Pathology,
Departments of Obstetrics and Gynecology and Pathology,
University of Louisville School of Medicine,
Louisville, Kentucky

Marcello Pietrantoni, M.D.
Assistant Professor,
Department of Obstetrics and Gynecology,
University of Louisville School of Medicine,
Louisville, Kentucky

Dwight D. Pridham, M.D.
Assistant Professor,
Department of Obstetrics and Gynecology,
University of Louisville School of Medicine,
Louisville, Kentucky

Kirk D. Ramin, M.D.
Fellow, Maternal-Fetal Medicine,
Department of Obstetrics and Gynecology,
University of Texas Southwestern Medical Center,
Dallas, Texas

Susan M. Ramin, M.D.
Assistant Professor,
Department of Obstetrics and Gynecology,
University of Texas Southwestern Medical Center,
Dallas, Texas

William E. Roberts, M.D.
Associate Professor,
Department of Obstetrics and Gynecology,
University of Mississippi Medical Center,
Jackson, Mississippi

Daniel W. Skupski, M.D.
Assistant Professor,
Department of Obstetrics and Gynecology,
The New York Hospital;
Director of Fetal Assessment,
Division of Maternal-Fetal Medicine,
Cornell University School of Medicine
New York, New York

Joseph A. Spinnato, M.D.
Professor of Obstetrics and Gynecology,
Department of Obstetrics and Gynecology,
University of Louisville School of Medicine;
Director, Division of Maternal-Fetal Medicine,
University of Louisville Hospital,
Louisville, Kentucky

Joanne Stone, M.D.
Assistant Professor of Obstetrics, Gynecology, and Reproductive Science,
Mt. Sinai University School of Medicine;
Assistant Professor,
Department of Obstetrics, Gynecology, and Reproductive Science,
Mount Sinai Medical Center,
New York, New York

Deward H. Voss, M.D.
Assistant Professor,
Division of Maternal-Fetal Medicine,
Department of Obstetrics and Gynecology,
University of Louisville School of Medicine,
Louisville, Kentucky

Jonathan W. Weeks, M.D.
Assistant Professor,
Department of Obstetrics and Gynecology,
University of Louisville School of Medicine,
Louisville, Kentucky

Katharine D. Wenstrom, M.D.
Associate Professor,
Director, Prenatal Diagnosis,
Department of Obstetrics and Gynecology,
University of Alabama at Birmingham School of Medicine,
Birmingham, Alabama

This book is dedicated to my wife Flo, who has been a constant source of support. This book reminds me of the stillborn delivery of Flo's co-twin and the studies we have made since that event.

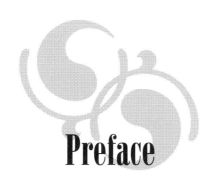

Preface

Multiple gestation is such a frequently encountered experience by obstetricians that it must be considered an epidemic. There is hardly a day that goes by on a busy Labor and Delivery Service that at least one patient with a multiple gestation is not present. The euphoria following the diagnosis of a multiple gestation by the patient and obstetrician is replaced by a realistic approach when the risks of the multiple gestation are explained to the patient and contemplated by the obstetrician.

The development of this publication was given impetus by a lack of complete clinical information regarding multiple gestation in a readable format easily accessible and affordable by the obstetrician and resident. This textbook discusses singleton gestations only as they compare and relate to multiple gestations. The various sections of this textbook are written by clinicians with extensive experience in the management of multiple gestation. In areas of management where there is no difference between the management of singleton and multiple gestations, the detailed management is not discussed, since it may be found in standard textbooks of obstetrics.

The epidemiology of multiple gestation is extensively discussed. Importantly, the bad news is that preterm delivery, intrauterine growth retardation, and congenital anomalies are occurring at a constant rate without signs of decreasing incidence. The good news is that survival, intact survival, and days in the neonatal intensive care unit are decreasing. We currently are more successful with multiple gestations than even 5 years ago.

The embryogenesis and placentation of multiple gestation may be associated with teratogenic events that predispose the pregnancy to disaster. The events that include the twinning process may be associated with abnormal development. This concept is developed more fully in the text.

An important etiology of the multiple gestation epidemic is the contribution by assisted reproductive technologies. The physicians utilizing these potent medications to induce ovulation or those involved in the variety of gamete manipulation must be knowledgeable in the ability to obtain a singleton pregnancy rather than a multiple gestation. This chapter discusses the impact of assisted reproductive technologies and how they should be used to minimize higher order gestations.

The section on ultrasound utilization is extensive and helpful in assessing multiple gestations. The changes in maternal physiology in multiple gestation, antepartum assessment, and fetal abnormalities is nicely discussed.

The outcomes of multiple gestations should be well known to all obstetricians and are discussed in detail. Despite improving statistics for multiple gestation, the fetuses and neonates remain at a significant increased risk of not surviving or surviving with a handicap.

An area that should be emphasized is the need for timely consultation with a maternal fetal medicine specialist. A multiple gestation is a high risk pregnancy, and personnel such as nurse midwives and family physicians do not have either the training or the experience to care for a patient with a multiple gestation. Obstetrics would likewise be advised that timely consultation could be rewarding. A well-developed game plan by the obstetrician may allow management by the obstetrician. However, if an adverse event occurs, such as preterm labor, discordant growth, diabetes mellitus, toxemia, or others, the referral lines are established and an effortless transport can occur. It is imperative that the patient with a multiple gestation deliver her infants in a facility with proper equipment and skilled personnel. A health maintenance organization (HMO) should not be allowed to dictate an inferior facility in the cause of financial expediency.

It is hoped that this textbook will live up to the goal of assisting the obstetrician in caring for multiple gestation. The goal of every obstetrician is a continuing improvement in the outcome of multiple gestations.

Stanley A. Gall, M.D.

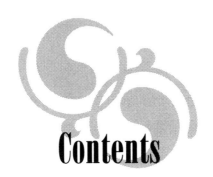

Contents

1 Epidemiology

Stanley A. Gall

The epidemiology of multiple gestation has taken on a new urgency for clinicians, since they are being subjected to an epidemic of multiple gestations. Multiple gestations have held a fascination for obstetricians, as well as historians and philosophers throughout history. Since 1980, the development of a variety of assisted reproductive techniques (ARTs) has made not only twins but multiple gestations of a higher order more common. When the euphoria of the knowledge of a multiple gestation has quieted, it is replaced by somber facts related to significant increases in morbidity, mortality, and severe disabilities that occur in multiple gestations compared with singleton gestations. Clinicians caring for women with multiple gestations need a broad knowledge base and must have access to adequate facilities and consultants for these mothers and infants. A twin or higher-order pregnancy truly constitutes a high-risk condition, and appropriate consultation is in order.

Etiology

The etiology of multiple gestation must be approached in several different ways. There is the endogenous, or natural, rate of twin, triplet, and other multiple pregnancies, and there is the exogenous multiple gestation created by ART. The differences caused by the two methods of conception are discussed wherever possible throughout this chapter.

In the natural setting or in the endogenous setting, twin fetuses result from the fertilization of two separate ova, thus creating dizygotic, or fraternal, twins. Two thirds of all natural twins are dizygotic, and their incidence depends on geography, race, maternal age, maternal past, and size. One third of twins result from a single fertilized ovum that subsequently divides at some time within the first 2 weeks of embryonic life. These twins are monozygotic, or identical. The same processes that produce the dizygotic or monozygotic twins can be repeated in the formation of higher-order gestations (such as triplets and quadruplets).

Monozygotic Twinning

Monozygotic twinning is usually considered to be a chance phenomenon associated with implantation delay and possibly with a lack of oxygen and nutrients. This theory is attractive because it could explain the higher incidence of malformations in monozygotic twins compared with

TABLE 1-1

Types of Monozygotic Twins and Mortality Rates

CHORION	AMNION	TIME TO DIVISION (DAYS)	RATE OF OCCURRENCE (%)	MORTALITY RATE (%)
Dichorionic	Diamniotic	0-3	30	9
Monochorionic	Diamniotic	4-8	68	25
Monochorionic	Monoamniotic	>8	5	>50

From Hollenbach KA, Hickok DE: Clin Obstet Gynecol 33:3-9, 1990.

that of dizygotic twins. However, accepted theories of monozygotic twinning are not available.

Because of the lack of monozygotic twin specimens from the earliest days of gestation, current knowledge of embryology is derived from the classic contributions of Hertig and Rock[15,16] and of Corner.[11] In 1955, Hertig and Rock postulated that monozygotic twins are formed by the splitting of the conceptus at any time between day 2 through day 15 or 17 of gestation. Corner added that ultimate morphologic differentiation depended on the embryonal developmental stage at the time the splitting took place. He proposed three critical stages at which distinct characteristic morphogenesis may result: (1) separation of early blastomeres about day 2 after fertilization, (2) duplication of the inner cell mass about day 5, and (3) duplication of the embryonal rudiment of the germ disk about day 15. This concept by Corner is translated into a practical understanding of the chorionicity of the twin pregnancy.

The separation of the blastomeres at the two-cell stage presupposes that each cell is capable of development into a morula, blastula, and embryo with its corresponding membranes (the chorion and amnion), so each conceptus may be implanted

at a different site. The resulting placenta is dichorionic-diamniotic, and the septal membrane is composed of four layers: amnion-chorion–chorion-amnion. This type of development results from division within the first 72 hours after fertilization. This form of division accounts for 30% of monozygotic twins (Table 1-1).

Division of the fertilized ovum between 4 and 8 days after fertilization results in the division of the inner cell mass and the trophoblast, which is differentiating to form the chorion. The amnion has not been formed at this time, but it will eventually be covered by chorion. This type of twin pregnancy is monochorionic-diamniotic, and the septal membranes have two layers, amnion-amnion, without an intervening chorion. This accounts for 68% of monozygotic twins.

Division of the fertilized ovum between 8 and 13½ days after fertilization results in a monochorionic-monoamniotic twin pregnancy. The amnion is formed at day 8, and division after this results in two embryos with a common amniotic sac. This accounts for less than 5% of monozygous twins.

If separation of the ovum is delayed beyond 13½ days, duplication of the embryonic forming cells may be incomplete and lead to a variety of bizarre twins, such as conjoined twins. The occurrence of con-

TABLE 1-2

Twinning Rates by Zygosity/1000 Births in Different Countries			
	MONOZYGOTIC	DIZYGOTIC	TOTAL
Nigeria	5	49.0	54.0
United States			
Black	4.7	11.1	15.8
White	4.2	7.1	11.3
England and Wales	3.5	8.8	12.3
India (Calcutta)	3.3	8.1	11.4
Japan	3.0	1.3	4.3

From MacGillivray I: Semin Perinatol 10:4-8, 1986.

joined twins is 1/500 twin pregnancies or 1/50,000 to 80,000 deliveries.

MacGillivray[32] feels that the recording of the incidence of twinning has been inaccurate and is based on hospital statistics that have significant errors because abortions, early fetal losses, or vanishing twins are not taken into consideration. He quotes the Weinberg formula, which calculates the number of pairs of monozygotic twins. This formula states that the number of monozygotic pairs is equal to the total number of pairs minus 2 times the number of pairs of unlike sex. Apparently this formula is accurate for total populations but not for hospital statistics.

Dizygotic Twinning

Dizygotic twinning results from multiple ovulation, which is the result of overstimulation by follicle-stimulating hormone (FSH) and the surge of luteinizing hormone (LH). The administration of exogenous gonadotropins or clomiphene citrate used for infertility therapy causes a rise in serum FSH levels, which causes multiple ovulation and multiple births. Women who

have delivered twins have been found to have higher levels of FSH and LH than those women who have delivered singletons.[33] These twins have dichorionic-diamniotic placentas, and the septal membranes have all four layers.

Incidence

Twinning rates have been published that compare many countries in the world (Table 1-2).

MacGillivray[32] indicates that the triplet rate in Nigeria is also high (1.78/1000 deliveries) when compared with the rates in the United States (0.9/1000 of all deliveries to white parents; 13.4/1000 of all deliveries to black parents), in England and Wales (1/1000 of all deliveries), and in Japan (0.056/1000 of all deliveries). The rate of monozygotic twinning is remarkably similar throughout the world (3.5/1000 deliveries). In contrast, the dizygotic twinning rate varies from 4 to 50/1000 deliveries.

The twinning rate is usually stated as 3 to 5/1000 deliveries for monozygotic twins and 4 to 50/1000 deliveries for dizygotic twins. Spellacy, Handler, and Ferre,[47] using data on 101,506 deliveries from the University of Illinois Perinatal Network, reported the overall incidence of twinning to be 12/1000 deliveries. This data included similar rates for white and black patients (13/1000) and lower rates for Hispanic (10/1000) and Asian patients (9.5/1000). Another study reported higher rates of twinning among blacks than among whites.[40]

The quoted incidences for twin pregnancy are based on hospital discharges rather than on the total number of twin or higher-order conceptions. Landy et al.[24] reported that serial ultrasonographic examinations could demonstrate the "disappearance" of at least one of two gestational rings and that the number of twins observed at delivery was markedly less than the number of twin pregnancies identified sonographically in the first trimester. A disappearance rate of 21.2% was observed and is comparable to reported spontaneous-loss rates for singleton pregnancies. Although the true loss rate is unknown, the spontaneous-abortion rate in the first trimester of pregnancy is thought to be approximately 15%.[9]

The only apparent complication associated with the vanishing fetus is vaginal bleeding or spotting. Landy et al.[24] reported that 25% of patients with a vanishing fetus experience vaginal bleeding, whereas 18.5% of women (10/54) with continuing twin gestation and 7.2% of women (68/946) with singleton pregnancies experience vaginal bleeding.

The prognosis for continuing the pregnancy in association with a vanishing fetus appears to be good, although the rate of future fetal death is 14.3%. This confirms the standard obstetric teaching that a pregnancy complicated by first trimester bleeding is associated with an increased risk of spontaneous loss or other complications.

The use of drugs to induce ovulation increases the incidence of multiple gestation. The incidence of multiple conception ranges from 6.8% to 17% after treatment with clomiphene citrate and from 18% to 53.5% after treatment with gonadotropins.[43] Schneider, Bessis, and Simonnet[45] used first trimester sonography as the diagnostic modality and reported early ovular resorption occurred in 63% of spontaneous gestations and in 64% of clomiphene-induced gestations. Landy et al.[24] reported that 32.1% of patients (9/28) with twin pregnancies caused by ovulation induction experienced a vanishing fetus.

Andrews et al.[1] reported on 125 consecutive pregnancies in which the fetus was conceived in vitro that resulted in 155 total pregnancies and the delivery of 100 babies. The clinical abortion rate was 14.8% (23/155) and the preclinical spontaneous abortion rate was 18% (28/155), giving a pregnancy loss rate of 33% (51/155). It is of importance to note that vaginal bleeding occurred in 59% of the pregnancies and was as common among patients with single transfers as those with multiple transfers. They also reported that 26 of their 100 pregnancies (26%) were multiple, as determined by sonography before 12 weeks' gestation. Sixty-nine patients had two or more conceptuses transferred; therefore a pregnancy loss occurred in 62.3% of the patients (43/69).

Kilby, Govind, and O'Brien,[23] using data on 34,804 live deliveries, examined the outcome of twin pregnancies complicated by a single uterine death after 20 weeks' gestation. This occurred in 20/342 twin gestations (5.8%). There was an increase in congenital structural anomalies in pregnancies with a death in utero compared with uneventful twin pregnancies (25% versus 0.3%; P = <.001). A significant proportion of the twin pregnancies with a death had monochorionic placentas (35% versus 9%; P = <.001). Additionally, more of these pregnancies resulted in neonates being admitted to special care units (70% versus 5.6%), compared with neonates from the normal twin sample.

The study by Kilby, Govind, and O'Brien[23] demonstrates that the death of a fetus after 20 weeks' gestation significantly increases the risk of the remaining fetus either dying or having a severe abnormality. This is in contrast with twin pregnancies exhibiting a vanishing fetus at less than or equal to 12 weeks' gestation, where there is a smaller risk of subsequent adverse effects. Kilby, Govind, and O'Brien[23] reinforced the concept that there is an increased risk of fetal death in twin pregnancies that have either a monochorionic placenta or a *de novo* structural abnormality in one fetus. Monochorionic placentas are associated with a significantly increased perinatal mortality rate (PMR) than dichorionic placentas (26% versus 9%).

Mortality

Multiple gestations have a PMR that is significantly higher than singleton pregnancies, although the rate has been decreasing over the last 20 years. Using data from the National Collaborative Perinatal Project of the mid-1960s, which included 53,518 mother-baby pairs that were studied until children were 5 years old, Naeye et al.[39] reported a PMR for twins of 139/1000 births, compared with the PMR for singletons of 33/1000 births. The deaths of

twins were caused by the following conditions: 16% from amniotic fluid infections, 11% from premature rupture of membranes, 8% from monovular twin transfusion, 8% from large placental infarcts, 7% from congenital anomalies, and 50% from over 20 other disorders. The PMR for monozygotic twins was 2.7 times the PMR for dizygotic twins. Each of the diagnoses was significantly greater in twin pregnancies than in singleton pregnancies.

McCarthy et al.[34] reviewed 7001 liveborn twins in Georgia from 1974 to 1978. The rate of twins delivered after 20 weeks' gestation was 0.8% (1/112 pregnancies). A comparison of neonatal mortality rates for twins and singletons is shown in Table 1-3.

The weight-specific mortality rate was equivalent to that of singletons, but the overall relative risk of neonatal death for twins compared with singletons was 6.6. Spellacy, Hander, and Ferre[47] compared the outcomes of 1253 twin pregnancies with a random control group of 5119 singleton pregnancies from a regional network data base of 101,506 deliveries from 1982 to 1987. The PMR and fetal death rate are listed in Table 1-4. When all twins who weighed 500 gm were compared, the risk of death for Twin B during the fetal and neonatal periods exceeded that for Twin A. However, when the comparison was limited to twins who weighed 2500 gm, the risk for Twin A exceeded that for Twin B during the neonatal period. The fetal mortality rate for twins was lower than that for singletons at birth weights less than or equal to 2500 gm but higher for singletons at weights greater than 2500 gm. At weights greater than 2500 gm, the neonatal death rate for both twins was higher than for singletons; Twin A had the greater disadvantage.

TABLE 1-3

Comparison of Neonatal Mortality Rates for Twins and Singletons

	TWINS	SINGLETONS	RR OF TWINS VS. SINGLETONS* (95% CI)
Neonatal deaths	543	4585	
Live births	7001	391,401	
NMR	78	12	6.6 (6.1-7.1)†

*RR, relative risk; CI, confidence interval; NMR, neonatal mortality rate/1000 live births; †p=<.001.
From McCarthy BJ et al: Am J Obstet Gynecol 141:252-256, 1981.

TABLE 1-4

Risk of Death for Singleton and Twin Infants/1000 Births

	FETAL DEATH	NEONATAL DEATH	PERINATAL DEATH
ALL INFANTS			
Twin A	16.0	33.4	48.8
Twin B	25.6	39.9	64.1
Singleton	5.7	4.9	10.4
INFANTS <2500 GM			
Twin A	27.6	60.5	86.6
Twin B	41.4	72.9	111.4
Singleton	53.7	62.2	112.7
INFANTS >2500 GM			
Twin A	4.7	7.9	12.6
Twin B	7.0	1.8	8.7
Singleton	1.3	1.1	2.3

From Spellacy WN, Handler H, Ferre CD: Obstet Gynecol 75:168-171, 1990.

Seoud et al.[46] reviewed the PMRs for twins, triplets, and quadruplets in patients undergoing in vitro fertilization. The PMR for twins was 72.7/1000 births (16/220 twin pregnancies); for triplets, it was 22.2/1000 births (1/45 triplet pregnancies); and for quadruplets, it was 0% (0/4 quadruplet pregnancies). Sassoon et al.[42] reported a similar PMR for twins and triplets of 100/1000 births and 95/1000, births respectively. Collins and Bleyl[10] investigated the outcome of 71 quadruplet pregnancies occurring between 1980 and 1989 and found that 67 (94%) of the 71 quadruplet pregnancies occurred after ovulation induction. There were 6 first-trimester losses, 10 stillbirths, and 33 neonatal deaths in 284 fetuses. The neonatal mortality rate was 119.5/1000 births, and the PMR was 155.5/1000 births.

Luke and Keith[28] determined the risks for infant mortality and postneonatal morbidity and handicap using data from the National Infant Mortality Surveillance (NIMS) project and from birth-weight–specific postneonatal handicap rates from the Office of Technology Assessment's report titled *Healthy Children* for a 1988 birth cohort.[50] These rates were compared with the United States' health objectives for the year 2000 for race-specific birth weight and infant mortality (Table 1-5).

The information in Table 1-5 indicates that neither black nor white infants meet the target health objectives. The failure to meet target goals is magnified in twins and particularly in triplets. Infants from multiple births are at greater risk for neonatal mortality because of their birth weight distributions, and the postneonatal survivors are at higher risk for a birth-related handicap. Birth weight appears to be a major contributing factor to the excess morbidity and mortality rates of twins and triplets.

The data already presented indicate a decrease in perinatal mortality in both singletons and multiple generations over the last 30 years. Kiely, Kleinman, and Kiely[22] have compared infant mortality rates of infants from high-order multiple births and singletons born between 1983 and 1985 with those born in 1960. The information for 1972 through 1989 was obtained from the National Center for Health Statistics (Tables 1-6 and 1-7).

The infant mortality rate is much higher in infants of high-order multiple births than in singletons. It is to be noted that the infant mortality rate has decreased significantly for infants from high-order multiple births as well as for singletons. Most of the higher mortality rates in high-order births are related to a much higher rate of low birth weight (LBW) infants. It is important to note that birth-weight–specific mortality among infants of multiple gestation compares favorably with that of singletons. For infants weighing 500 to 999 gm the mortality rates are about the same, but for infants weighing 1000 to 2499 gm, the mortality rates of infants from multiple gestations are much lower than those of singletons.

An obvious hypothesis is that infants from a multiple gestation are more mature at the same weights as LBW singletons; therefore their survival rates will be better. Kiely, Kleinman, and Kiely[22] found that for infants weighing 1250 to 1499 gm, the median gestation was 31 weeks for singletons, twins, and higher-order multiple gestations. When they added gestation to the regression analysis in Table 1-6, they changed the relative risk by 1% to 5%. They concluded that gestation maturity was the main reason for the difference in mortality. Record, Gibson, and McKeown[41] had postulated the same conclusion earlier by the observing that large birth-weight–specific mortality differences between triplets and singletons occurred when comparison was restricted to infants delivered during the same period of gestation.

The data also support the concept that infant mortality rates have dramatically decreased between 1960 and 1983-1985.

TABLE 1-5

Rates of Adverse Health Outcomes and Relative Risk by Race and Plurality/1000 Live Births in the United States, 1988

RACE AND PLURALITY	BIRTH WEIGHT			INFANT MORTALITY
	VLBW* (RR)	LBW (RR)		
WHITE				
U.S. Health Objective	10.0	50.0		7.0
Singletons	7.5 (1.0)	46.8 (1.0)		9.4 (1.0)
Twins	82.0 (10.9)	470.9 (10.1)		49.4 (5.3)
Triplets	327.6 (43.7)	906.2 (19.4)		166.1 (17.7)

	HANDICAP		
	SEVERE (RR)	MODERATE (RR)	OVERALL (RR)
Singletons	19.4 (1.0)	70.3 (1.0)	89.7 (1.0)
Twins	32.4 (1.7)	90.3 (1.3)	122.7 (1.4)
Triplets	56.6 (2.9)	120.9 (1.7)	177.5 (2.0)

	BIRTH WEIGHT			INFANT MORTALITY
	VLBW (RR)	LBW (RR)		
BLACK				
U.S. Health Objective	20.0	90.0		11.0
Singletons	24.0 (1.0)	116.6 (1.0)		20.8 (1.0)
Twins	166.2 (6.9)	621.7 (5.3)		86.8 (4.2)
Triplets	386.7 (16.1)	946.7 (8.1)		193.3 (9.3)

	HANDICAP		
	SEVERE (RR)	MODERATE (RR)	OVERALL (RR)
Singletons	21.6 (1.0)	73.6 (1.0)	95.2 (1.0)
Twins	40.5 (1.9)	100.5 (1.4)	141.0 (1.5)
Triplets	62.0 (2.9)	128.1 (1.7)	190.1 (2.0)

*VLBW, very low birth weight; LBW, low birth weight; RR, relative risk.
Modified from Keith L et al: Am J Obstet Gynecol 138:781-789, 1980; Luke B, Keith L: J Reprod Med 37:661-666, 1992; and U.S. Congress, Office of Technology Assessment: Pub No OTA-H-345, Washington, D.C., U.S. Government Printing Office, 1988.

TABLE 1-5

Rates of Adverse Health Outcomes and Relative Risk by Race and Plurality/1000 Live Births in the United States, 1988—cont'd

| | BIRTH WEIGHT | | |
	VLBW (RR)	LBW (RR)	INFANT MORTALITY
ALL RACES			
U.S. Health Objective	10.0	50.0	7.0
Singletons	10.3 (1.0)	59.2 (1.0)	8.6 (1.0)
Twins	98.7 (9.6)	502.0 (10.3)	56.6 (6.6)
Triplets	336.3 (32.7)	911.8 (18.8)	166.7 (19.4)

| | HANDICAP | | |
	SEVERE (RR)	MODERATE (RR)	OVERALL (RR)
Singletons	19.7 (1.0)	70.6 (1.0)	90.4 (1.0)
Twins	34.0 (1.7)	92.3 (1.3)	126.3 (1.4)
Triplets	57.5 (2.9)	121.6 (1.7)	179.1 (2.0)

The 1983-1985 infant mortality rates in very low birth weight (VLBW) infants of multiple gestation were about half as high as they were in 1960. Mortality rates of infants from multiple gestations who weighed 1500 to 2499 gm were one fifth to one fourth as high as they were in 1960. A similar trend is present for singletons as well.

It would seem that improved obstetric and nursery care, as well as the development of the subspecialty areas of maternal fetal medicine and neonatal medicine, have had a substantial impact on the survival rates of singletons, twins, and infants of higher-order multiple gestations. The coincidental development of the neonatal intensive care unit (NICU) and techniques to deal with the altered physiology of the VLBW infant has had a significant impact on survival rates.

Morbidity

NEONATAL

Morbidity and the subsequent development of moderate and severe handicapping conditions are related to LBW and short gestational ages. It is well recognized that the mean gestational age at delivery of twins is 36 weeks; for triplets, it is 34 weeks; and for quadruplets, it is 31 weeks. In a University of Illinois twin study,[14] 42% of twins were born after 37 weeks of gestation or earlier, compared with 8% of singletons. Birth weights of infants from multiple gestations are lower than birth weights of infants from singleton gestations. In the Northwestern University Multi-Hospital Twin Study,[21] 48.9% of first-born twins had birth weights less than 2500 gm, whereas 52.6% of second-born twins weighed less than 2500 gm. The

TABLE 1-6

Birth-Weight–Specific Infant Mortality Rates in High-Order Multiple Births and Singleton Births in the United States for Whites from 1983 to 1985

BIRTH WEIGHT GM	INFANT MORTALITY RATE/1000 LIVE BIRTHS*		RR† OF HIGH-ORDER MULTIPLE BIRTHS VS. SINGLETON BIRTHS (95% CI)
	HIGH-ORDER MULTIPLE BIRTHS	SINGLETON BIRTHS	
500-599	888.9	862.7	1.03 (0.95-1.12)
600-699	800.0	731.9	1.09 (0.97-1.23)
700-799	585.4	580.5	1.01 (0.84-1.21)
800-899	431.6	445.2	0.97 (0.77-1.22)
900-999	304.0	353.7	0.86 (0.66-1.12)
1000-1249	145.1	222.4	0.65 (0.51-0.83)
1250-1499	57.8	131.5	0.44 (0.29-0.65)
1500-1999	20.5	68.3	0.30 (0.20-0.44)
2000-2499	8.8	23.7	0.37 (0.20-0.69)
≥2500	6.1	3.9	1.56 (0.50-4.81)

*High-order multiple birth deaths=567; singleton deaths=71,802; †RR, relative risk.
From Kiely JL, Kleinman JL, Kiely M: Am J Dis Child 146:862-868, 1992.

University of Illinois twin study by Ghai and Vidyasagar[14] revealed that 47% of twins exhibited some form of neonatal morbidity, compared with 27% of singletons. They also indicated that clinical and objective evidence of intrauterine growth retardation (IUGR) is present in as many as 66% of twin infants. Admission to NICUs can be taken as a measure of morbidity and recently has been reported to occur in 22.7% of twins, 64.1% of triplets, and 75% of quadruplet infants.[46] The reported length of stays in the NICU were 12.0 days, 17.4 days, and 57.8 days for infants from twin, triplet, and quadruplet pregnancies, respectively. Most multiple gestation morbidity is related to prematurity and its associated complications, such as asphyxia, neurologic depression, and chronic respiratory disease. However, IUGR and an increased incidence of con-genital anomalies are represented at a significant rate.*

Most multiple gestation studies have reported an increase in the incidence of congenital anomalies.[38] The incidence rate of any single anomaly is the number of affected conceptuses expressed as a percentage of the total number of conceptuses alive during the period of development when that anomaly may be manifest. The true incidence of anomalies is difficult to determine, because not all conceptuses are examined. If a conceptus is examined, the anomaly may not be detected. Additionally, the anomaly may be altered by tissue regeneration concealing the damage that occurred in earlier fetal development, or it may be missed because of delayed manifestation of the anomaly. Because of these

*References 18, 21, 29, 44, 52, 53

TABLE 1-7

Infant Mortality in High-Order Multiple Births, in 1960 and in 1983-1985

BIRTH WEIGHT AND RACE	INFANT MORTALITY RATES/1000 LIVE BIRTHS		% CHANGE	95% CI
	1960	1983-1985		
< 1500 GM				
Whites	682.9	350.9	−49	−43 to −54
Blacks	940.5	423.3	−55	−48 to −61
1500-2499 GM				
Whites	74.6	15.0	−80	−69 to −87
Blacks	128.6	35.3	−73	−42 to −87
> 2500 GM				
Whites	0	6.1		
Blacks	66.7	0		
TOTAL				
Whites	269.6	130.3	−52	−42 to −58
Blacks	383.7	224.5	−42	−28 to −53

Modified from Kiely JL, Kleinman JL, Kiely M: Am J Dis Child 146:862-868, 1992.

conditions, it would be more appropriate to consider prevalence rather than incidence at various stages of development. However, the current literature reports anomalies in both modes and no consensus is apparent.

Spellacy, Handler, and Ferre,[47] in a study of 1253 twin pregnancies, found that both A twins and B twins had significantly more congenital anomalies than found in the control group of singletons. Congenital anomalies were found in 7.3% of Twin A infants and 9.4% of Twin B infants, compared with 2.4% of singletons.

Several authors have reported abnormality rates among abortuses of twin pregnancies.[26,49] Livingston and Poland[26] found that 46/52 twin embryos (88%) had anomalies, with the majority exhibiting growth disorganization and that 11/54 twin fetuses (21%) had anomalies, with most showing cardiac defects. Uchida et al.[49] found that 5/29 twin abortuses (17%) had chromosomal anomalies.

Reports that deal with anomalies in neonates only address a smaller, and therefore underreported, proportion of the anomalies occurring in conceptuses in general. In most studies, malformations have been found to be more common in multiple gestations than in singleton gestations. However, some studies have reported no difference. The following list gives several explanations for the difference in reporting[25,35,37]:

1. The proportion of conceptuses surviving to any specific gestational age differs between multiple gestations and singletons, because the rate of intrauterine survival of multiple conceptuses is less than it is for singletons. Therefore liveborn infants and stillborn fetuses represent original populations that differ.

2. There are differences in the range of anomalies included in studies; therefore some anomalies could be excluded, particularly those that seem to occur more often in multiple gestations.

3. The timing and thoroughness of the examination, as well as the careful recording of the findings, can significantly affect the final conclusions.

4. The type of twinning affects the risk of malformation, and the risk of abnormalities is higher in monozygotic twins than dizygotic twins.[8] The risk of malformation increases with maternal age, as does the dizygotic twinning rate; however, when adjusting for maternal age and parity, there does not seem to be an excessive risk in twins.[35]

5. The analysis may be skewed by ascertainment of the proportion of unlike-sex twins. Malformations tend to be higher in twins of like sex than of unlike sex.[33,35] Therefore the rate of malformations is expected to be lower if the proportion of unlike-sex twins is high.

Schinzel, Smith, and Miller[44] studied 660 like-sex twin pairs with a structural defect. The incidence of structural defects in twin pairs was 6%. They calculated that 46% of monozygotic twins had a defect. The structural defects in monozygotic twins may be attributed to: (1) poor formation of tissue (that is, a malformation plus secondarily derived defects); (2) defects that are the result of disruptions of previously normal tissues—disruptions in monozygotic twins are commonly based on vascular interchanges that occur in the monochorionic placenta, which is present in a majority of monozygotic twins; and (3) defects that are the result of in utero crowding.

The excess of malformations in monozygotic twins or triplets predominately represents patients with a single localized defect causing the malformation or malformation complex and not those with chromosomal abnormalities or mutant gene disorders. There is an excessive association of monozygotic twinning with defects determined in early embryogenesis, such as exstrophy of the cloaca; sirenomelia; expanded vertebral defects, imperforate anus, tracheoesophageal fistula, and radial and renal dysplasia (VATER) association with renal agenesis, anal atresia, or tracheoesophageal fistula; anencephaly; situs inversus viscerum, and holoprosencephaly. The most likely explanation for findings that associate monozygotic twinning and early structural defects is that the same cause of the formation of monozygotic twins also causes the malformation in one or more of the fetuses.[44] The frequency of early malformations is implied to be highest 10 to 15 days after conception and suggests that duplication at this period of development is especially likely to cause problems of morphogenesis beyond monozygotic twinning alone.

Schinzel, Smith, and Miller[44] also reported that conjoined twins and amorphous fetuses occur more often in triplet pregnancies. They found that 6/91 conjoined twins (6.5%) and 19/158 amorphous fetuses (12%) were from triplet pregnancies.

If both twins have the same defect, it is considered to be concordant; if only one has the defect, it is nonconcordant. The concordance of malformation in monozygotic twins ranges from 5% to 50% and is commonly thought to be as high as 10% to 20%. Therefore the majority of affected monozygotic twins are nonconcordant. The concordance frequency in monozygotic twins is higher than it is in dizygotic twins, who have the same concordance frequency as singleton siblings. Therefore malformations are nonrandomly associated with monozygotic twinning but not with dizygotic twinning. The same circumstances that give rise to monozygotic twinning may be responsible for malformation in one or both monozygotic twins.

The notion of structural defects resulting from vascular interchanges among multiple fetuses is an important concept. The majority of monozygotic twins have a conjoined monochorionic placenta, which may contain a vascular anastomosis of the vein-to-vein, artery-to-artery, or artery-to-vein type.[6] Reverse flow in early embryogenic life in monozygotic twins may lead to amorphuses or acardiac twins. The acardiac twin is found to have artery-to-artery and vein-to-vein anastomoses with the monochorionic twin. Benirschke and de Roches Harper[6] have postulated that early pressure flow in the placental artery of one twin exceeds that of the other and results in a reversal of flow at the artery-to-artery anastomosis. The recipient is perfused preferentially to the lower segment rather than to the cranial segment.

The consequences of the reversed flow for the recipient twin are all gradations of disruption of circulation. Variable missing or deficient tissues commonly include the head, heart, limbs, lung, liver, pancreas, and small bowel. All gradations may occur, and the acardiac twin may appear as an amorphous twin.

The death of a monozygotic twin can cause problems for the surviving twin.[5] It has been postulated that thromboplastin may enter the circulation of the surviving twin and cause disseminated intravascular coagulation. It is also possible for clots and debris from the dead twin to embolize the circulation of the surviving twin and give rise to areas of ischemia, necrosis, and disruption with loss of tissue. The impact on the development of the brain must also be considered. The consequences of ischemia or debris embolization include porencephaly or hydrocephalus with microcephaly, mental deficiency with spasticity, and seizures. Microcephaly may often be a result of ischemia or debris embolization. Durkin et al.[12] found that 9/281 individuals (3.2%) with severe mental deficiency and spasticity of unknown cause had a history of a macerated stillborn twin. Melnick[35] noted that 7/188 monozygotic twins (3.7%) had a history of a deceased twin. All seven survivors had microcephaly; four had porencephaly, and one with hydrocephalus died of brain necrosis in infancy. The occurrence of these defects in an implied vascular mode of pathologic development allows us to better understand the genesis of the defects and provides a vascular basis for other defects.

Another clinical problem with its basis in aberrant placental vascularization is an artery-to-vein anastomosis that allows one twin to transfuse the other. In this syndrome the transfusing twin usually develops hypovolemia with a decreased renal blood flow, oligohydramnios anemia, a small size, and advanced pulmonary maturity caused by stress. The recipient twin develops hypervolemia, a high hematocrit, an enlarged heart, an increased renal blood flow with polyhydramnios, and an increased size. The recipient fetus is at risk for intravascular coagulation in utero, as well as in neonatal life. The incidence of an unusual discrepancy in size and hematocrit count in monozygotic twins is estimated to be 18%.[48]

Structural deformities may occur as a consequence of intrauterine crowding. Multiple fetuses grow at singleton growth rates until they are approximately 31 weeks old. The impact of uterine crowding can give rise to mechanically induced malformations of the extremities. These deformities are more common in infants of multiple gestations than in singletons and occur in monozygotic and dizygotic twins at the same rate. Most deformities are transient and return to normal growth and form after birth.

An important area of discussion is neonatal depression at the time of birth and subsequent neurologic morbidity. Twin and higher-order multiple infants are more likely to suffer neonatal depression than singletons. This increased incidence can be primarily attributed to prematurity, a greater likelihood of IUGR, abnormal presentation, and operative delivery, as well as to acute and chronic uteroplacental insufficiency. Apgar scores between 0 and 3 occur in approximately 5% of neonates. Neonatal depression is more common in second-born twins and triplets because of additional birth-related problems such as delayed delivery, cord prolapse, and premature placental separation. The neonatal depression is usually not prolonged, and 5-minute Apgar scores and 15-minute capillary blood pH measurements have been found not to differ significantly among the twin pairs.

Twins and infants from higher-order multiple gestations have a higher prevalence of neurodevelopmental disease (cerebral palsy and seizures) than singletons. Bejar et al.[3,4] studied 89 twins and 12 triplets (101 infants) with a gestational age of less than 36 weeks. Three days after delivery, all had had a full pathologic assessment of the placenta and one or more echoencephalographic studies. The purpose of the study was to determine the influences of abnormal vascular connections in the placenta and of the antenatal diagnosis of necrosis of cerebral white matter on cerebral palsy and developmental delay. Antenatal necrosis of cerebral white matter was present in 14/101 infants (13.9%). The incidence of antenatal necrosis of cerebral white matter was significantly higher in infants with a monochorionic placenta—12/40 infants examined (30%). This is highly significantly different from infants with dichorionic placentas; in this group, only 2/61 (3.3%) were diagnosed with antenatal necrosis of cerebral white matter. The placental studies in the same report found vascular anastomoses in 36 of the 40 infants with monochorionic placentas (90%). Antenatal necrosis of cerebral white matter occurred more often in infants with multiple anastomoses. The type of anastomosis was a critical factor in determining which infants developed antenatal necrosis of cerebral white matter. Vein-to-vein anastomoses occurred alone in seven placentas and six of the seven infants (89%) who had antenatal necrosis of

TABLE 1-8

Distribution of Monochorionic Infants by the Presence of Feto-Fetal Transfusion Syndrome, Antenatal White Matter Necrosis, and Placental Anastomosis (n = 36)

| | FETO-FETAL TRANSFUSION SYNDROME | | | | |
| | PRESENT | | ABSENT | | |
PLACENTAL ANASTOMOSES	WITH AWMN*	WITHOUT AWMN	WITH AWMN	WITHOUT AWMN	TOTAL
Artery-to-vein	1†	3	0	8	12
Artery-to-vein	0	0	2	6	8
Artery-to-vein, artery-to-artery	1†	0	2	6	9
Artery-to-vein, artery-to-artery, vein-to-vein	3	1	3	0	7
Total	5	4	7	20	36

*AWMN, antenatal white matter necrosis; †Intrauterine fetal death of a co-twin; p=<.003
From Bejar R et al: Am J Obstet Gynecol 159:357, 1988.

cerebral white matter. This was followed by 16 infants with multiple anastomoses in which 9/26 (56%) had antenatal necrosis of cerebral white matter. Only 3/20 infants with artery-to-vein or artery-to-artery anastomoses (15%) had antenatal necrosis of cerebral white matter.

The feto-fetal transfusion syndrome was diagnosed in monochorionic twins with documented vascular anastomosis by using such clinical manifestations as hydrops fetalis, polyhydramnios, oligohydramnios, intrauterine fetal death of one twin in the absence of cord entanglements or knots in the umbilical cord, and 20% or greater discordance in birth weights (Table 1-8). An analysis by Bejar et al.[3,4] suggests that cavitary lesions in the white matter and cerebral atrophy develop 2 or more weeks after the acute stage of necrosis of the cerebral white matter. The demonstration of cavitary lesions in the white matter and cerebral atrophy during the first 3 days after birth indicates that the ischemic results to

the fetuses' brains occurred during the antenatal period.[2] The finding of a 13.8% incidence of antenatal necrosis of cerebral white matter in infants of multiple gestations is higher than the 8.8% incidence of antenatal necrosis of cerebral white matter found in preterm singletons. Infants of monochorionic gestations had a significantly higher incidence (30%) of antenatal necrosis of the cerebral white matter than singletons (p<.005) or infants (p=<.001) of dichorionic gestations.

The cerebral necrosis in twins and higher-order gestations may be explained by several hypothesis. Fetal death of one of the twins may be explained by placental vascular connections leading to a transfusion syndrome. The death of one twin predisposes the survivor to disseminated intravascular coagulation produced by the generation of thromboplastin-enriched blood. Thromboembolic debris and clots from the dead twin can reach the surviving fetus through vascular connections and can cause necrotic lesions in the brain, skin, intestine, liver, lungs, and kidneys.[5]

Respiratory distress syndrome as manifested by hyaline membrane disease (HMD) occurred in 51/177 premature twins (29%) and in 8.5% overall in twin deliveries.[18] No differences were found between first-born and second-born twins. In the University of Illinois twin study,[14] twins had a higher incidence of HMD compared with singletons (11% versus 2%). There was no statistically significant difference between first-born (10.2%) and second-born (12.1%) twins. In the same study there was no difference in the incidence of HMD in male twins (11.5%) and female twins (11.0%). There were no differences in the incidence of HMD when the twins were segregated into male-male, male-female, female-male, and female-female pairs. The presence of a girl in the twin pair did not protect the boy from HMD. Additionally, no difference was present when comparing female-female, male-female, and female-male twin pairs with male-male twin pairs.

The incidence of respiratory disorders other than HMD is strikingly increased in twins. The group weighing 500-1499 gm showed no differences between twins and singletons, but the birth weight groups of 1500-2999 gm and greater than 3000 gm showed a significant increase in respiratory disease in the twin group.[18] These data indicate that larger twins are more prone to develop respiratory disease in the neonatal period. It may indicate that these disorders are causally related or aggravated by intrauterine stress and birth asphyxia, and it may indicate a greater tendency of larger twins to in-utero stress and birth asphyxia.

IUGR is a major factor in neonatal morbidity in multiple gestation. Compared with singletons, twin infants are more than twice as likely to have LBWs and a relative risk of 6.6 of dying before their first birthday; the survivors have a relative risk of 1.4 of having a handicapping condition.[28] The important concern is how much of the excess neonatal morbidity is the result of LBW, preterm birth, IUGR (birth weight at or below the tenth percentile for gestational age), or twinning itself. Luke, Minoque, and Witter[29] studied 490 twins and 17,879 singleton infants who were nonanomalous, had a gestational age of 28 weeks or more, and had a birth weight of 1000 gm or more. The authors evaluated the association between length of gestation and IUGR, as well as the role of IUGR in excessive morbidity as measured by length of hospital stay.

The data presented in Table 1-9 indicate that twins with IUGR had significantly lower mean birth weights, longer mean gestations, and twice the mean length of stay ratio compared with nonIUGR twins. Significantly, more nonIUGR twins were born at 28-32 weeks and 33-35 weeks; however, more IUGR twins were born at 39-41 weeks. Additionally, the combination of IUGR with immaturity magnifies the adverse effect of IUGR on length of stay. Myers and Ferguson[37] demonstrated that the fetal death rate increased exponentially as birth weight decreased at each gestational age, indicating that IUGR at any gestational age is associated with an increase in adverse perinatal outcome.

The risk of IUGR is greatly increased after 38 weeks. Singletons and twins have similar growth patterns until 30 weeks' gestation, when they begin to diverge; sig-

TABLE 1-9

Comparison of Selected Characteristics and Perinatal Outcome by Fetal Growth Status of Twins

CHARACTERISTIC	FETAL GROWTH STATUS		P
	NON-IUGR (N = 410)	IUGR (N = 80)	
Race (black)	58.3%	67.5%	—
Cesarean birth	69.8%	72.5%	—
Gestational age (wk)	34.8	37.8	<.0001
28-32 wk	23.9%	1.3%	<.0001
33-35 wk	28.5%	11.3%	.001
36-38 wk	38.0%	43.8%	NS
39-41 wk	9.5%	43.8%	<.0001
Length of stay (days)	12.8	14.6	—
Length of stay ratio* (Mean)	1.75	3.94	<.0001
Length of stay by gestational age (days)			
28-32 wk	28.8	63.0	<.0001
33-35 wk	10.3	32.6	<.0001
36-38 wk	6.3	14.4	<.0001
39-41 wk	5.9	8.7	.004
Birth weight (gm)	2391	2023	<.0001
Discharge weight (gm)	2399	2148	<.0001
Discordancy (mean %)	10.2	17.5	<.0001
≥15%	22.4	52.5	<.0001
≥20%	13.2	36.3	<.0001
≥25%	8.3	26.3	<.0001

*Ratio of the twin length of stay divided by the fiftieth percentile singleton length of stay for the same gestational age.
Modified from Luke B, Minoque J, Witter F: Obstet Gynecol 81:949-953, 1993.

nificant differences are observed at 35 weeks and later.[31] In a large California study of more than 2.28 million births, Williams et al.[51] concluded that the peak growth rate was about 250 gm per week at 33 weeks for singletons, compared with 31 weeks for twins. After 31 weeks' gestation the average twin's birth weight falls progressively behind that of singletons. By 38 weeks, the tenth percentile for singletons is equivalent to the fiftieth percentile for twins, and the fiftieth percentile for singletons is equivalent to the ninetieth percentile for twins. Since the maturation process is accelerated in twin gestation, as manifested by the more rapid aging of the placenta and earlier lung maturation, neonatal morbidity in twins is comparable to singletons in the absence of IUGR. Therefore early recognition of IUGR should be a primary goal in reducing immediate and long-term adverse outcomes.

TABLE 1-10

Maternal Antepartum Complications in Twin Versus Singleton Pregnancies

COMPLICATION	TWINS (N = 1253)	SINGLETONS (N = 5119)	ODDS RATIO	95% CI
Hypertension	12.9%	5.6%	2:5	2.1-3.2
Abruptio placentae	2.2%	0.8%	3:0	1.9-4.7
Anemia	9.4%	4.1%	2:4	1.9-3.0
Urinary tract infection	8.7%	6.7%	1:4	1.1-1.7
Pyelonephritis	0.7%	0.3%	2:1	0.9-4.5
Post-dates	1.2%	3.1%	2:6	1.6-4.4

From Spellacy WN, Handler H, Ferre CD: Obstet Gynecol 75:168-171, 1990.

The prevention of IUGR at any stage of gestation has been shown to significantly reduce hospitalization rates of newborn twins to a level comparable to that of singletons.[29] Several studies have shown an association between maternal weight gain patterns, total weight gain, and twin birth weight.[29,30] These studies show that the best outcomes in twin gestation were achieved with a 24-pound maternal weight gain by 24 weeks' gestation and a total weight gain of 40 to 45 lb. In triplet gestations, better outcomes were achieved with weight gains of 45-51 pounds by 32-34 weeks and 46 to 68 lb by 31 weeks' gestation in quadruplet gestations.[13,27,46]

Maternal Morbidity

Maternal medical complications are significantly increased in multiple gestations compared with singleton gestations. This increase is present in twins and higher-order multiple gestations (Table 1-10).

Mothers of twins are 2.5 times as likely to have hypertension than mothers of singletons. The increased risk of maternal hypertension is independent of age, race, weight gain, or weight at delivery. Abruptio placentae was diagnosed 3 times as often in mothers of twins; adjustment for hypertension, age, and race did not modify the effect. Mercer et al.[36] studied clinical characteristics of twin gestations complicated by preterm premature rupture of membranes (PROM). They found that preterm PROM occurs more often in twin gestations than in singleton gestations (7.4% versus 3.7%, p=—<.001, odds ratio 2:1) and that mid-trimester (less than 26 weeks' gestation) preterm PROM also occurs more often in twin gestations (1.37% versus 0.52%, p=<.001, odds ratio 2:71). The mean latency period to delivery was 1.1 days for twins and 1.7 days for singletons. Ninety-one percent of twins and 90% of singletons were delivered within 7 days of rupture of membranes.

Sassoon et al.[42] reviewed 15 triplet and twin pregnancies matched for maternal age, race, type of medical insurance, delivery mode, parity, and history of previous preterm delivery. Their prenatal and

TABLE 1-11

Prenatal and Neonatal Complications of Triplet versus Twin Pregnancies				
COMPLICATION	TRIPLET (N = 15)	TWIN (N = 15)	P	RELATIVE RISK
Anemia	2 (13.3%)	1 (6.7%)	—	0.5
Preterm labor	12 (80.0%)	6 (40.0%)	.03	2.0
PPROM	4 (26.7%)	1 (6.7%)	—	4.0
Pregnancy-induced hypertension	1 (6.7%)	2 (13.3%)	—	0.5
Gestational diabetes	0 (0.0%)	1 (6.7%)	—	
Intrauterine fetal death	1 (6.7%)	1 (6.7%)	—	1.0
Gestational age of infants at delivery (wk)	33 ± 5.1	36.6 ± 3.4	.03	
Mean average birth weight of infants (gm)	1720 ± 700	2475 ± 683	.016	
Mean lowest birth weight of infants (gm)	1438 ± 599	2285 ± 628	.006	
Mean average hospital days	29 ± 46.2	8.5 ± 11.5	.05	5.0

From Sassoon DA et al: Obstet Gynecol 75:817-820, 1990

neonatal complications are shown in Table 1-11.

These authors reported that triplet pregnancies are complicated by a significantly higher incidence of preterm labor and delivery, growth retardation discordancy, and necessity neonatal intensive care. The perinatal mortality rate in this study was 95/1000 births.

Collins and Bleyl[10] reviewed the management and outcome of 71 quadruplet gestations and found the mean gestational age of the infants at delivery was 31.4 weeks and the mean birth weight was 1482 gm. The mean maternal weight gain was 45.8 pounds. All but one of the 71 patients experienced preterm labor. Other maternal complications included first trimester bleeding (35%), toxemia (32%), and anemia (25%).

Other Epidemiologic Considerations

MULTIPLE BIRTHS AND THE MATERNAL RISK OF BREAST CANCER

The current medical thinking about risk factors for breast cancer includes age at menarche or menopause and age at first pregnancy and breast feeding. Jacobson, Thompson, and Janerick[20] evaluated data from the Cancer and Steroid Hormone Study to determine whether pregnancies ending in multiple births affected the risk of subsequent breast cancer in the mother. The study group consisted of 3918 parous women ages 20 to 54 with newly diagnosed breast cancer and 4047 parous women selected randomly from the same geographic area. Multiple gestations were reported in 188 women in the study group and in 161 women in the control group. The authors found that a multiple last birth was protective against maternal breast cancer (odds ratio 0:60, 95% CI 0.43-0.85), whereas a multiple birth before the last birth was not protective against maternal breast cancer (odds ratio 1:11, 95% CI 0.79-1.57). In a subsequent study,[39] no association between multiple births and maternal risk of breast cancer was found. It would seem that, at this point, neither a positive nor a negative association between multiple gestation and breast cancer exists.

Summary

Epidemiologic data indicate a significant rise in the number of women with multiple gestations. This is almost entirely the result of the widespread use of fertility-enhancing drugs and ART. With this increase, the obstetrician will be encountering more maternal morbidity problems and significantly worse neonatal outcomes of multiple gestations compared with singleton gestations. The maternal complications include an increased incidence of hypertension, anemia, abruptio placentae, urinary tract infection, preterm PROM, preterm delivery, and IUGR. The neonatal complications are an increased incidence of admission to the NICU, respiratory distress syndrome, sepsis, and neonatal neurologic abnormality.

An exciting strategy, potentially preventive, is that of an adequate, early weight gain (24 pounds by 24 weeks) in a twin gestation and a total weight gain of greater than 45 pounds. An increase in fetal weight of as little as 500 gm can significantly improve outcome.

References

1. Andrews M et al: An analysis of the obstetric outcome of 125 consecutive pregnancies conceived in vitro and resulting in 100 deliveries, *Am J Obstet Gynecol* 154:848-854, 1986.
2. Banker BQ, Lanoche JC: Periventricular leukomalacia of infancy, *Neurology* 7:386-410, 1962.
3. Bejar R et al: Antenatal origin of neurological damage in newborn infants, *Am J Obstet Gynecol* 159:357-363, 1988.
4. Bejar R et al: Antenatal origin of neurologic damage in newborn infants with multiple gestations, *Am J Obstet Gynecol* 162:1230-1236, 1990.
5. Benirshke K: Twin placenta in perinatal mortality, *N Y State J Med* 61:1499-1507, 1961.
6. Benirschke K, des Roches Harper V: The acardiac anomaly, *Teratology* 15:311-316, 1977.
7. Benirschke K, Driscoll SG: The placenta in multiple pregnancy, *Handbuch Pathol Histol* 7:187, 1967.
8. Cameron AH et al: The value of twin surveys in the study of malformations, *Eur J Obstet Gynecol Reprod Biol* 14:347-356, 1983.
9. Can first trimester diagnosis be reliably evaluated? *Lancet* 1:735-736, 1985 (Editorial).
10. Collins MS, Bleyl JA: Seventy-one quadruplet pregnancies: management and outcome, *Am J Obstet Gynecol* 162:1384-1392, 1990.
11. Corner GW: The observed embryology of human single-ovum twins and other multiple births, *Am J Obstet Gynecol* 70:933-951, 1955.
12. Durkin MV et al: Analysis of etiologic factors in cerebral palsy with severe mental retardation. I. Analysis of gestational, parturitional and neonatal data, *Eur J Pediatr* 123:67-81, 1976.
13. Elster AD, Bleyl JL, Craven TL: Birth weight standards for triplets under modern obstetrical care in the United States, 1984-1989, *Obstet Gynecol* 77:387-393, 1991.
14. Ghai V, Vidyasagar D: Mortality and morbidity factors in twins: an epidemiological approach, *Clin Perinatol* 15:123-140, 1988.
15. Hertig AT, Rock J: Two human ova of the pre-

villous stage having a development age of seven and nine days respectively, *Centr Embryol* 557:65-84, 1945.

16. Hertig AT, Rock J, Adams EC: A description of 34 human ova within the first 17 days of development, *Am J Anat* 98:435-93, 1956.

17. Heuser CH: Monozygotic twin human embryo with an estimated ovulation age of 17 days, *Anat Rec* 118:310, 1954.

18. Ho SK, Wu PK: Perinatal factors and neonatal morbidity in twin pregnancies, *Am J Obstet Gynecol* 122:979, 1975.

19. Hollenbach KA, Hickok DE: Epidemiology and diagnosis of twin gestation, *Clin Obstet Gynecol* 33:3-9, 1990.

20. Jacobson HI, Thompson WD, Janerick DT: Multiple births and maternal risk of breast cancer, *Am J Epidemiol* 129:854-873, 1989.

21. Keith L et al: The Northwestern University multihospital twin study: a description of 588 twin pregnancies and associated pregnancy loss, 1971 to 1975, *Am J Obstet Gynecol* 138:781-789, 1980.

22. Kiely JL, Kleinman JL, Kiely M: Triplets and higher-order multiple births, *Am J Dis Child* 146:862-868, 1992.

23. Kilby MD, Govind A, O'Brien PM: Outcome of twin pregnancies complicated by a single intrauterine death: a comparison with viable twin pregnancies, *Obstet Gynecol* 84:107-109, 1994.

24. Landy HJ et al: The "vanishing twin": ultrasonographic assessment of fetal disappearance in the first trimester, *Am J Obstet Gynecol* 155:14-19, 1986.

25. Layde PM et al: Congenital malformations in twins, *Am J Hum Genet* 32:69-78, 1980.

26. Livingston JE, Poland BJ: A study of spontaneously aborted twins, *Teratology* 21:139-148, 1980.

27. Luke B: The changing pattern of multiple births in the United States: maternal and infant characteristics, 1973 and 1990, *Obstet Gynecol* 84:101-106, 1994.

28. Luke B, Keith LG: The contributions of singletons twins and triplets to low birth weight, infant mortality, and handicap in the United States, *J Reprod Med* 37:661-666, 1992.

29. Luke B, Minoque J, Witter F: The role of fetal growth restriction and gestational age on length of hospital stay in twin infants, *Obstet Gynecol* 81:949-953, 1993.

30. Luke B et al: Gestation age-specific birth weights of twins versus singletons, *Acta Genet Med Gemollol (Roma)* 40:69-76, 1991.

31. Luke B et al: The ideal twin pregnancy patterns of weight gain, discordancy, and length of gestation, *Am J Obstet Gynecol* 169:588-597, 1993.

32. MacGillivray I: Epidemiology of twin pregnancy, *Semin Perinatol* 10:4-8, 1986.

33. Martin NG et al: Gonadotropin levels in mothers who had two sets of DZ twins, *Acta Genet Med Gemellol (Roma)* 33:131-139, 1984.

34. McCarthy BJ et al: The epidemiology of neonatal death in twins, *Am J Obstet Gynecol* 141:252-256, 1981.

35. Melnick M: Brain damage in survivor after in utero death of monozygous co-twin, *Lancet* 2:1287, 1977 [letter].

36. Mercer BM et al: Clinical characteristics and outcome of twin gestation complicated by preterm premature rupture of membranes, *Am J Obstet Gynecol* 168:1467-1473, 1993.

37. Myers SA, Ferguson R: A population study of the relationship between fetal death and altered fetal growth, *Obstet Gynecol* 74:325-331, 1989.

38. Myrianthopoulus NC: Congenital malformations: the contribution of twin studies, *Birth Defects* 14:151-165, 1978.

39. Naeye RL et al: Twins: causes of perinatal death in 12 United States cities and one African city, *Am J Obstet Gynecol* 131:267-272, 1978.

40. Newton ER: Antepartum care in multiple gestation, *Semin Perinatol* 10:19, 1980.

41. Record RG, Gibson JR, McKeown T: Fetal and infant mortality in multiple pregnancy, *J Obstet Gynecol Br Empire* 59:471-482, 1952.

42. Sassoon DA et al: Perinatal outcome in triplet versus twin gestations, *Obstet Gynecol* 75:817-820, 1990.

43. Schenker JG, Yarkoni S, Granat M: Multiple pregnancies following induction of ovulation, *Fertil Steril* 35:105-123, 1981.

44. Schinzel A, Smith DW, Miller JR: Monozygotic twinning and structural defects, *J Pediatr* 95:921-930, 1979.

45. Schneider L, Bessis R, Simonnet T: The frequency of ovular resorption during the first trimester of twin pregnancy, *Acta Genet Med Gemellol (Roma)* 28:271-272, 1979.

46. Seoud M et al: Outcome of twin, triplet and quadruplet in vitro fertilization pregnancies: the Norfolk experience, *Fert Steril* 57:825-834, 1992.

47. Spellacy WN, Handler H, Ferre CD: A case-control study of 1253 twin pregnancies from a 1982-1987 perinatal data base, *Obstet Gynecol* 75:168-171, 1990.

48. Tan KL et al: The twin transfusion syndrome: clinical observations on 35 affected pairs, *Clin Pediatr (Phila)* 18:111-114, 1979.

49. Uchida IA et al: Twinning rate in spontaneous abortion, *Am J Hum Genet* 35:987-993, 1983.

50. U.S. Congress, Office of Technology Assessment: Healthy children: investing in the future, Pub No OTA-H-345, Washington, D.C., 1988, U.S. Government Printing Office.

51. Williams RL et al: Fetal growth and perinatal viability in California, *Obstet Gynecol* 59:624-632, 1982.

52. Windham GC, Bjerkedal T: Malformations in twins and their siblings, Norway 1967-1979, *Acta Genet Med Gemellol (Roma)* 33:87-95, 1984.

53. Wittle J, Bryan E: Congenital anomalies in twins, *Semin Perinatol* 10:50-64, 1986.

2

Classification, Placentation, and Pathology

Dennis M. O'Connor and Alexandra Gerassimides

But Semele's mortal frame could not endure the exaltation caused by the heavenly visitant, and she was burned to ashes by her wedding gift. Her child, still not fully formed, was snatched from his mother's womb and, if the tale be believed, the feeble baby was sewn into his father's thigh till the months for which his mother should have carried him were fulfilled. . .

Metamorphoses Book III, 306-313[17]

At first glance, the mythologic gestation of Bacchus on the thigh of Jupiter may be another example of the vivid imaginations of the storytellers from ancient Greece and Rome. It is possible, however, that a parasitic conjoined twin could represent the phenomenon described above by Ovid. It would be encouraging to think that clinicians have become more sophisticated in their understanding of abnormal pathologic conditions in multiple gestations; this is unfortunately not the case. Rare events, such as conjoined twins and other anomalies, are often reported in tabloid newspapers and magazines. In the scientific literature, it is easy to sensationalize these events in case reports.

In the past, abnormalities of twinning were considered too obscure to be of any significant clinical relevance. Nevertheless, the pathology of multiple gestations can be extremely important to the clinician. The introduction of assisted reproductive techniques (ART) has increased the number of multiple pregnancies, as well as associated perinatal loss, prematurity, and congenital malformations. Additionally, gross and microscopic examination of the placenta from a multiple gestation can result in identification of the type of placentation. This can be a potentially inexpensive method to determine zygosity.

All multiple gestations are at risk for fetal and placental abnormalities. However, the degree of risk increases significantly for both monochorionic and monoamniotic types.

As the majority of information available on abnormalities of multiple gestation focuses on twin pregnancies, this discussion of placentation and pathologic states concentrates on this type of multiple gestation. Triplet and higher-order multiple pregnancies demonstrate the same anomalies. Any features unique to these high-order gestations are discussed in sections pertaining to the specific abnormalities.

Embryology and Etiology

There are two major types of twin gestations. Dizygotic twins, or nonidentical (fraternal) twins, occur as a result of polyovulation. This may involve ovulation of multiple follicles from the same or both ovaries, or there may be ovulation of multiple oocytes from the same follicle (polyovular follicle). Monozygotic, or identical twins, occur as a result of the conceptus splitting at various times during embryogenesis. Splitting can occur randomly and at any time during the first 2 weeks of gestation. To appreciate how the different types of monozygotic twin gestations can develop, a review of early embryogenesis is necessary.

Once fertilization has occurred, the resulting zygote travels through the fallopian tube. The zygote divides by cleavage, forming blastomeres. After 4 days, or in the morular stage, all the daughter cells are of equal size and remain surrounded by the zona pellucida. Compaction, involving the migration of certain blastomeres, then occurs. The central cells be-

come the embryoblast, and the peripheral blastomeres become the trophoblastic precursors. By day 5, an influx of extracellular fluid results in the formation of a cyst cavity, and the conceptus, now called a blastocyst, hatches from the surrounding zona pellucida. Implantation occurs at day 6 or 7. By day 8, the embryoblast, or inner cell mass, separates into the epiblast, or primitive ectoderm, and the hypoblast, or primitive endoderm. Peripheral epiblastic cells are separated from the remaining embryoblast by cavitation. These cells form the primitive amnion. Ten days after fertilization, the hypoblast extrudes into the blastocyst cavity to form both the primary and definitive yolk sacs. Both the yolk sac surface and the primitive trophoblast form the extraembryonic mesoderm, although the true origin of this mesoderm is disputed.[23] The extraembryonic mesoderm differentiates into the chorion and the extraembryonic vasculature. By day 15, the embryo is now a disk-shaped oval, and a central groove appears along its longitudinal midline. The resultant primitive streak becomes a landmark for embryo symmetry. Gastrulation, or migration of the epiblast along the primitive groove, occurs around day 16. These cells first replace the hypoblast and then form the definitive endoderm; continued migration of these cells results in development of the embryonic mesoderm. The epiblastic cells that migrate into the superior portion of the primitive streak continue cephalad. By day 21, these cells form the notochord.[23]

Figure 2-1 summarizes the various landmarks of embryogenesis and the types of monozygotic twins formed if separation occurs before these events. Although

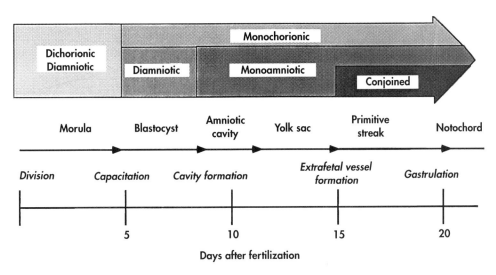

FIGURE 2-1   Embryologic landmarks and associated types of monozygotic twins.

monozygotic twinning can result from separation of either the blastomeres or the embryoblast, separation of embryonic cavities does not occur. In other words, if separation occurs after formation of the blastocyst cavity, the gestation is always monochorionic. If separation occurs after formation of the amnionic cavity, the gestation is monoamniotic.

Figure 2-2 illustrates the type of placentation seen in twin pregnancies. In dizygotic twinning, the embryos may implant separately, resulting in two disks (dichorionic, diamniotic, separate disks), or they may implant close enough together to cause disk fusion (dichorionic, diamniotic, fused discs). In monozygotic twinning, the timing of blastocyst division determines the type of placenta. Early division of a two- to eight-cell blastocyst results in two separate embryos and a dichorionic-diamniotic twin placenta. Such a placenta may be separate or fused. Placentas of this type can be found in 30% of monozygotic

twin pregnancies. Division of the inner cell mass of the blastocyst results in a monochorionic-diamniotic placenta. This is characterized by a single disc, a single chorion, and two amniotic sacs. Fusion of the overlapping chorion occurs where the amniotic sacs are adjacent. Seventy percent of monozygotic twin pregnancies are of this type. In fewer than 2% of monozygotic twins, the inner cell mass of the blastocyst separates, and a monochorionic-monoamniotic twin placenta forms. This placenta has two embryos in one cavity. If the division is incomplete, conjoined twins result. Figure 2-3 outlines the relative incidences for the different placentations and zygosity.[27]

The origin of dizygotic multiple gestations is partially understood.[6] The incidence is generally 1/80 pregnancies and varies with different populations. The mechanism is multiple ovulation events that occur during the same menstrual cycle. Therefore it is most likely that the

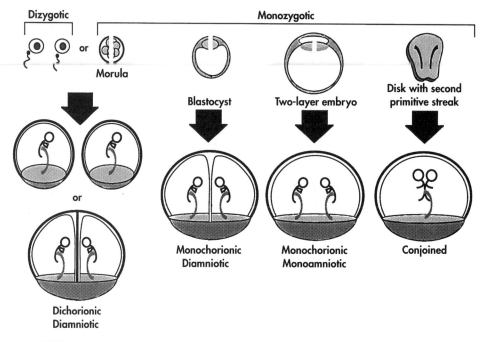

FIGURE 2-2   Types of twinning and placentation in relation to theoretic embryonic origin.

inciting cause is increased gonadotropin activity, specifically follicle-stimulating hormone (FSH) and luteinizing hormone (LH).[35] The use of medications such as clomiphene citrate (Clomid) and human menopausal gonadotropin (HMG) (Pergonal) to enhance ovulation can result in an increased incidence of twin and higher-order multiple gestations.[46] Other factors that support the presence of increased gonadotropin activity include the increased risk of twinning in older women, a variable risk for twinning in different races, a hereditary predisposition for twinning, a seasonal incidence of twinning, and a potential increase in twinning immediately after the cessation of oral contraceptives.[5] It is unknown whether the abnormal production of pituitary gonadotropins is the result of increased hypothalamic produc-

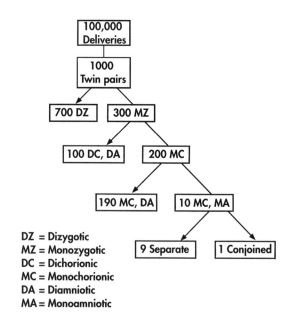

FIGURE 2-3   Relative incidence of twin types. *(From Machin GA: Birth Defects 29:141-179, 1993.)*

tion of gonadotropin-releasing hormone (GnRH), increased GnRH receptor activity in the pituitary gland, or a direct increased synthesis of gonadotropins by the pituitary cells themselves. Additionally, other factors may interact with an increase in gonadotropic hormones. Multiple gestations formed after ovulation induction are not always exclusively dizygotic.[10] There is also an increased incidence of like-pairs in dizygotic twins.[18]

The cause of monozygotic twinning is more obscure. The incidence is quoted at approximately 1/250 pregnancies, and it does not vary for race, age, or family history.[6] The mechanism for monozygosity is a random separation of a formed conceptus, or an abnormal event. The inciting cause may be detrimental environmental conditions, chronic hypo-oxygenation, or yet unidentified teratogenic agents. Benirschke[5] has named this the *twinning impetus*. An intact zona pellucida may also be necessary to prevent early fission. Experimental removal of portions of the zona pellucida has resulted in an increase in monozygotic twinning.[34]

Monozygotic twins that form late in gestation are more likely to be female. There is a preponderance of females in monoamniotic multiple gestations, including acardiac fetuses and conjoined twins. It is postulated that the inactivation of one X chromosome (lyonization) may be abnormal, leading to delayed embryonic maturation and subsequent fission of the germinal disk.[19]

A third type of multiple gestation has been described and categorized as an "intermediate type" between dizygotic and monozygotic twinning. The mechanism of formation is a multiple ovulation event, but the secondary oocytes originate from a single precursor oocyte. It is thought that many like-sex dizygotic twins originate in this manner. Polyovular follicles are most likely the source of this phenomenon. This idea also includes the possibility of simultaneous fertilization of a polar body and its associated oocyte. The finding of fraternal twins with a single corpus luteum may represent evidence of this type of unusual gestation.[4]

Superfecundation is defined as fertilization of more than one oocyte by spermatozoa from different sources. Occasional documentation of cases of dizygotic twins, one white and one black, is an example of this type of twinning.[47] Considered a rare event, the true incidence may be greater than previously reported.

Superfetation is defined as the fertilization of two oocytes from temporally spaced ovulation events. This infers a second fertilization event during a developing pregnancy, a highly unusual occurrence because of hormonal suppression of ovulation. Although it is possible that some discordant dizygotic twins may represent superfetation, this type of twin pregnancy has never been confirmed in humans.

Pathology

The pathology of multiple gestations can be separated into two general categories: abnormalities associated with high-risk singleton pregnancies and abnormalities unique to twinning.

Conditions seen in high-risk singleton pregnancies, including chorioamnionitis, prematurity, preeclampsia, and hemorrhage, can occur in twins; because of the increase in placental mass and accelerated

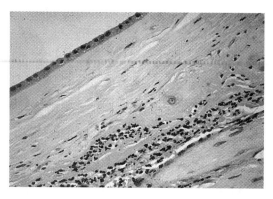

FIGURE 2-4   Section of fetal membranes with chorioamnionitis, characterized by an infiltrate of neutrophils within the chorioamnion (hematoxylin and eosin [H & E] × 40).

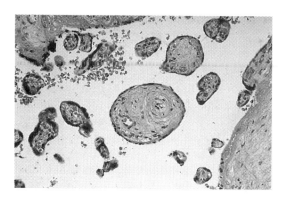

FIGURE 2-5   Photomicrograph of a placenta demonstrating hypertensive vasculopathy (H & E × 40).

uterine growth, multiple gestations are at increased risk for these problems. Twins weigh an average of 800 gm less than singletons at birth; this is most likely the result of early delivery for premature labor or premature membrane rupture.[31] Chorioamnionitis occurs more often in multiple gestations because of premature cervical dilation (Figure 2-4). The gross and microscopic abnormalities found in these disorders are no different from the abnormalities in singleton pregnancies. In chorioamnionitis, the decidual surface and the reticular portion of both the chorion and amnion contain large numbers of polymorphonuclear neutrophil leukocytes (PMNs). In advanced infections, an influx of PMNs from the fetus into the umbilical cord results in vasculitis or funisitis. The presence of a nonspecific villitis, characterized by mononuclear cells within or surrounding a focus of chorionic villi, is associated with a threefold increase in the rate of stillbirths.

A twin placenta associated with severe preeclampsia demonstrates hypertensive changes. Grossly, hemorrhage or infarction can be seen along the maternal surface. The placenta may be smaller than average for a fused multiple gestation, and it may be thinner. Microscopically, the placenta has evidence of intervillous thrombosis, fibrous obliteration of the villi, basement membrane thickening, hypovascularity, and fibromuscular sclerosis of the vessel walls (Figure 2-5). The subsequent adjacent areas of asphyxia show an increase in clumping of syncytiotrophoblastic cells (syncytial knotting or Tenney-Parker changes). There is an indication that perfusion of the placental bed in multiple gestations may be less than in singleton placentas. Placental infarction is therefore not uncommon. Abruptio placentae can occur randomly along the maternal surface of either a separate or fused placenta. Its effect is not preferential for the presenting or subsequent fetus.[32]

The pathologic abnormalities unique to twinning are strongly related to the type of placentation; zygosity type is not a factor. The overall morbidity in monochorionic twins is 191/1000 pregnancies, which is a twofold increase over dichorionic

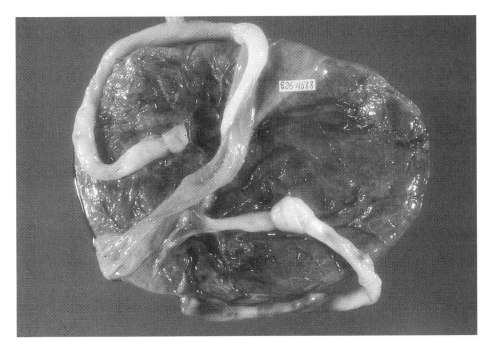

FIGURE 2-6 A dichorionic placenta. The disks are asymmetrical in size, and separated by a thickened opaque membranous septum. Both fetal circulations are independent.

twinning.[31] Morbidity and psychomotor impairment are also higher in monochorionic twinning. Abnormal vascular development and the presence of anastomotic channels is the underlying cause of most of these abnormalities.

DICHORIONIC PREGNANCIES

There may be two separate placentas, or fusion of the two disks may occur if the placentas develop in proximity to each other. Aberrant folding of the developing membranes, similar to extrachorial placental formation, may result in an unequal separation of each gestational sac by the transverse membranous septum. Dichorionic placentas that fuse have a greater discordancy in infant birth weights (Figure 2-6). It is possible that the proximity of the

two placentas may modify fetal development. Whereas the surface area of each placenta is usually different, the smaller placenta is not always associated with the smaller fetus. More important are the qualitative areas of infarction and the number of vascular lesions found in each placenta. The effects are similar to intrauterine growth retardation (IUGR) seen in singleton fetuses.[11] Naeye et al.[32] have shown that perinatal death from placental infarction is twice as common in the second twin, which is often the smaller of the two fetuses. The vascular abnormalities appear confined to the fetal microvasculature; the maternal vessels within the endomyometrium are not affected.[15]

A single case of amniotic rupture of one gestational sac within the transverse septum and extrusion of a foot and hand into the extraamniotic space has been reported.[14] Amniotic bands subsequently developed. The fused chorion and the amnion of the other gestational sac remained intact.

Marginal and velamentous cord insertions occur in 14% of dichorionic placentas. This can lead to increased risk of fetal vessel rupture from vasa praevia.[3]

MONOCHORIONIC-DIAMNIOTIC PREGNANCIES

Monochorionic-diamniotic gestations are subject to specific abnormalities, all of which arise from anomalous vascular development along the fetal surface of the placenta. Normally, trophoblastic growth results in about 200 primary stem villi that anchor the major placental lobules. Aggregates of lobules become the placental cotyledons.[54] The extraembryonic mesoderm, in conjunction with the yolk sac, generates the placental vessels. As stated previously, development of these vessels begins early in embryogenesis. The extrafetal circulation is established by the end of the second week of gestation. Although each fetus contributes to development of an autonomous distribution of vessels (since they have separate yolk sacs), numerous anastomoses develop between each circulation. These probably occur as a result of the formation of a single placenta and chorion; separate placentas in monochorionic-diamniotic gestations are extraordinarily rare. Anastomoses can be of three types, artery-to-artery, vein-to-vein, and artery-to-vein; the first two are typically superficial and, depending on their size and flow rate, are of little consequence (Figure 2-7). The third type usually involves the deep circulation within a cotyledon and is responsible for the ma-

jority of the morbidity and mortality seen in monochorionic-diamniotic twins. These can be divided into three major pathologic entities, the vanishing twin syndrome, fetus papyraceus, and the twin-twin transfusion syndrome. The cause of each is related to the timing of a potential fetal loss.

Marginal and velamentous insertions of the umbilical cord are found in 27% of monochorionic-diamniotic placentas.[3] The cause of this is unknown, but it may be related to the abnormal development of the separate fetal circulations and loss of some vessels through thrombosis. Single umbilical arteries are also common in these gestations.[3]

Vanishing twin syndrome

The *vanishing twin syndrome* is defined as a documented multiple pregnancy that loses one or more fetuses. The diagnosis is made sonographically, usually before the fifteenth week of gestation. The loss may be spontaneous or assisted; the latter involves directed reduction of pregnancy size in higher-order multiple gestations following ovulation induction (OI) techniques. In a recent series reported by Blumenfeld et al.,[8] 221 fetuses originally diagnosed by ultrasound decreased to 112 survivors. Of those fetuses that were lost, two were directly reduced, and three were spontaneously aborted. The remaining 46% vanished without documented evidence of a gestation beyond sonography (Table 2-1). Other investigators[25,48] have reported an incidence of vanishing twins in the range of 50% to 70%. The incidence is probably difficult to establish; many early gestational sacs are resorbed before documentation of their presence, and hematomas or exaggerated decidual growth can be falsely identified as an early gesta-

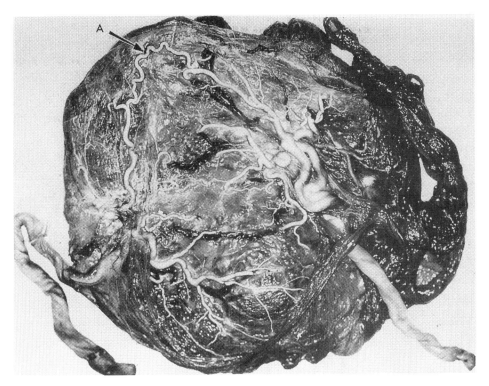

FIGURE 2-7   A monochorionic-diamniotic placenta demonstrating vascular surface anastomoses (A). *(From Benirschke K, Kaufman P: Pathology of the human placenta, ed 2, New York, 1990, Springer-Verlag.)*

tional sac. The phenomenon is common before the fifteenth week of gestation. The earlier a multiple gestation is diagnosed sonographically, the higher the risk for spontaneous fetal loss.

A vanished twin can occasionally be found on the surface of the placenta as a thickened yellow-white plaque, usually 3 to 4 cm in length. It is often visible peripherally in the chorionic plate or within the fetal membrane (Figure 2-8). Careful inspection may identify an umbilical cord remnant. The insertion is typically marginal.[20] The plaque may have an embryonic shape; transillumination may identify retinal pigment.[4] Vanishing twins can occasionally be identified as acardiac fe-

tuses. Microscopically, the plaque is encapsulated by collapsed fetal membranes. The central area consists of fibrinoid with entrapped degenerated chorionic villi. Fetal structures, such as somites, may be recognized (Figure 2-9). The surviving fetus usually demonstrates no pathologic anomaly, but there is an increase of marginal and velamentous cord insertions. In most cases, this may be the only confirmatory evidence of a vanished embryo.[20]

Fetus papyraceus

The *fetus papyraceus*, also known as fetus compressus, is formed by a process similar to mummification. Fetal death usually occurs around 16 to 20 weeks of ges-

TABLE 2-1

Outcome of Multiple Gestations Derived from Assisted Reproduction Techniques

ORIGINAL DIAGNOSIS (SETS)	FOLLOW-UP DIAGNOSIS (SETS)					
	QUINTUPLETS	QUADRUPLETS	TRIPLETS	TWINS	SINGLETONS	ABORTIONS
3 Quintuplets			2*	1*		
5 Quadruplets			2	1	1	1
26 Triplets				12	12	2
54 Twins				51	3	

*One fetus reduced intentionally
From Blumenfeld Z et al: Br J Obstet Gynaecol 99:333-7, 1992.

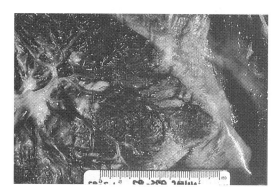

FIGURE 2-8　Peripheral disk of a twin placenta. A thickened plaque is found along the fetal membranes, consistent with a vanished twin.

tation. Body fluids are resorbed, and the fetus is flattened by the continued growth of the second survivor (Figure 2-10). Causes of fetal loss include placental insufficiency from hypertensive vasculopathy, abnormal cord insertions, vascular anastomoses, and reversed twin perfusion. Although fetus papyraceus can occur in dichorionic placentas, they are more common in monozygotic placentas. The incidence is quoted as 1/12,000 live births or 1/184 twin gestations;[26] however, the true incidence may be underreported from lack

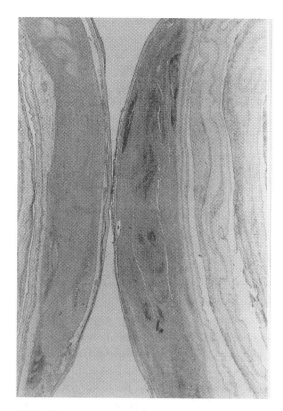

FIGURE 2-9　Membrane roll demonstrating hyperchromatic cell clusters representing compressed embryonal tissue. These findings are consistent with a vanished twin (H & E × 16). (*From Benirschke K, Kaufman P: Pathology of the human placenta, ed 2, New York, 1990, Springer-Verlag.*)

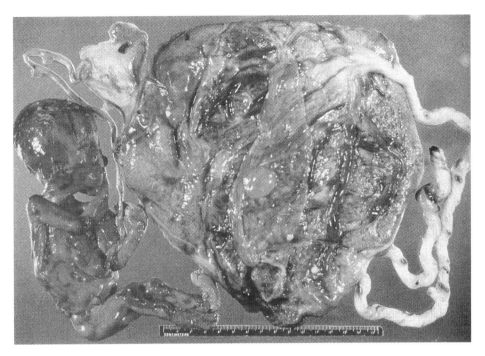

FIGURE 2-10   Fetus papyraceus. The collapsed and dehydrated nature of the fetus is evident. The cord insertion is velamentous. *(From Benirschke K, Kaufman P: Pathology of the human placenta, ed 2, New York, 1990, Springer-Verlag.)*

of recognition. These fetal losses are usually not registered as a birth.

Optimal conditions for the formation of a fetus papyraceus occur at the early-to-mid–second trimester. The typical dehydration and compression cannot develop in a large fetus. Nevertheless, the mummified fetus may be large enough to cause dystocia.[24] The appearance is variable, ranging from an amorphous mass to a recognizable but macerated fetus. Careful dissection is necessary to identify fetal parts or the umbilical cord; radiologic examination may be useful to identify bony structures. Calcification of the entire fetus can result in formation of a lithopedion. However, because of the abbreviated period between death and delivery, this

event is extremely rare. The associated placental parenchyma, if recognizable, shows evidence of infarction and fibrosis. The cord insertion is commonly marginal.

The survivor also has increased morbidity and risk for antepartum death.[26] The fetuses have skin lesions, ranging from focal areas of necrosis to aplasia cutis congenita,[52] and bowel atresias.[41,52] The origin of these defects is obscure, but vascular anastomoses between the two fetuses seem to play a role. One mechanism proposes that circulating tissue thromboplastins from the dead fetus or placenta cross the septum, leading to a hypercoagulable state in the survivor. Thrombosis of various fetal vessels leads to end-organ infarction.[29] Wagner et al.[52] described a case of fetus papyraceus complicated by polyhydramnios in the second twin. After premature delivery, the surviving fetus was found to have colonic atresia, ascites, and hepatomegaly. Multiple thrombi were identified in the microvasculature of the surviving placenta. It is also possible that acute exsanguination of the survivor into the dead fetus may lead to hypovolemia with poor tissue perfusion, necrosis, and death.[4]

Twin-twin transfusion syndrome

A wide variety of fetal weight and hemoglobin discordancies can be found in monochorionic-diamniotic twin gestations. Various disease states, including infections, congenital malformations, and hypertensive diseases that variably affect the placenta, have been implicated.[53] By far the most acutely concerning to the clinician and the pathologist, however, is the twin-twin transfusion syndrome (TTS). This syndrome can occur in either an acute or a chronic state.

Although vascular anastomoses in twin placentas were first identified in the seventeenth century, their significance was first described in the nineteenth century by Schatz, who attributed the possibility of a "third circulation" to explain the presence of simultaneous polyhydramnios and oligohydramnios in a twin pregnancy.[7] As stated, vascular anastomoses can be superficial, deep, or a combination of both. The superficial connections, in order of frequency, are artery-to-artery alone (28%) or in combination with artery-to-vein (28%) and 11% artery-to-vein without other connections. The remaining 33% are vein-to-vein anastomoses and other combinations.[7] The overall in-

cidence of vascular anastomoses is reported to range between 50% and 100%.[9,40] The latter number may be more correct, since injection studies are limited by the type of media used and the size of the anastomotic bridge. Additionally, many channels are lost by placental thrombosis. The type of shunting associated with TTS is the deep type; an artery from one twin supplies a cotyledon drained by the venous system of the other twin. The cotyledon is shared by the two fetal circulations, and the flow is directly from one twin (the donor twin) to the other (the recipient). Depending on the degree of flow from one twin to the other, there is a net loss of blood in one direction. The blood loss may be compensated by back flow through superficial anastomoses, but this is limited by their size and number. If TTS is to develop, the circulation between fetuses must thus be unbalanced.[7] These arteriovenous anastomoses may develop at the time of extrafetal angiogenesis (day 15). This may explain some of the early fetal losses that are diagnosed as vanishing twins or fetus papyraceus. A case of TTS documented by discordant cardiac sizes at 11 weeks has been reported by Benirschke.[5] Although differences in blood volume contribute to twin discordancy, other factors may be important. Growth factors produced by either placenta may modify the development of either fetus. Low placental weight or poor uteroplacental perfusion can cause an increase in fetal hemoglobin.[30]

The incidence of reported TTS ranges from 5% to 30% in surviving monochorionic twins.[38] This number varies according to the criteria used for diagnosis. TTS has been defined as a 5 gm/dl difference of

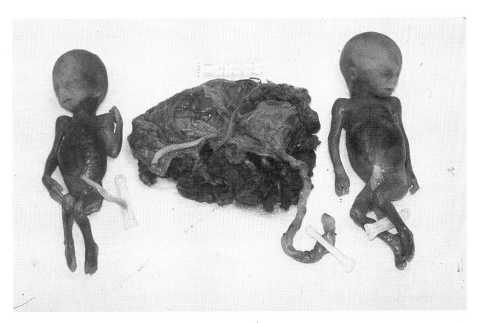

FIGURE 2-11   Twin fetuses with the TTS. Note the marked discrepancy in size. The larger twin also has marked ascites.

fetal hemoglobin or a 20% difference in fetal weight.[38,49] Although these criteria are arbitrary, they have generally been accepted.[12]

The pathologic features seen in chronic TTS are strikingly different for each fetus. The donor, or pump twin, is the smaller of the two (Figure 2-11). It is usually pale and anemic. Hypotension and hypovolemia result in oliguria and oligohydramnios. A lack of amnionic fluid restricts fetal movement (the "stuck twin" phenomenon), and the fetus may demonstrate facial and limb deformities similar to fetuses with renal agenesis. Additionally, compensatory hematopoiesis and cardiac failure may result in changes similar to nonimmune fetal hydrops. This may lead to paradoxical concordance in fetal weight.[7] The placenta is pale and thin. Microscopically, the villi may show trophoblastic proliferation (Tenney-Parker changes) and small villi with empty vessels. The vessels themselves have thinning of the muscularis. In some cases, the placenta may show changes compatible with hydrops. The villi are immature; Langhans' layer persists, and erythroblasts can be found within fetal vessels. Chronic oligohydramnios may result in the formation of amnion nodosum.

In contrast, the recipient twin is usually large and plethoric. The internal organs are also larger (Figure 2-12). Specifically, the kidneys show marked enlargement from renal cortical hyperplasia and glomerular proliferation.[7] The cause of this is unknown, although it has been shown that elevated levels of atriopeptin, a natriuretic substance, have been found in a small series of recipient twins with TTS.[33] The modification of kidney function prob-

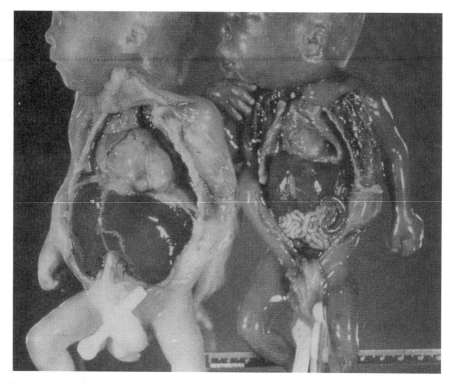

FIGURE 2-12   Autopsy specimens of two fetuses with TTS. Note the marked discrepancy in organ sizes. *(From Benirschke K, Kaufman P: Pathology of the human placenta, ed 2, New York, 1990, Springer-Verlag.)*

ably contributes to the associated polyhydramnios. Cardiomegaly is universally present. Popek et al.[36] have documented three cases of calcified pulmonary valves in stillborn twin fetuses. All three were associated with a volume overload state. Two were pump fetuses associated with acardiac twins, and one was a recipient fetus associated with TTS. The valves were otherwise structurally normal. They postulate that a chronic increase in cardiac output resulted in this valvular alteration.

The acute form of TTS is usually a result of rapid volume shifts after the death of one fetus or at the time of delivery. It is important to note that changes associated with either twin may be modified by this fluid shift. For example, rapid influx of blood into the donor fetus gives it a reddish plethoric appearance; conversely, blood loss of the recipient twin gives it an anemic appearance. The use of other changes, such as organ sizes, fetal weights, amnionic fluid volumes, and placental appearance may help determine which twin was the original donor and which was the original recipient.

Perinatal mortality in TTS is high. In the series of nineteen cases reported by Rausen, Seki, and Strauss,[38] four cases (19%) had survival of both twins and 5 cases (26%) had survival of one fetus. Factors predisposing a fetus to death include prematurity, the size of the anastomotic bridges, and the length of gestation. When one fetus dies, an equilibrium is established, and amniotic fluid volumes return to normal amounts. Nevertheless, the surviving fetus is at risk for subsequent morbidity. This is related to the size of the dead fetus and the length of gestation at the time of death. Specific effects include central nervous system abnormalities, renal cortical necrosis, skin anomalies including aplasia cutis, and limb defects.[5,6] As with fetus papyraceus, it is postulated that there is a release of thromboplastins that cross to the surviving fetus, causing infarction at specific organ sites. More recently, Benirschke[3] has postulated that the exsanguination from the survivor into the other twin can result in the same effect. The surviving fetus can maintain the circulation of the placenta associated with the dead fetus, and the morphologic changes of death in the placenta may not be seen.[12]

Twin reversed arterial perfusion

The twin reversed arterial perfusion (TRAP) sequence is a more recent term used to indicate the presence of an acardiac twin. Other names used to describe these peculiar entities include chorioangiopagus parasiticus, hemicardius, acardius homosomius, and hemisomus.[51] These fetuses are characterized by marked deformities and an absence of a normally formed cardiac structure. Circulation in an acardiac twin is maintained by vascular anastomoses from the other, or pump twin, and the flow in the perfused twin is essentially reversed, that is, flow is from the umbilical artery to the umbilical vein. The incidence is estimated at 1/100 monozygotic twins, but many cases are probably unrecognized.[5]

In TTS, a placental artery of one twin perfuses a placental vein in the other through a shared cotyledon. In the TRAP sequence, the connection from one fetus to the acardiac fetus is artery-to-artery and vein-to-vein. The connection is superficial and can develop within shared vessels in partially joined umbilical cords. Therefore the necessary requirement for the formation of an acardiac twin is not a volume difference but a difference in arterial pressure from one twin to the other. Two theories may explain the evolution of an acardiac twin, although the exact mechanism is unknown. In the first theory, development of both fetal hearts may not be simultaneous. If one heart forms before the other, the fetus with the hemodynamic advantage becomes the pump twin, and vascular anastomoses allow it to perfuse the second twin. The premature establishment of a circulation in the second twin may interrupt induction of the primary cardiac tube, and no heart is formed.[51] An alternative explanation supposes the primary absence of the cardiac tube in one twin.[5] It is, nevertheless, salvaged through perfusion by the second twin. Chromosomal abnormalities have been found in some acardiac twins, lending support to this second theory.[51] In either event, the dependent circulation is predicated on the adequacy of the intraarterial and intravenous anastomoses. Inadequate perfusion results in early fetal loss.

In the perfused, or acardiac twin, there are multisystem malformations and an unusual body form. The appearance can be striking in some cases (Figure 2-13). The mythologic Gorgon Medusa ("whom no man shall behold and draw again the breath of life. . .") may reflect the description of an acardiac twin.[16a] Numer-

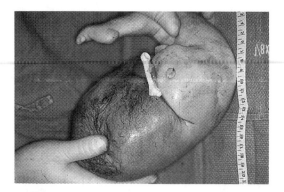

FIGURE 2-13   An acardiac twin. Excepting one leg, no recognizable body structure is present. The umbilical cord contained a single umbilical artery.

ous classifications have been developed to categorize so-called patterns, but the abnormalities are all part of a morphologic spectrum. Commonly seen are absence of a cardiac structure and a lack of body development, starting in the upper body and ending with a total loss of organogenesis and body form. A predominance of acardiac twins is female. Their size is variable, ranging from small placental surface nodules to a term fetus. A 3000 gm acardiac twin causing dystocia during delivery has been described.[6]

The heart demonstrates anomalies ranging from a single tube to a folded common chamber and truncus.[51] A persistent vitelline artery may also be found, confirming abnormal vascular development. The presence of liver tissue in acardiac twins has been disputed.[5,51] The lower extremities and abdomen may be minimally deformed. This reflects preferential perfusion of the abdomen and lower extremities through the iliac arteries by poorly oxygenated blood. Internal organs may be well formed or absent. Malformed or absent organs have an associated lack of vascular development.[51] Polyhydramnios can

sometimes be seen. In these cases, the acardiac twins are large and have developed kidneys. Single umbilical arteries are common.

The survival rate for the perfusing twin is 50%. Death is usually the result of prematurity.[51] This twin demonstrates changes consistent with volume overload. Cardiomegaly with right ventricular hypertrophy is commonly present. In the series of pulmonic valvular calcifications reported by Popek et al.,[36] two such calcifications were found in pump twins from acardiac pregnancies. Hepatomegaly, ascites, and edema similar to hydrops may be present.[51] This may indicate an overall hypoalbuminemic state. Infarction from embolic phenomenon or circulating thromboplastins, commonly seen in TTS, is not seen in the TRAP sequence.

MONOCHORIONIC-MONOAMNIOTIC PREGNANCIES

The incidence of monochorionic-monoamniotic gestations is 1/100 twin gestations or 1/60,000 pregnancies.[5] The placenta is characterized by two or more umbilical cords within a single amniotic sac (Figure 2-14). Fusion of fetal yolk sacs may lead to partial or complete fusion of the cords. Velamentous insertion of one or both cords can also occur. The death rate of one or both fetuses in such cases is 50% to 70%.[5] The cause of death is typically cord entanglement or knotting. The location of both cords has no direct relation to the incidence of cord complications. It is important to identify the proper umbilical cord associated with the presenting fetus before the cord is cut. This can be difficult in situations where the fetus has a nuchal cord.[5]

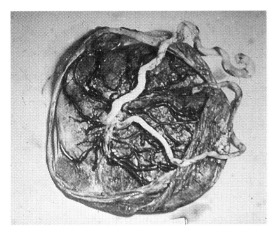

FIGURE 2-14   A monochorionic placenta. The two umbilical cords are closely approximated within a single chorioamniotic sac.

Although anastomoses of fetal vessels can occur between the two fetuses, the incidence is less than it is in twins with diamniotic placentas.[5] In these monoamniotic placentas, fetal death can occur as tissue thromboplastins transfer from one fetus to the other. The survivor is also at increased risk because of acute exsanguination.

Occasionally, monochorionic placentas contain chorionic folds along the fetal surface. The plicae typically traverse between the two umbilical cords. They probably represent remnants of membrane septa that ruptured early in pregnancy. Amniocentesis has been cited as a cause of septal rupture.[14]

CONJOINED TWINS

The rarest of all twin abnormalities, the occurrence of conjoined twins has been recorded throughout history as an event of great importance. It is likely that Janus, the god of good beginnings who had two opposite heads, and satyrs and centaurs (half human and half four-legged animals)

represent examples of conjoined twins. The birth of a craniopagus in Germany in 1495 was considered a sign from God and resulted in preparations for war by both Christians and Muslims.[55] During the 19th century, the exhibition of Chang and Eng Bunker by P.T. Barnum as "Siamese twins" has resulted in the lay use of the latter term to represent conjoined twins.[44] The incidence is approximately 1/300 monozygotic pregnancies.[27] There is a preponderance of females.

The formation of conjoined twins is not well understood. If there is a delay of growth in the germinal disc, a second growth center may be established and two gastrulation events occur. This may be initiated by organizer sites within certain not-yet-identified inducer genes; axiation genes then mediate the orientation of the two notochords.[27] Fetal movements may also contribute to alignment.[55] Separation is then incomplete, and the fetuses share common organs. In some conjoined twins, secondary fusion may occur after separation of the two embryonic disks, but this is unlikely.[45] The following features are common for conjoined twins: (1) the majority have two complete notochordal axes; (2) the twins are equidistant in a longitudinal axis and match somite for somite; and (3) shared organs are often distorted, malaligned, or absent.[27,45,55]

The classification of conjoined twins is confusing. Most can be grouped into a few main anatomic types. General categorizations of Guttmacher and Nichols[16] emphasize the area of duplication, whereas those of Potter and Craig[37] are based on the site of union. Table 2-2 lists the various forms of conjoined twinning and their incidences.[27]

The thoracopagus is the most common

TABLE 2-2

Types of Conjoined Twins

TYPE	SITE OF UNION	INCIDENCE (%)
Thoracopagus	Chest	33
Thoracoomphalopagus	Chest and abdomen	16
Dicephalus	Lower body	11
Cephalothoracopagus	Head and chest	6
Craniopagus	Head	5
Pygopagus	Sacrum	4
Ischiopagus	Pelvis	3
Other combinations		22

From Machin GA: Birth Defects 29:141-179, 1993.

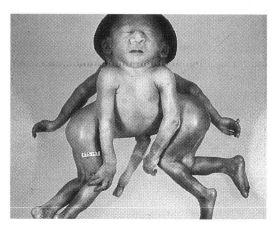

FIGURE 2-15 The cephalothoracopagus type of conjoined twins. A unified face is 90 degrees to the fused heads. If the notochordal rotation is completely symmetrical, another face can be found on the opposite side. *(From the American Society of Clinical Pathologists.)*

type of conjoined twin. The twins are fused at the front, and they are supplied by a single umbilical cord. The number of vessels within the cord, however, can vary widely. Because of the proximity of the two notochordal systems, the shared organs can be markedly distorted or absent. If the heart is shared, the heart of the right twin usually has the worse anomalies.[5] The twins always face each other; however, in one reported case, the twins were rotated 180 degrees.[45]

In ischiopagous and cephalothoracopagous twinning, organs formed at the site of fusion can be rotated laterally.[27,45] In the case of the former, the bladders and lower genital tracts are 90 degrees from the midline. A kidney from each fetus supplies the midline bladders. In the cephalothoracopagus, the two notochords are probably aligned at the superior poles and rotated in a caudad fashion. Symmetrical rotation results in facial features on either side, 90 degrees to the head and body (the *janiceps* formation) (Figure 2-15). Asymmetrical rotation results in abnormal facial fea-

tures and cranial anomalies (holoprosencephaly) of one twin.

Parasitic twinning is a variant of conjoined twinning in which one twin (the parasite) is small and malformed and the other (the autosite) demonstrates normal development. The pathogenesis is obscure. It is likely that the parasite dies during embryologic or fetal development and is subsequently vascularized by the autosite.[45] Additionally, abnormal transfetal anastomoses can also result in chronic ischemia and maldevelopment of the parasite. The attachment is typically midline; those documented have been connected to the face, chest, abdomen, and pelvis.[5]

Fetus in fetu is a condition whereby one twin is internalized into the other. It may represent a type of parasitic twinning. The location is usually in the superior retroperitoneum. Its vascular supply is the superior mesenteric artery, which is a derivative of the vitelline artery.[5,6] Karyotyping may be necessary to differentiate between fetal development of this type and a retroperitoneal teratoma with homunculus formation.

OTHER ABNORMALITIES

Congenital abnormalities are more common in monozygotic twinning. This is probably related to the teratogenic event that caused the initial embryonic fission. Other causes include asymmetrical splitting of the blastomeres or abnormal vascular development in one or both twins. The most common abnormalities seen are a single umbilical artery and esophageal atresia. Both the vertebral, anal, tracheoesophageal fistula, renal anomalies (VATER) and the addition of cardiac and limb anomalies (VACTERL) syndromes have been reported in twins. Anencephaly, sirenomelia, holoprosencephaly, and cleft deformations are seen less often.[5]

Twin ectopic pregnancies have been described; the vast majority are monochorionic.[5] It is possible that delayed uterine implantation may result in embryonic splitting and tubal implantation. The size of the gestational sac may also hinder passage through the isthmic portion of the fallopian tube.

Heterotopic twin pregnancies (embryonic development in both the uterus and fallopian tube) are seen in 1/30,000 pregnancies. Because of potential resorption of either the intrauterine or ectopic pregnancy, the true incidence is difficult to determine. The number of cases has recently increased with the introduction of various ovulation induction (OI) techniques.[39]

It is possible that craniopharyngeal and sacrococcygeal teratomas may, in some cases, represent a malformed second twin.[5] They are seen more often in females, and the babies with these tumors have an increased incidence of congenital anomalies. The appearance of these tumors is similar to the immature teratoma seen in the older child and adult, but the malignant potential is much less than that seen in the latter type.

Pathologic Examination

PLACENTAL EXAMINATION

Placental examination is gaining importance as the role of the placenta in infant morbidity and mortality is being recognized. How placentas should be handled by surgical pathology laboratories has been disputed.[1,42] A reasonable compromise is gross examination of all placentas. Certain subgroups are triaged for microscopic examination (Table 2-3).[21] Fortunately, the importance of examining the placentas in multiple pregnancies is not a new idea. The pathologist has a twofold mission: to help determine zygosity and to discover any pathologic condition that is present (general or twin-related).

All placentas should be examined with as much available clinical data as can be provided. Most institutions where examinations are done routinely provide an information sheet. This is filled out by the clinician and submitted with the placenta (Figure 2-16). The handling of the specimen should be determined by the examining pathologist. Some prefer to examine the placenta in the fresh state; others prefer formalin-fixed specimens. Significant gross lesions are identifiable in either state. Formalin-fixed organs present less of an infectious hazard. However, care must be taken to fix the organ flat without distortion. Additionally, adequate

TABLE 2-3

Indications for Placental Microscopy

FETAL	MATERNAL	PLACENTAL
Stillborn	Preexisting condition (hypertension, diabetes, drug abuse)	Abnormal fetal/placental weight ratio
Possible infection	Poor reproductive history	Extensive infarction
Multiple gestation	Possible infection	Single umbilical artery
Prematurity (<36 weeks)	Abruption	Retroplacental hemorrhage
Postmaturity (>42 weeks)	Repetitive bleeding	Excessive fibrin deposition
Intrauterine growth retardation (IUGR)		Villous atrophy
Congenital anomalies		Chorioangioma
Hydrops		Possible infection
Meconium staining		
Oligohydramnios		
"Fetal distress"		
Admission to neonatal intensive care unit (NICU)		
Apgar <3 at 5 minutes		

From Kaplan CG: Color atlas of gross placental pathology, New York, 1994, Igaku-Shon.

amounts of formalin must be used, and this can be a considerable expense. Fresh placentas can be stored at 4° C for several days without significant tissue deterioration. The fresh state preserves the tissue for chromosomal studies. Care should be taken not to freeze the tissue before examination, because this can lead to distortion of the histologic sections.

At delivery, the umbilical cords should be clamped and marked for easy identification. As an example, the umbilical cord of Twin A can be singly clamped, and Twin B's umbilical cord can be doubly clamped. If infection is suspected and the amniotic fluid has not been cultured, placental tissue should be taken in the delivery room for appropriate microbiologic studies.

Gross evaluation

Multiple gross presentations may be encountered with twin placentas. For example, a dizygotic placenta may have fused or separate disks. Monozygotic placentas may be monochorionic or dichorionic. The monozygotic dichorionic placenta, like the dizygotic dichorionic placenta, may have fused or separate disks. The monozygotic monochorionic placenta has a single disk with two amniotic sacs.

When there are two separate disks, the placenta is classified as dichorionic and diamniotic. In this case, the zygosity of like-sex twins cannot be determined by examination of the placenta. Each disk is examined as a singleton. The following informa-

University of Louisville Hospital

PLACENTA REGISTRY
ANATOMIC/SURGICAL PATHOLOGY

PATIENT IDENTIFICATION

Date	Unit/Bed	Service □ OBSTETRICS □ OTHER: _____

This form is to be completed for all placentas.

For Unknown History, Person to Call	Phone Number	Infection Warning/Special Requests

INFANT

□ LIVE BIRTH   □ STILL BIRTH

Delivery □ SVD □ FORCEPS □ VBAC □ CS □ EMERGENT CS

| Gestation Age weeks | Birthweight gm | Sex □ M □ F |

Presentation □ VERTEX □ BREECH

Apgars 1 _____ 5 _____

Length of Cord NOT Submitted _____ cm

Gases AA _____ VV _____

	Yes	No	
Congenital abnormalities	□	□	Type: _____
Intrauterine growth retardation	□	□	_____
Multiple gestation	□	□	_____
Other studies inititated	□	□	Specify: _____

MATERNAL HISTORY

Age	G	P Term	Preterm	Spont. Ab.	VIP

Stillbirths _____
Neonatal Loss _____

	Yes	No	
Prenatal care	□	□	_____
Amniocentesis	□	□	_____
Abnormal fetal tracing	□	□	_____
Meconium	□	□	_____
Premature rupture of membranes	□	□	_____
Prolonged rupture of membranes	□	□	_____
□ Oligohydramnios □ Polyhydramnios	□	□	_____
Fever > 100.4 (or treated during labor)	□	□	_____
Cervical cultures done	□	□	_____
Known infections	□	□	Specify: _____
Cord abnormality/prolapse/knot	□	□	_____
Bleeding/Impression of	□	□	Abruption: _____ Previa: _____
Anemia Hg <10 gr/dl	□	□	_____
Essential hypertension/diabetes	□	□	_____
Pre-eclampsia/Eclampsia	□	□	_____
Medications/Antibiotics	□	□	_____
Tobacco	□	□	_____
Alcohol	□	□	_____
Illicit drugs	□	□	_____
Toxic screen	□	□	_____

PREVIOUS INFANT/FETAL PROBLEMS

□ HHUofL   □ OTHER HOSPITAL _____

	Yes	No	
Intrauterine growth retardation	□	□	_____
Intrauterine death	□	□	_____
Malformations	□	□	Type: _____
Prolonged hospital stay	□	□	Due to: _____
Autopsy results	□	□	

Physician's Signature MD	Resident's Signature MD	Lab Number

FIGURE 2-16   Clinical form for placental pathologic evaluation.

tion should be obtained: (1) placental weight after trimming the fetal membranes and umbilical cord; (2) the disk shape and measurements; (3) the length, insertion site, vessel number, and presence of knots in the umbilical cord; (4) the type of insertion, presence of velamentous vessels, color, and opacity of the fetal membranes; (5) the color, vascularization, presence of nodules, and cysts in the chorionic plate; and (6) the color, completeness, and presence of adherent clot in the maternal surface.

Placental weight in twin gestations offers a clue to fetal growth. In separate disks, the relative weights of the placentas should be compared with the relative size of the babies. Fused disks usually weigh less than the sum of their separate disk counterparts.[2] Unusual disk shape may occur secondary to uterine structural abnormalities (leiomyomata) or implantation abnormalities (placenta previa).

The normal range for cord length is 35 to 65 cm and partially determined by fetal movement.[30] Marginal and velamentous cord insertions are more common in twin placentas and should be noted. A single umbilical artery is three to four times more common in multiple gestations and is associated with fetal malformations.[15]

The fetal membranes and chorionic plate may be opacified from ascending infection, or they may be stained with meconium. With the latter, the intensity and color depend on the temporal sequence since the time of meconium passage. The presence and integrity of any velamentous vessels should be recorded. The type of membrane insertion should be noted, since both circummarginate and circumvallate placentas can be found in multiple gestations. The clinical significance of these abnormal membrane insertions is related to the decrease in size of the amniotic cavity and the increased risk of placental bleeding from the exposed extrachorial villi.[43] Subchorionic fibrin plaques, nodules of squamous metaplasia, amnion nodosum, cysts, and yolk sac remnants can be found on the fetal surface. The surface vascular pattern should show three to four large vessel systems arborizing over the chorionic plate.

The maternal surface should be examined for completeness and for the presence of indentations that indicate chronic abruption secondary to a retroplacental hematoma.

Each disk should then be sliced at 1-cm intervals (from maternal to fetal surface) in a "bread loaf" manner, and the pathologist should search for infarcts, chorioangiomas, and recent hemorrhage. The color of the cut surface (pale or red-purple) should also be recorded. Histologic sections should be submitted from each disk and should include the three levels of the umbilical cord, the maternal surface, and the fetal surface, as well as a full-thickness section. The peripheral fetal membranes are rolled to the edge of the chorionic plate and sectioned. The parenchyma sections should be taken in an area away from the periphery of the disk. Any lesion noted grossly should also be sampled.

When there is a single disk, attention is first directed to the dividing membrane, if present. In most cases, it is possible to determine grossly whether the membrane represents a monochorionic or dichorionic placenta. A thin, translucent membrane that separates easily in two represents a monochorionic placenta, and it is always

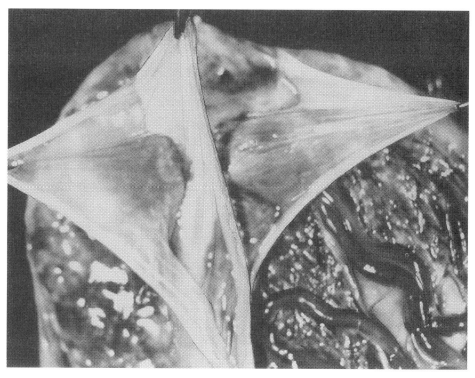

FIGURE 2-17   The membranous septum (dividing membranes) of a dichorionic-diamniotic placenta. Teasing apart the two amnions demonstrates a fused chorionic center. Thus three distinct layers can be discerned. *(From Benirschke K, Kaufman P: In Pathology of the human placenta, ed 2, New York, 1990, Springer-Verlag.)*

derived from a monozygotic pregnancy. A thick, opacified dividing membrane that cannot be easily teased apart represents a dichorionic placenta. When carefully separated, three individual membranes representing the two amnions and a central fused chorion can be identified (Figure 2-17). There is also a raised ridge of fibrin along the placental disk where the dividing membrane inserts onto the chorionic plate. A histologic section of rolled portion of the dividing membranes, including their insertion point into the placenta, should be submitted. If the placenta is dichorionic, the remainder of the examination is similar to that for twins with separate placentas. The percentage of the

disk occupied by each placenta should be recorded.

If the placenta is monochorionic, vascular anastomoses between the two sides must be sought. A simple technique involves the injection of air into the large vessels of the fetal surface. Opaque substances, such as milk or water colored with food dye, may be used. The path of the injected material can then be traced across the disk. The type of vessel can usually be identified because arteries always run over the surface of veins. However, many anastomoses are found within the parenchyma and are difficult to recognize grossly. Unbalanced anastomoses can lead to TTS. If this is suspected, the thickness and coloration of each placental disk should be recorded. Peripheral fibrinous plaque-like structures could represent a small fetus papyraceus or a vanishing twin, and they should be carefully dissected. Histologic sections submitted from each disk are the same as those from a singleton placenta, and they include the umbilical cord, fetal membranes from each sac, the maternal and fetal surfaces, full-thickness sections, and all gross lesions. The sections should be designated as arising from Twin A or Twin B (Figure 2-18).

If there is no dividing membrane present, the placenta is monoamniotic. A careful search should be done to ensure that the dividing membranes have not been accidentally stripped off the fetal surface. The length, thickness, coloration, and insertion site of each cord should be recorded. Vascular anastomoses should be sought by injection of air or opaque materials. Except for the addition of the second umbilical cord, histologic sections are similar to those of a singleton placenta.

For high-order multiple gestations, each separate disk is handled as a singleton placenta. In areas with fused disks, each dividing membrane is examined separately, as summarized in the gross description of a monochorionic twin placenta. Submitted sections include portions of each placenta, peripheral membranes and cord, and sections from each dividing membrane (Figure 2-19).

Histologic examination

In a fused twin placenta, a carefully obtained roll of dividing membranes is immensely useful in confirming the type of placentation and, in many cases, the zygosity. In monochorionic placentas, the two amniotic surfaces, each composed of

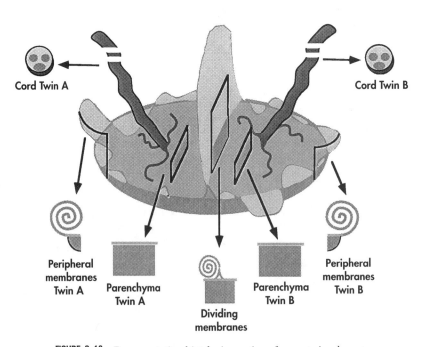

Cord Twin A

Cord Twin B

Peripheral membranes Twin A

Parenchyma Twin A

Dividing membranes

Parenchyma Twin B

Peripheral membranes Twin B

FIGURE 2-18   Representative histologic sections from a twin placenta.

a single layer of cuboidal to columnar cells, are juxtaposed. A sparsely cellular myxoid matrix separates them; no chorion is present (Figure 2-20, *A*). In dichorionic placentas, the two chorions usually fuse, leading to a layer of compressed villi and trophoblast between the two amniotic membranes (Figure 2-20, *B*). The fetal surface at the site of the dividing membrane insertion demonstrates the union of the chorion from each gestational sac. This is identifiable as a raised triangular protuberance of trophoblastic cells. Oth-

erwise, histologic findings in the twin placenta are the same as those found in a singleton placenta.

Examination of each umbilical cord should confirm the number of vessels documented grossly. Occasionally an involuting artery may be seen on section. Other structures found histologically in the cord include hemangiomas and embryonic remnants such as omphalomesenteric ducts, allantoic stalks, and vitelline vessels. Inflammation in the cord, a fetal response to infection,[28] should be documented as either a vasculitis or a true funisitis (neutrophils within Wharton's jelly).

Examination of the fetal membranes should document the presence of any maternal vasculopathy. Inflammation should be noted, and the type (acute or chronic) and site (decidua, chorion, or amnion) should be included. Meconium-laden histocytes, if present, should be noted as located in the amnion or chorion; the finding of meconium within the chorion indicates its existence within the amnion fluid for at least 3 to 4 hours.

The placenta parenchyma should be ex-

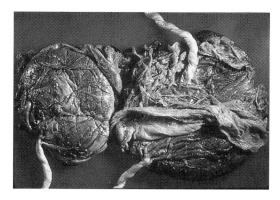

FIGURE 2-19 A triplet placenta. There is one separate disk and a fused dichorionic-diamniotic placenta with discordancy in disk size. Note the thickened dividing membranes.

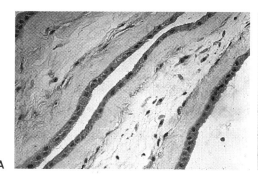
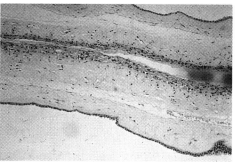

A   B

FIGURE 2-20 Microscopic appearance of the dividing membranes. A is an example of monochorionic-diamniotic membranes; there is an absence of trophoblast in the center. B is an example of dichorionic-diamniotic membranes. The central trophoblastic layers have not quite fused in this section.

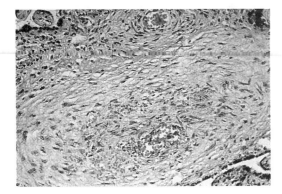

FIGURE 2-21 Hemorrhagic endovasculitis. Note the extravasation of red blood cells into the vessel wall (H & E × 200).

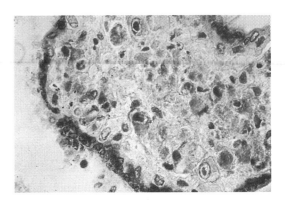

FIGURE 2-22 Cytomegalovirus infection of a villus. There is an enlarged nuclear inclusion present (H & E × 200).

amined for fetal vascular lesions, including thrombosis, basement membrane thickening, and hemorrhagic endovasculitis. The latter is characterized by obliteration of the vessel lumen and extravasation of red cells into the vessel wall and surrounding stroma (Figure 2-21). In stillborn fetuses, this change is probably regressive; when it occurs in liveborn infants, some observers feel that the lesion results from thrombosis of stem vessels and may indicate thrombosis elsewhere within the fetal circulation.[22] The villus size, vessel number, and presence of syncytial knots can be used to assess placental maturity. If acute or chronic villitis is recognized, a search for specific organisms (such as cytomegalovirus) is mandated (Figure 2-22). Villitis with abscess formation can represent *Listeria* infection.[13] Specific placental tumors are usually represented by chorioangiomas.

FETAL EXAMINATION

If one or both fetuses is submitted with the placenta as a stillbirth, the gross and microscopic evaluation is no different from that described in standard perinatal autopsy protocols.[50] If the fetus is classified as an abortus and therefore submitted as a surgical pathology specimen, a "mini-autopsy" can be performed at the bench. Fetal weights and measurements must be obtained, since the differentiation between twin discordancy and TTS depends on these values. External examination should focus on identification of cranial abnormalities, midline defects, or renal anomalies, since these malformations are commonly seen in twins. Fetal congestion or pallor reflect a potential hemorrhage from one twin to the other. Internal inspection should include the location, weights, and size of identifiable organs. Fresh material from the skin and spleen can be used for karyotyping and other tissue analysis, if appropriate. Minimum sections to be submitted include portions of lung, kidney, liver, and gonad; these organs usually show the least amount of autolysis. Microscopic examination should include a search for potential infectious agents.

Summary

Careful pathologic evaluation of both the fetus and placenta can help clarify many of the abnormalities unique to twin and higher-order multiple gestations. It is the only way that clinicians can better understand the pathophysiology of these otherwise exceptionally rare events. It is important, as with all specimens sent for surgical pathologic evaluation, that the clinician submit all pertinent clinical information, including relevant sonographic and radiologic findings. The pathologist must then issue a report that is detailed and complete. It should include information on the type of placentation, abnormalities peculiar to multiple gestations, and any findings reflecting other high-risk conditions, if applicable.

References

1. American College of Obstetricians and Gynecologists, Committee on Obstetrics, Maternal and Fetal Medicine: ACOG Committee Opinion: Placental Pathology, Washington, D.C., 1993, author.
2. Baldwin VJ: *Pathology of multiple pregnancy.* In Dimmick JE, Kalousel DK, editors: *Developmental pathology of the embryo and fetus,* Philadelphia, 1992, Lippincott.
3. Benirschke K: The contribution of placental anastomoses to perinatal twin damage, *Hum Pathol* 23:1319-1320, 1992.
4. Benirschke K: Intrauterine death of a twin: mechanisms, implications for surviving twin, and placental pathology, *Semin Diagn Pathol* 10:222-231, 1993.
5. Benirschke K, Kaufmann P: *Multiple pregnancy.* In *Pathology of the human placenta,* ed 2, New York, 1990, Springer-Verlag.
6. Benirschke K, Kim CK: Multiple pregnancy, *N Engl J Med* 288:1276-1284, 1973.
7. Blickstein I: The twin-twin transfusion syndrome, *Obstet Gynecol* 76:714-722, 1990.
8. Blumenfeld Z et al: Spontaneous fetal reduction in multiple gestations assessed by transvaginal ultrasound, *Br J Obstet Gynaecol* 99:333-337, 1992.
9. Chescheir NC, Seeds JW: Polyhydramnios and oligohydramnios in twin gestations, *Obstet Gynecol* 71:L882-884, 1988.
10. Derom C et al: Increased monozygotic twinning rate after ovulation induction, *Lancet* 1:1236, 1987.
11. Eberle AM et al: Placental pathology in discordant twins, *Am J Obstet Gynecol* 169:931-935, 1993.
12. Galea P, Scott JM, Goel KM: Feto-fetal transfusion syndrome, *Arch Dis Child* 57:781-794, 1982.
13. Gersell D: Chronic villitis, chronic chorioamnionitis and maternal floor infarction, *Semin Diagn Pathol* 10:251-266, 1993.
14. Gilbert WM et al: Morbidity associated with prenatal disruption of the dividing membrane in twin gestations, *Obstet Gynecol* 78:623-630, 1991.
15. Giles W et al: Placental microvascular changes in twin pregnancies with abnormal umbilical artery waveforms, *Obstet Gynecol* 81:556-559, 1993.
16. Guttmacher AF, Nichols BL: Teratology of conjoined twins, *Birth Defects* 3:3-9, 1967.
16a. Hesoid, *The theogeny.* In Speert, H: *Obstetrics and gynecology: a history and iconography,* San Francisco, 1994, Norman Publishing.
17. Innes MM, editor: *The metamorphoses of Ovid,* New York, 1957, Penguin Books.
18. James WH: Excess of like sexed pairs of dizygotic twins, *Nature* 232:277-278, 1971.
19. James WH: A further note on the sex ratio of monoamniotic twins, *Ann Hum Biol* 18:471-474, 1992.
20. Jauniaux E et al: Clinical and morphological aspects of the vanishing twin phenomenon, *Obstet Gynecol* 72:577-581, 1988.
21. Kaplan CG: *Color atlas of gross placental pathology,* New York, 1994, Igaku-Shon.
22. Kraus FT: Placental thrombi and related problems, *Semin Diagn Pathol* 10:275-283, 1993.
23. Larsen WJ: *Human embryology,* New York, 1993, Churchill Livingstone.
24. Leppert PC, Wartel L, Lowman R: Fetus papyraceus causing dystocia: inability to detect blighted twin antenatally, *Obstet Gynecol* 54:381-384, 1979.
25. Levi S: Ultrasonic assessment of the high rate of human multiple pregnancy in the first trimester, *J Clin Ultrasound* 4:3-5, 1976.
26. Livnat EJ et al: Fetus papyraceus in twin pregnancy, *Obstet Gynecol* 51:41s-45s, 1977.
27. Machin GA: Conjoined twins: implications for blastogenesis, *Birth Defects* 29:141-179, 1993.
28. Macpherson T: Fact and fancy: what can we really tell from the placenta? *Arch Pathol Lab Med* 115:672-681, 1991.
29. Moore CM, McAdams AF, Sutherland J: Intrauterine disseminated intravascular coagulation: a syndrome of multiple pregnancy with a dead twin fetus, *J Pediatr* 74:523-528, 1990.

30. Naeye RL: Functionally important disorders of the placenta, umbilical cord and fetal membranes, *Hum Pathol* 18:680-691, 1987.

31. Naeye RL: *Disorders of the placenta, fetus and neonate*, St. Louis, 1991, Mosby.

32. Naeye RL et al: Twins: causes of perinatal death in 12 United States cities and one African city, *Am J Obstet Gynecol* 131:267-272, 1978.

33. Nagoette MP et al: Atriopeptin in the twin transfusion syndrome, *Obstet Gynecol* 73:867-870, 1989.

34. Nijs M et al: A monozygotic twin pregnancy after application of zone rubbing on a frozen-thawed blastocyst, *Hum Reprod* 8:127-129, 1993.

35. Nylander PS: Serum levels of gonadotrophins in relation to multiple pregnancy in Nigeria, *Br J Obstet Gynaecol* 80:651-653, 1973.

36. Popek EJ et al: In utero development of pulmonary artery calcification in monochorionic twins: a report of three cases and discussion of the possible etiology, *Pediatr Pathol* 13:597-611, 1993.

37. Potter EL, Craig JM: *Pathology of the fetus and infant*, ed 3, Chicago, 1975, Mosby.

38. Rausen AR, Seki M, Strauss L: Twin transfusion syndrome: a review of 19 case studies at one institution, *J Pediatr* 66:613-628, 1965.

39. Reece EA et al: Combined intrauterine and extrauterine gestations, a review, *Am J Obstet Gynecol* 146:323-328, 1984.

40. Robertson EG, Neer KJ: Placental injection studies in twin gestation, *Am J Obstet Gynecol* 147:170-174, 1983.

41. Saier F, Burden L, Cavanagh D: Fetus papyraceus: an unusual case with congenital anomaly of the surviving fetus, *Obstet Gynecol* 45:217-220, 1975.

42. Salafia CM, Vintzileos AM: Why all placentas should be examined by a pathologist in 1990, *Am J Obstet Gynecol* 163:1282-1293, 1990.

43. Sander CH: The surgical pathologist examines the placenta. II. *Pathol Annu* 20:235-288, 1985.

44. Speert H: *Obstetrics and gynecology: a history and iconography*, ed 2, Norman Obstetrics and Gynecology Series no. 3, San Francisco, 1994, Norman Publishing.

45. Spencer R: Conjoined twins: theoretical embryological basis, *Teratology* 45:591-602, 1992.

46. Speroff L, Glass RH, Kase NG: *Clinical gynecologic endocrinology and infertility*, ed 5, Baltimore, 1994, Williams and Wilkins.

47. Stein IF: *Multiple pregnancy*. In Curtis AH, editor: *Obstetrics and gynecology*, vol 1, Philadelphia, 1933, WB Saunders.

48. Sulak LE, Dodson MG: The vanishing twin: pathologic confirmation of an ultrasonographic phenomenon, *Obstet Gynecol* 68:811-815, 1986.

49. Tan KL: The twin transfusion syndrome, *Clin Pediatr (Phila)* 18:111-114, 1979.

50. Valdes-Dapena M, Huff D: *Perinatal autopsy manual*, Washington, D.C., 1983, Armed Forces Institute of Pathology.

51. Van Allen MI, Smith DW, Shepard TH: Twin reversed arterial perfusion (TRAP) sequence: a study of 14 twin pregnancies with acardius, *Semin Perinatol* 7:285-293, 1983.

52. Wagner DS et al: Placental emboli from a fetus papyraceus, *J Pediatr Surg* 25:538-542, 1990.

53. Wenstrom KD et al: Frequency, distribution, and theoretical mechanisms of hematologic and weight discordance in monochorionic twins, *Obstet Gynecol* 80:257-261, 1992.

54. Wigglesworth JS: Vascular anatomy of the human placenta and its significance for placental pathology, *Br J Obstet Gynaecol* 76:979-989, 1969.

55. Winston KR: Craniopagi: anatomical characteristics and classification, *Neurosurgery* 45:769-781, 1987.

3

The Biology of Twinning and Assisted Reproduction

Dwight D. Pridham

Twin and higher-order multiple gestations have always attracted interest, in part because of their novelty, but also because of the dramatic increase in risk to both the mother and the neonates. The study of twinning is also fascinating as a natural experiment for the elucidation of processes of early embryonic development.

The incidence of multiple gestation varies by geographic and ethnic regions, from a high of 1/22 pregnancies in the Yoruba tribe in Nigeria to a low of 1/150 pregnancies in Japan. In the United States, in spite of some regional variation, the historic rate of twins is 1/80 pregnancies. Triplets have been considerably less common, occurring once in every 6750 live births in the United States. Gestations of higher order should occur only once or twice in every million pregnancies. Although multiple gestations historically account for only about 1% of births, they generate more than 10% of perinatal mortality and a great deal of morbidity.[25,75] It is for this reason that an adequate understanding of etiologies, developmental mechanisms, and possible preventative measures remains an important component of obstetric knowledge.

The advent of ovulation induction (OI), ovarian hyperstimulation, and assisted reproductive techniques (ART) (in vitro fertilization, gamete intrafallopian transfer, and others) has in recent years had a large impact on the incidence of multiple gestation, particularly gestations of high order.

As many as 80% of triplets and nearly all higher-order multiple gestations are initiated through such treatments.[20] Although the causes of twinning related to fertility therapies are not fully understood, it seems likely that polyovulation is the most common cause. This should mean that as the percentage of all twins resulting from such intervention increases, the previous understanding of the proportion of monozygotic to dizygotic twins (and triplets) may become outdated, with an increasing dominance of polyzygotic multiple pregnancies.

Many of the risks inherent in multiple gestation occur at dramatically different rates in dizygotic as opposed to monozygotic pregnancies. Some complications, such as twin-to-twin transfusions, almost never occur in dichorionic gestations and are therefore exceedingly rare in polyzygotic conceptions. Consequently, with increasing dominance of iatrogenic multiple gestations, the current appreciation of the patterns and incidences of perinatal risk to infants from multiple pregnancies may be altered. Zygosity has little effect on prematurity, the dominant risk of multiple gestation, so that strategies to reduce the risk of iatrogenic multiple gestation remain important.

This chapter first focuses on the biology of natural multiple gestations, then on the contribution of OI and ART to the current understanding and risk of multiple gestation, and finally on strategies for reducing this risk. Readers interested in exploring the biology and pathology of natural twinning in greater depth are referred to several excellent texts.[7,9,83,86]

Definitions

Before the mechanisms of twinning are discussed, a variety of terms should be defined. Many of these terms have been used interchangeably; however, their relationships are not always as predictable as might be desired. The terms *identical* and *fraternal twins*, which are commonly used in lay literature, are imprecise and are avoided in this discussion.

Monozygotic twinning refers to a gestation derived from a single fertilized zygote. Such twins should therefore be genetically identical, although phenomena such as mitotic crossing over, postzygotic nondisjunction, differential genetic imprinting, and differential inactivation of the X chromosome may yield slight genetic and particularly phenotypic differences. The environments (that is, placentation and intrauterine environment) of each twin cannot be considered identical and may cause substantially different phenotypes. The Collaborative Perinatal Project found that in a study of monozygotic twins in which both twins in each set had anomalies, the anomalies were the same in only 69% of twin pairs, thus illustrating the importance of development or environment in the expression of such defects.[81] Depending on the timing of embryonic separation, placentation of monozygotic twins may produce a *monoamniotic gestation* (one chorion with a single amniotic sac containing two embryos), a *monochorionic-diamniotic gestation* (single chorion but two amniotic sacs, each containing a single embryo), or a *dichorionic gestation* (separate chorions and amniotic sacs for each embryo). The presence of two chorions does not exclude monozygosity, and a single chorion does not necessarily indicate monozygosity, as is discussed in the following paragraphs. Therefore the terms *monoamniotic* and *monochorionic* should not be used interchangeably with *monozygotic*.

Other forms of *monovular conceptions* are possible, including fertilization of the primary or secondary polar body along with the secondary oocyte, which yields a *monovular dispermic conception*. These embryos are genetically less similar than monozygotic twins but somewhat more so than conceptions derived from two completely separate mature oocytes. A *binovular dispermic conception* is also possible and occurs when two mature oocytes are closely associated within a single follicle (and presumably the same zona pellucida). Both of these situations, with the developing blastocysts closely associated within the same zona, could yield a monochorionic gestation.

Dizygotic twins, or twins resulting from two separately fertilized zygotes, may be a result of *polyovulation* (mature oocytes from multiple follicles), or of a binovular follicle as described in the preceding paragraph. This should almost invariably result in a dichorionic gestation, except in the situation of a shared zona in a binovular dispermic conception. Although *unlike-sex twins* are usually presumed to be dizygotic and therefore dichorionic, this is not always the case. A monovular dispermic conception or a binovular dispermic conception could result in unlike-sex twins sharing the same chorion, as could monozygotic twinning with postzygotic mitotic nondisjunction (an example might be a twin pair with 46XY and 45X karyotypes). Thus even unlike-sex twins cannot be unequivocally categorized as dizygotic.

These terms should be used carefully and conservatively to indicate the degree of information available about a given gestation. When any doubt exists regarding zygosity (fetal sex and placental membranes allow tentative assignment about 50% of the time), it should be established by any of the methods of placental isoenzymes, placental cytogenetics, major and minor blood cell antigens, human leukocyte antigen (HLA) typing, chromosome analysis, and deoxyribonucleic acid (DNA) analysis.[7]

Even the term *twinning* can have various meanings. Newman[83] argues that *twinning* should really be applied only to monozygotic gestations, or to the production of two individuals from one. He suggests that dizygotic twins are no more special than any other siblings, reflecting his academic interest in the embryologic level of twinning. From a clinical perspective, the presence of two (or more) fetuses concurrently in the same uterus, regardless of their embryologic origin, is the determinant factor for much of the maternal fetal risk and justifies a broad use of the term.

With the advent of in vitro fertilization, cryopreservation, and the recent creation in human (abnormal) embryos of intentionally separated blastomeres replaced in artificial zonas (the functional equivalent of monozygotic twins), the definition of twinning has been altered still further. Already children exist whose conception occurred during the same cycle (dizygotic) but who were born years apart. In spite of the general public's fascination with these cases, they are no different in a medical sense than any other siblings and carry none of the increased risk of multiple gestation. They certainly should not be classified as twins. When monozygotic human embryos can be carried in separate gestations (as has been done in animals), they will from an obstetric perspective be no different than singleton gestations. However, they will fit Newman's concept of two individuals created from one. The term *clone* may carry too many negative connotations to be used in this situation, but *twins* in the usual sense does not really apply. A new word will probably need to be coined when this theory becomes reality.

Mechanisms of Twinning

MONOVULAR TWINS

In his fascinating treatise on monozygotic twinning, written in 1923 and based on extensive observation of lower animal phyla, Newman suggested that the stimulus for such twinning is primarily environmental. Trauma, aging of the oocyte, and perhaps hormonal influences result in a retardation of embryonic development and loss of the axis of polarity. When conditions improve and growth resumes, two new axes can form, allowing the development of two completely or partially separate embryonic plates.

Another potential mechanism for monozygotic twinning could be early separation and splitting of the preembryotic cell mass into two separate blastocysts before any formation of embryonic plates. This might occur because some blastomeres escape through a weakened or abnormal zona, or it could occur within the zona if differences in cell surface proteins caused by different genetics in two cell populations (resulting from mitotic crossing over, nondisjunction, or differential inactivation of the X chromosome) cause separation because of lack of adhesion.

A number of illustrative points can be drawn from animal studies. Newman[83] notes that many of the lowest animal phyla, including Mollusca, Nemertinea, Nemathelminthes, Rotifera, Ctenophora and Tunicata never form monozygotic twins. These organisms undergo determinate cleavage of the oocyte. The uncleaved egg is already highly organized into prospective regions, and even the first cell division is distinctly uneven, leaving two cells that are not totipotent. Separation of even these first two blastomeres uniformly results in failed development. Arthropods and annelids can undergo monozygotic twinning at an intermediate rate, whereas echinoderms and vertebrates have a relatively high rate of this type of twinning (of course, dizygotic twinning is meaningless in most lower animals). These last four groups all undergo indeterminate cleavage for a considerable time (up to the early blastocyst), allowing any separated cells or

reorganized axis within the blastocyst to be totipotent.

Newman's experiments with echinoderm oocytes and embryos revealed high rates of twinning accompanied by retarded growth in parthenogenic, hybrid, and crowded embryo cultures. These abnormal eggs exhibited slower division times, discordance between blastomeres, and early (abnormal) separation of blastomeres. Newman hypothesized that most, if not all, monozygotic twinning might be the result of some form of insult, whether it is a decreased developmental rate (such as parthenogenesis or hybridization) or a decreased metabolic rate (such as crowding). This hypothesis is strengthened by the observation that mice exposed to chemotherapy agents have an increased rate of monozygotic twinning.[63] In theory, the initial insult leads to a loss of developing polarity within the blastocyst. With continued growth, it is possible that two or more areas of the blastocyst might be equally favorable for formation of new axes of polarity, leading to development of two embryonic plates. This should be feasible up to the point of gastrulation, at which time clear axes of symmetry and polarity are physically present in the developing embryo.

An interesting association has been noted between Down syndrome, twinning, and theoretically aged oocytes in the orthodox Jewish population.[104] Because of strict religious practices regarding menstruation, fertilization of the oocyte might more commonly occur at a more distant time after ovulation, perhaps resulting in a suboptimal zygote that might not develop normally. It has long been noted in human gestations that an excess of anomalies occurs in monozygotic twins compared with dizygotic twins or singletons. Anomalies may not be caused by the twinning process, but they may in fact be the initiators. Some of the genetic abnormalities seen should lead to slow mitosis, increasing the likelihood of subsequent separation into monozygotic twins.

Another fascinating animal model studied by Newman is the armadillo. In this mammal, implantation lags behind fertilization by as much as 2 to 3 weeks. During this time the embryonic vesicle is suspended at the blastocyst stage in a state of reduced metabolic activity. Subsequently, under normal circumstances, the armadillo gives birth to quadruplets. These siblings are a pair of mirror-image "identical" twins, and all four can be shown to be monozygotic in origin, suggesting a controlled two-stage splitting of the embryo that is presumably initiated by the suppressed growth of the embryo. This model may also have the potential for interesting studies of decidual-to-embryo signaling.

Placentation of monozygotic twins (dichorionic, monochorionic-diamniotic, and monoamniotic) is thought to depend on the timing of separation relative to implantation and formation of the amnion. If separation occurs before implantation (postovulatory day 3 or 4), then a dichorionic gestation should result. A splitting later than this but before separation of the amnion from the embryo (postovulatory day 8) should yield a monochorionic-diamniotic pregnancy. Division after this date causes a monoamniotic gestation, and theoretically about 12 to 14 days after ovulation, disruptive stimulations may produce incomplete separation of the embryonic poles, with conjoined twins as a consequence.

Although most studies of humans have concluded that monozygotic twinning is not familial, a few have found some clustering among families.[57,101,103] However, there are several theoretical mechanisms by which a family tendency for monozygotic twinning might occur. Chromosomal anomalies that cause a slowing of mitosis and therefore retard embryonic development might increase the risk of twinning by mechanisms outlined in the preceding paragraph. An association has been noted between Down syndrome and twinning,[104] although Down syndrome is not familial in most cases (unless it is associated with a translocation). At least 14 pairs of heterokaryotic monozygotic twins have been reported,[10] all with an infant that has either Turner's or Down syndrome and a normal infant. The zygosity in many of these cases was confirmed only by placental membrane studies, which may be misleading (see the discussion of polar body twinning in this chapter). This phenomenon suggests that a postzygotic nondisjunction occurred, either just after or perhaps stimulating the twinning. Certainly nondisjunction tends to slow embryonic development, allowing axis reorganization as theorized earlier in this discussion, but this does not explain why only one of the two resulting embryos contains all of the abnormal cell line. Another theory holds that altered cell surface recognition factors cause segregation of the two cell lines and splitting into two embryonic cell masses. Abnormalities such as balanced translocation, inversion, or ring chromosomes can be familial and have been associated with an increased incidence of abnormal gametes and habitual abortion. Most of the effect of this type of chromosomal anomaly occurs during meiosis, as abnormal chromosomes try to line up with their normal counterparts.

They should have little effect on mitosis, and thus they probably do not cause an inheritable risk of twinning.

There is another chromosomal mechanism that has been documented to increase the risk of monozygotic twins, although it occurs with normal chromosomes. Females make up an increasing percentage of the spectrum of monozygotic twins that are delivered; 48.6% of singleton and dizygotic infants, 50.4% of all monozygotic twins, 58% of monochorionic twins, and 77% of conjoined twins are female. The same progression occurs with increasing size of the gestation; 49% of twins, 50% of triplets, and 54% of quadruplets are female.[92] This is hypothesized to be the result of either the increased mass of the X chromosome or perhaps of the random inactivation of one copy, which slows the mitotic process. Superior survival of female twins versus male twins may be an alternative explanation, but the slight excess of males in dizygotic twins and singletons argues against this. Certainly if a family had a tendency to produce more female embryos, which may occur if abnormalities of Y-bearing sperm are present or with severe X-linked disease, then a concurrent slight increase in the rate of monozygotic twins should also exist. This has yet to be proven, but it may be difficult to demonstrate, given the rarity of monozygotic twins. Potential single-gene mechanisms that might predispose a family to monozygotic twinning include abnormal transcription of zona proteins and cellular adhesion molecules such as integrins. Such defects have yet to be demonstrated.

Most studies of twinning epidemiology find that the regional variations in incidence are explained by increases in the dizygotic rate. The frequency of monozygotic twinning, 3.5 to 4/1000 births, is surprisingly constant.[19] This suggests that the dominant factor in monozygotic twinning is not genetic, familial, or probably even environmental, but rather it is some more uniform and random biologic phenomenon.

A few studies do suggest a possible hormonal influence on monozygotic twinning (which can then allow a hypothetical link to familial conditions or OI and ART). One of these, a retrospective survey conducted in Australia in the late 1970s that covered over 1000 twin deliveries found a possible link between conceptions occurring shortly after oral contraceptive use (with the greatest effect at 0 to 6 months) and an increased percentage of monozygotic versus dizygotic twins (the overall rate of twinning was also increased).[73] The authors recognized the methodologic problems of the study, but it remains an interesting observation. A prospective study of over 17,000 women in Britain, 56% of whom were using oral contraceptives, did not find any consistent relationship between any contraceptive method and twin pregnancies, but it did demonstrate an unusually high percentage of twins (9.5% of all pregnancies) in parous women experiencing an unplanned pregnancy while taking oral contraceptives.[113] In spite of the large population enrolled, this finding was related to two pregnancies, limiting the statistical significance. A third study also found a higher rate of twinning shortly after discontinuing oral contraceptives, but zygosity was not addressed.[96]

CONJOINED TWINS

At one end of the spectrum of monozygotic twins lies the interesting but disconcerting phenomenon of conjoined twins. They are rare, occurring in between 1/150 and 1/800 monozygotic twin births.[10] In his 1923 treatise, Newman[83] relates the then current debate over whether such gestations represent a collision of two separately developing embryos or an incomplete fission of a single embryonic cell mass. It is now generally accepted that the second theory is probably correct. This version, involving a partial disorganization of the embryonic axis with two new axes developing at one end (or parallel but too close together) is confirmed by zygosity studies of delivered twins and explains such findings as mirror imaging and situs inversus viscerum in some organ systems. Whether conjoined twins simply represent a milder (partial) disruption of the embryonic polarity with only partial duplication of embryonic axes or whether the degree of separation is dependent on the timing of the divisive impulse relative to embryonic development remains unclear. Whereas embryonic development is thought to proceed in a linear and predictable fashion, many patterns of conjoined twins are recognized. Fusion of the upper or lower torso, head, or pelvis are all possible, as are a variety of positions: head to head, back to back, front to front, side to side. It would seem that if timing were the critical issue, a distinct spectrum of progressively less separation in either a caudal or cephalad direction would result. Since this is not the case, the other theory that conjoined twins represent a similar (in timing) but less complete reorganization of embryonic axial polarity seems more appropriate. It is not within the scope of this chapter to enter into greater detail on this intriguing topic; interested readers are referred to later chapters on abnormalities of twinning and other references on twin pathology (such as Baldwin[7] and Newman[83]).

POLAR BODY TWINNING

Fertilization of both the primary and secondary polar body has been proven by HLA typing, DNA fingerprinting, and polymerase chain reaction techniques in several case reports.[7,12] Although this phenomenon is probably rare, it can lead to unusual twin combinations. Since the first polar body is diploid, its fertilization with a sperm leads to triploidy. Cases have been reported of twin gestations with one anomalous fetus or partial mole with triploid karyotype coupled with a normal twin.[12] Analysis of HLA haplotypes can establish the double maternal contribution. Because of the close association of these embryos within the same zona, monochorionic gestations are possible (and have occurred).

The secondary polar body is haploid; it is genetically identical to the mature oocyte but usually has much less cytoplasm. Existence of a "tertiary" polar body, which means only a normal secondary polar body that has received a higher percentage of cytoplasm than usual, has been hypothesized. Fertilization of a secondary or tertiary polar body results in a euploid embryo that is not identical to the fertilized oocyte (because a different sperm accomplished the fertilization) but more genetically similar than a polyovular twinning.

With a relative paucity of cytoplasm and slower development, these polar body embryos might not be capable of producing their own extraembryonic membranes and might survive only if coupled with a normal conceptus, thus sharing a chorion.

They would thus always be monochorionic but should be diamniotic, since the amnion is derived from the embryonic cell mass. Such twin pairs may be overlooked if they are of like sex, and if they are of unlike sex, they may be presumed to be dichorionic unless a careful study of membranes is made. This phenomenon may be more common than expected. In one study of 12 monochorionic twins, 3 pairs were found to differ in minor blood groups.[80] In the case of the larger tertiary polar bodies, or if cytoplasmic volume is not important in the ability of a developing blastocyst to generate extra embryonic membranes, polar body twinning could result in dichorionic or monochorionic gestations.

CHIMERISM

Two types of chimerism have been identified in humans: whole body and blood. Although many of the reported pairs were previously presumed to be dizygotic because of unlike sex,[10] both types imply a monochorionic gestation—the former because only one individual is present and the latter because placental vascular anastomoses are required, which have been demonstrated only in monochorionic gestations. Since chimeric individuals contain two genetically different cell lines, either two initial embryos or a postmeiotic nondisjunction must be necessary. In the case of two karyotypically normal cell lines, two separately fertilized embryos are necessary. For the close association necessary for either fusion of the early embryonic cell masses (whole body chimeras) or placental vascular anastomoses (blood chimeras), monochorionic gestations are required. Thus the most plausible explanation of this rarely reported event is either

a binovular follicle (two eggs sharing a zona) or a monovular dispermic (polar-body twin) conception. A case reporting unlike-sex twins, each having circulating lymphocyte populations of equally mixed 46XX and 46XY karyotypes, establishes blood chimerism as a rare but possible occurrence in humans.[7] Whole body chimerism seems to be exceedingly rare, since one half of such chimeric individuals should have a mixture of 46XY and 46XX cell lines, a situation that is rarely reported.[8]

CAPP TWINS

Another unusual form of monozygotic twinning is the chorangiopagus parasiticus (acardiac acephalus). This twinning aberration may also be related to polar body fertilizations, in that a normal fetus is coupled to a genetically or developmentally abnormal fetus. The poorly developed fetus, usually lacking normal cardiac development, clearly would not have survived independently without the vascular support of its normal twin. Many of these abnormal fetuses are karyotypically abnormal, suggesting either separate fertilizations or early splitting of an embryo after establishment of an aberrant cell line, perhaps through nondisjunction. The concept that fertilized polar bodies may lack sufficient cytoplasm to proceed with normal development may also play a role. This topic also cannot be adequately covered within this chapter; additional details can be gained from texts on twin pathology (for example, Baldwin[7] and Newman[83]).

POLYOVULAR TWINS

Polyovular (dizygotic) twinning accounts for nearly 70% of naturally occurring twins in Europe and the United States.[21] A simpler mechanism than in monovular twinning is involved, namely the fertilization of two or more separate oocytes during either one ovulatory cycle or conceivably during sequential cycles. Twins formed in this fashion share no more genetic similarity than any other siblings, but still retain considerably more risk than infants of singleton pregnancies because of the crowded uterine environment. This form of twinning seems to account for most of the variation noted in geographic and ethnic twinning rates, as well as for the familial risk of twinning. It is also the probable mechanism of increased risk in fertility therapies, although monozygotic twinning may also contribute to a much smaller extent. A variety of natural risk factors for polyovular twins have been identified,[7] including a family history, a dietary risk (vegetable gonadotropins or phytohormones), seasonal variations in incidence, narcotic addiction, and advanced maternal age. Most of these factors probably act through the common pathway of altered pituitary-ovarian axis interactions in a fashion similar to exogenous gonadotropins. Increased coital frequency[61] and the first 3 months of a marriage[19] have also been associated with a risk of dizygotic twinning.

Four potential varieties of polyovular twins have been either proposed or demonstrated, but with the exception of superfetation, the end result and management are all exactly the same, warranting little attention to these details in most cases.

Unifollicular binovular ovulation has been documented and occurs when a single follicle contains two oocytes, presumably within one zona.[50] This caveat is added because the only way to be completely certain of the actual presence of two *mature* oocytes in a preovulatory follicle is their discovery during an in vitro fertilization oocyte aspiration. Pathologic specimens of ovaries may occasionally suggest double oocyte follicles, but they are evident in a sense much more removed from functional ovulation and maturation. During in vitro fertilization oocyte retrievals, with rare exceptions, it is usually impossible to be certain whether two eggs found within an aspirate came from a single follicle or two follicles. The exceptions would be the presence of only one follicle on an ovary, or the presence of two oocytes within the same zona. An unusually large polar body (previously mentioned as a tertiary polar body) might also give this appearance of a binovular follicle. With surrounding granulosa cells, the presence of two or even one primary polar body can be hard to ascertain. Thus the incidence of this event is impossible to estimate, but it is probably rare. As mentioned, this form of dizygotic twinning might allow a monochorionic gestation with genetically different or even unlike-sex twins.

Multifollicular ovulation is presumably the most common form of twinning, accounting for 1/80 pregnancies and about 70% of all twin pregnancies. The presence of several preovulatory follicles is certainly a common occurrence during ovulation induction cycles, and it is not uncommon during ultrasound-monitored natural cycle ovulations. Factors contributing to multiple ovulations (apart from fertility therapies) may include a familial predisposition, diet, endogenous and environmental hormones, and iatrogenic causes (for example, cycles occurring after the discontinuation of oral contraceptives). The biology of this twinning event is otherwise rather uninteresting, since it is the same as it is for singletons with the following few exceptions.

Heterotopic twins can occur from polyovular conceptions; in other words, an intrauterine pregnancy may be coupled with an ectopic tubal pregnancy. Although this is extremely rare in natural circumstances (estimates are usually in the range of 1/30,000 pregnancies), this is a common enough occurrence in fertility therapy (perhaps 1/100 pregnancies) that nearly every established ART program has experienced this outcome. A high level of suspicion for heterotopic pregnancies must be maintained in OI or ART cycles. A similar circumstance reported several times in the literature is a twin bilateral ectopic pregnancy.[24,33,94]

Superfecundation is defined as the fertilization of two oocytes within the same ovulatory cycle but by coitus on two different occasions. Of course, this is impossible to document unless fertilization occurs by two different partners; although this has been documented, it is clearly more of social than medical interest, since management (apart from legal repercussions) is no different than for any other dizygotic gestation.[56,108]

Superfetation, another extremely rare form of gestation, involves conception on two subsequent ovulatory cycles. This might theoretically occur if ovulatory medications were given during an early pregnancy, overcoming pituitary suppression caused by the ongoing pregnancy at a time before the complete occlusion of the uterine cavity by the enlarging choriodecidual sac.[18]

For superfetation to occur the therapy would almost always have to involve clomiphene citrate, since the usual monitoring in gonadotropin stimulations generally detects pregnancy through higher-than-expected estrogen levels or visualization of a gestational sac by ultrasound. This concept seems somewhat improbable for a variety of reasons, including the inhibitory nature of progesterone on sperm penetration of cervical mucus and oocyte receptivity to fertilization, as well as the low likelihood that clomiphene citrate could competitively reverse the pituitary inhibition of the high levels of estrogen seen even in early pregnancy.

A second theory suggests that breakthrough ovulation might occur during a transient decrease in pituitary suppression as estrogen and progesterone production is shifting from the corpus luteum to the placenta.[79] This also seems unlikely because of the usually smooth and overlapping nature of this transition. The most plausible explanation for dizygotic twins of markedly different sizes that are occasionally seen is severely discordant growth, perhaps caused by differences in placentation. These theories are hard to prove or disprove by postpartum assignment of gestational age, since such techniques are relatively inaccurate. Adequate proof is early ultrasound visualization of a clear singleton pregnancy followed by later documentation (still in early pregnancy) of a second sac of markedly different size. This must occur in the first or early second trimester (when discordant growth will not yet have become apparent). This does not yet seem to have been demonstrated.

TRIPLETS AND HIGHER-ORDER MULTIPLE GESTATIONS

Multiple gestations greater than twin gestations seem to result from a combination of the phenomena of polyovulation and monozygotic twinning. Although monozygotic and monochorionic anomalies occur at a greater rate in high-order multiple gestations than in twin pregnancies (demonstrating the contribution of this mechanism), the rate of triplets within populations varies in concordance with twinning rates, from 1/612 in the Yoruba tribe[90] to 1/9524 in Japan.[60] As most of the variation in twinning between populations is thought to be related to polyovulation, this factor must also be important in higher-order multiple gestations.

Zygosity is often poorly studied in triplets, but estimates show differing patterns in various countries. In Nigeria (home to the Yoruba tribe), the pattern reflects the high propensity to polyovulation, with trizygotic gestations being most common, followed by dizygotic and then monozygotic gestations. In Japan, just the opposite pattern seems to hold (monozygotic gestations are more common than dizygotic gestations, and trizygotic gestations are least common). In the United States, dizygosity is the most common state, followed by monozygotic and then trizygotic gestations.

Whether triplet and higher-order multiple gestations are the result of polyovulation or monovular splitting, their risk factors are higher than even the already elevated risk for twins. Chord insertion abnormalities occur at a high rate (46%) even in trichorionic-triamniotic gestations, suggesting a compounding of the space and crowding problems seen in twins.[7] The median gestational age of triplets is also substantially lower than twins at 31 to 35 weeks.[84,98,114] This median gestational age drops to 30.2 weeks in quadruplets.[38] The contribution of OI and ART to triplet gestations and higher-order multiple pregnancies is substantial, as is discussed in later sections of this chapter.

Contributions of ART to Understanding Twinning Biology

Fertility therapies have certainly contributed to the incidence of multiple gestations, but they have also modified the current understanding of the biology of such pregnancies. Careful observation of oocytes and early embryos in the in vitro fertilization laboratory and the opportunity to observe many singleton and multiple gestations serially and from an early date with ultrasound have added to clinicians' knowledge of twinning mechanisms.

The occurrence of fertilized polar bodies is a phenomenon that should be observable in the laboratory. However, for a variety of reasons it might easily be missed. Oocytes are invested with a thick coat of granulosa cells (corona and cumulus) that can make identification of the polar bodies difficult, especially on the day of oocyte aspiration. The small size of polar bodies might render identification of their division difficult. Such division could easily be mistaken for "fragmentation" of blastomeres of the dividing fertilized main zygote. Finally, although such a phenomenon has been reported only rarely (in one clinic, there has not been a recognized fertilized polar body in over 4000 inseminated oocytes), most laboratories are probably not routinely watching for the event. Clinicians are unlikely to find evidence that is not actively sought. Tertiary polar bodies should be recognized more readily because of their large size. These are still an extremely rare finding, although there is no uniform reporting of oocyte anomalies within national data bases such as the Society for Assisted Reproductive Techniques (SART) annual survey.

Binovular follicles take one of two forms: two separate oocyte cumulus complexes within the same follicle or two oocytes within the same zona and cumulus. The former can only rarely be identified with any certainty during in vitro fertilization, namely in cases with only one follicle on an ovary. In most circumstances, the operator cannot be absolutely certain that more than one follicle has not been punctured or that an oocyte was not in the dead space in the aspiration needle before the puncture of a new follicle. Therefore although it is not at all uncommon to find two (or even three) oocytes in one aspiration during oocyte retrievals, this does not contribute to cumulative knowledge of the incidence of this event in nature; nor is it of particular interest, since the resulting pregnancy (in a natural cycle) is identical in all respects to one resulting from ovulation from two follicles.

Of more interest are binovular follicles in which the oocytes share the same zona. As mentioned, this might allow a dizygotic but monochorionic gestation. This should be identified by any qualified in vitro fertilization (IVF) technologist, but it is in fact extremely rare. In an evaluation of more than 4000 oocytes, this curiosity has been noticed only one or twice, or in about 0.025% of cases. Beyond the identification of a zona containing two oocytes, the odds of fertilization of both oocytes must be calculated. In an IVF program, fertilization occurs in about 60% to 70% of mature oocytes, whereas in spontaneous cycles the exact percentage is not known. Since the

likelihood of a clinical pregnancy when a single fertilized embryo transferred into the uterus during an IVF cycle is 15% to 20%, and since the cyclical rate of recognized conception (clinical pregnancy) in fertile couples is also about 15% to 20%, it can be assumed that fertilization of an oocyte occurs in a high percentage of ovulatory cycles. Using 70% as an estimate and presuming a loss rate of 15% per embryo, it is then possible to conservatively calculate the odds of a recognizable twin gestation from a binovular follicle (sharing a zona) as $0.7 \times 0.7 \times 0.85 \times 0.85 \times 0.00025$, or 1/11,300 pregnancies. With an incidence of twins of 1/80 pregnancies, this would be about 1/140 twin gestations.

Although ART has the potential to increase the rate of monozygotic multiple gestation, as is discussed in the following paragraphs, it may be difficult to identify such pregnancies within ART programs. Embryo transfer is accomplished at a two- to eight-cell stage (about 36 hours after fertilization), and separation of cell masses is not yet occurring. Occasionally after micromanipulation of the zona, a blastomere can be observed oozing through a tear in the zona at the time of embryo transfer. Whereas this could be an early step in twinning, it is felt to more realistically represent a poor prognosis for survival of that embryo.

Early ultrasound, usually performed at a gestational age of 6 to 7 weeks (4 to 5 weeks after embryo transfer), should allow delineation of monochorionic versus dichorionic implantations. Some monozygotic twins are dichorionic, so the finding of two chorionic sacs by ultrasound does not exclude monozygosity. However, since 70% to 80% of monozygotic twins are monochorionic, if any substantial numbers of ART-derived multiple gestations are monozygotic, at least some of these should be identified by ultrasound. In a study of 35 sets of twins and 9 sets of triplets, all have been dichorionic or trichorionic, respectively. The Survey '91 review of twins found that all known IVF triplets and all but one triplet gestation reported from clomiphene citrate therapy were trichorionic.[7] Other series from the literature have occasionally reported monochorionic twins,[54] but multiple gestations from OI and ART rarely seem to be monozygotic. This reasoning could be incorrect if monozygotic twinning in ART follows a different process than natural conceptions; for instance, there could be earlier separation of cell masses and a much higher ratio of dichorionic to monochorionic implantations.

Estimations of the rate of monozygotic twinning are sometimes based on Weinberg's differential, a calculation that stipulates that the percentage of monozygotic twins should equal the difference of like-sex pairs minus unlike-sex pairs divided by the total number of twin pregnancies. This calculation makes the presumptions that all unlike-sex pairs are dizygotic (previously discussed) and that the incidence of male and female conceptions and survival to delivery will be nearly equal. Although the calculation is somewhat robust (substituting rates of male to female fertilizations of $0.52:0.48$ or vice versa makes almost no difference to the calculated incidence of monozygosity), data from ART programs allow a controlled test of the validity of the calculation if we can presume that nearly all ART twins are dizygotic (discussed later in this chapter). Such data should exist in Society for ART (SART) data bases, but it is

not routinely reported in published summaries.[3] In one program (with limited experience) studying 37 pairs of twins, 16 were of like sex and 21 of unlike sex, yielding a somewhat meaningless calculated monozygosity rate of -14%.

One clear contribution of early ultrasound evaluation of pregnancies, which often occurs within the auspices of fertility programs, is to the understanding of the rate of early pregnancy loss and "vanishing twins." Benirschke[9] has advanced the proposition that fertilization and implantation of two embryos with the live birth of only a single infant is much more common than previously thought, with most such gestations being missed by inadequate evaluation of the placenta. He believes that careful pathologic evaluation would reveal the second gestational sac in most cases. Whereas this is probably true for twins lost at a more advanced gestational age (for example, after 10 weeks), careful ultrasound evaluation (especially with a vaginal transducer) can with reasonable certainty reveal earlier evidence of twin gestational sacs. Data from ART programs suggests that up to 25% of clinical pregnancies (gestational sac present) result in first trimester miscarriage,[3] whereas 2% to 5% of embryos with cardiac activity detected at 7 weeks fail to continue to develop. In singleton pregnancies, the result is miscarriage; in twin implantations with continued hormonal support from the thriving twin the result is usually a vanishing twin.

When early twin gestational sacs are encountered (before cardiac activity), it may be expected that there is a calculated chance of 2×0.25 (or 50%) for one sac to disappear. In slightly later gestations with dual cardiac activity noted, there is a 2×0.03 (6%) incidence of vanishing twins. These calculated numbers are supported by clinical findings. Some early studies suggest a rate of loss as high as 60% to 70%, but small numbers and less accurate sonographic capabilities may have influenced results.[67] More recent studies have suggested a 25% rate of loss of a single twin when twins were identified early in gestation after ART conceptions[30] or when two cardiac activities are noted initially.[66] One review of ultrasound findings in triplet implantations (with three heartbeats initially noted) found a 43% chance of demise of one embryo, a 15% risk of two embryos dying, and loss of the entire pregnancy before 20 weeks in 7.7% of cases.[102] If pregnancies in fertility programs (many of which are not the result of OI or ART) behave similarly to natural conceptions, then twin conceptions might be almost twice as common as recognized twin deliveries.

Fertility Therapy and the Risk of Multiple Gestation

POLYOVULAR GESTATIONS

The clearest increase in the risk of multiple gestation attributable to OI and ART is related to polyovular (dizygotic in the case of twins) conceptions. It is amply clear that most methods of OI produce multiple preovulatory follicles, and multiple embryos are intentionally returned to the uterus or fallopian tubes in ART procedures. Therefore the presumption is that most of these multiple gestations are polyzygotic.

In various ART techniques, the rate of twin deliveries ranges from 25% to 30%, whereas triplets account for 5% of deliveries. Higher-order multiple births are generally 0.5% to 1% of deliveries.[3] Statistics from OI programs using human menopausal gonadotropins are similar, with 18% to 54% of pregnancies resulting in twins, 5% in triplets, and usually 2% in quadruplets or more.[44,45,54,64] Many of the higher rates of multiple pregnancy in OI are associated with early protocols that are no longer used. OI with clomiphene citrate produces slightly fewer twins, with rates varying from 5% to 10%.[1,29,55] Clomiphene citrate therapy generally produces few triplets or quadruplets, but rates of 0.5% and 0.3%, respectively, have been reported, which are somewhat higher than the rates that are expected naturally.[76]

OI has a slightly greater risk of producing extreme high-order multiple pregnancies (more than quadruplets) than does ART, in which the number of embryos returned to the uterus or tubes can be limited. Maternal age and length of infertility are felt to be predictive of the likelihood of eventual conception, and they may also influence the risk of multiple conception. One study of 78 pregnancies resulting from OI found that in women with less than 3 years of infertility the rate of multiple gestation was 56%, for 3 to 4 years of infertility there was a rate of 47%, and in women with more than 4 years of infertility the rate of multiple pregnancies was 28%.[54]

MONOZYGOTIC GESTATIONS

Although multiple gestations resulting from ART and OI are generally felt to be polyovular, an increased risk of monovular twinning has also been postulated.[32,36,54,77] There are a variety of ways in which ART might theoretically be expected to increase the risk of monozygotic twinning. The initial hormonal stimulation, considerably greater than a natural cycle, may yield dysmature oocytes that are able to fertilize but are perhaps suboptimal for normal growth. Manipulation of embryos, laboratory culturing, and cryopreservation might be expected to be at least mildly traumatic, perhaps resulting in some retardation of embryonic growth. The somewhat empiric timing of embryo transfer to the uterine cavity (usually 2 days after oocyte retrieval) might place the embryo in an environment that is not normally expected to be suitable for it until several days later. All of these artificial alterations of normal oocyte maturation and fertilization can be supposed to create a situation in which suppression of normal embryonic axial polarity with subsequent reorganization into two codominant growth axes should be expected to occur, if the theory is correct. Perhaps though, the insults occurring with ART are so early that no polarity has yet been established in the blastocyst. With respect to teratogen exposure at this stage, the principle of "all or none" could apply: either an early embryo is so badly damaged that it fails to progress altogether, or if it survives, it has recovered sufficiently from any trauma by the time it is sensitive to twinning stimuli that nothing happens.

In addition to the artificial environment imposed on ART embryos, other biologic biases should theoretically lead to a higher rate of abnormal embryos and thus possibly to monozygotic twins. Many of the couples treated with OI and ART include women late in their reproductive years who are at higher risk of chromosomal abnormalities (primarily trisomies). Even young women with unexplained infertility

may have a tendency to produce oocytes with poor developmental potential, and male partners with poor sperm quality may also contribute suboptimal gametes. If the theory of delayed embryonic development as a cause of monozygotic twinning holds true, this population bias should contribute to a slight increase in risk for this type of twinning with these therapies.

Newer techniques of micromanipulation offer additional concerns for the risk of monozygotic twins by other mechanisms. Micromanipulation encompasses a variety of techniques of mechanical or chemical manipulation of the zona pellucida or oocyte that are aimed at enhancing fertilization or hatching. Partial zona dissection (PZD) is one of the earliest techniques attempted and consists of creating a rent in the zona with the goal of allowing sperm to penetrate more easily. Subzonal insertion (SUZI) places several sperm into the perivitelline space, necessarily violating the zona to do so. Intracytoplasmic sperm injection (ICSI) places a single sperm directly into the cytoplasm of the egg, again penetrating the zona as well. Assisted hatching techniques use either mechanical or acid disruption of the zona to encourage improved (and perhaps early) hatching of the blastocyst out of the zona. All of these techniques involve some weakening, if not frank disruption, of the zona. Depending on the degree of cellular adhesion between blastomeres, which increases rapidly from about the four-cell stage to the early blastocyst, separation of blastomeres may be more likely, and monozygotic twinning may be encouraged by the alternative mechanism of early splitting of the preembryonic cell mass.[31] In addition to zona damage, assisted hatching with acidic Tyrode's solution has the potential of damaging blastomeres if prolonged exposure occurs or if the zona is thinner than average.[27] ICSI, which involves placing an intact sperm into the ooplasm (a nonphysiologic event), might be expected to lead to prolonged or abnormal cell division, although clinical results to date indicate apparently normal early embryonic development and fetal anomaly rates no higher than the general population.

The 1992 AFS/SART survey[3] collected data on 1069 embryo transfers involving micromanipulated embryos (assisted hatching was not included). The transfers resulted in 189 deliveries with a twinning rate of 17.2% and a triplet rate of 2%. Cryopreserved embryos were involved in 5782 embryo transfers with 705 deliveries, 22% of which were multiple gestations. These rates are somewhat lower than expected for routine ART, suggesting that these additional manipulations do not appear to cause trauma beyond that of normal IVF techniques to increase the rate of monozygotic twinning by the previously mentioned theories.

An alternative explanation could be that the trauma of ART techniques does indeed cause an increased risk of monozygotic twinning, but that it still remains an unlikely rather than common outcome, and therefore cannot be demonstrated with the small numbers of deliveries attributable to these interventions.

In some recent interesting work on assisted hatching, Cohen et al.[26] found a higher rate of embryo implantation and multiple gestation with this technique. The initial trial yielded six pregnancies (including two twin and two triplet pregnancies) in 15 patients who were undergoing assisted hatching. Although these rates were higher than those of the control group (15 patients who had two pregnancies, both singleton), the treatment group received 3.3 embryos on average versus 2.3 in the control group. In a subsequent trial (reported in the same manuscript) with 25 treated patients and 24 controls, the number of embryos transferred was 2.8 per patient in each group. Pregnancy rates were comparable (32% versus 29%), and high rates of twins occurred in both groups (4/12 pregnancies in the treatment group and 2/7 pregnancies in the controls). The most interesting aspect was the report of one monochorionic twin pair. Another trial, reporting 33 cycles of ART with assisted hatching, documented a high pregnancy rate (64%) but also used ultrasound to note 40 gestational sacs with heartbeats in 21 pregnancies, suggesting a high rate of multiple gestation.[100] Although these reports do not clearly establish the advantages of assisted hatching, they do emphasize the risk of twinning in ART even if relatively low numbers of embryos are transferred. They are also interesting because they report one of the rare instances of monozygotic twins in ART. Although this may have been a random spontaneous event, its association with this technique is intriguing.

Monozygotic twinning has been reported in a few other pregnancies resulting from ART and OI, but it is rare.[16,54,116] As previously noted, early gestational sonographic evaluation of ART pregnancies suggests that almost all of these are polyzygotic. Additional evidence that monozygotic twinning is not a common occurrence with these techniques is derived from the rate of reported birth defects in liveborn infants whose parents underwent ART. In 1992, of 8902 infants who were delivered after ART and had available information regarding birth defects, 183 (2.1%) had birth defects (the status of an additional 65 infants was not reported). For cryopreserved embryo transfers that resulted in 619 deliveries, a birth-defect rate of 1.3% was reported.[3] Similar rates of birth defects have been reported for OI.[54] It is well established that monozygotic twins have a much higher than average rate of birth defects. The National Collaborative Perinatal Project[81] found the rate of major and minor anomalies in monoamniotic (all monozygotic) twins to be 17% each. These two facts, taken together, again suggest that monozygotic twinning cannot account for more than a few of the multiple gestations in ART or OI, or a higher rate of birth defects should be expected. This line of reasoning would be suspect if the mechanism of monozygotic twinning in ART was substantially different than in natural conceptions, with a higher degree of early splitting of cell masses versus retardation of embryonic growth and reorganization of polarity.

Another intriguing piece of information comes from one of the few OI series to report gender ratios. In twins, 69.6% of all infants were noted to be female.[54] As previously mentioned, older studies of naturally occurring twins show that males are usually slightly more common in dizygotic twins and females are more common in monozygotic twins, with the percentage of female infants increasing as monozygotic twins become more closely associated (the percentage of females is highest in conjoined twins). The relatively small number of twins (23) in this series lessens confidence in the reported figure, and the same study also found an unusual predominance of females in the singleton pregnancies (53.3%). Several other series have

commented on similar excesses of female infants in OI-related multiple gestations.[23] In an ART series of 37 twin sets and 9 triplets, male infants were found in 55% and 63% of pregnancies, respectively. Until larger series are available, gender ratios will not be able to suggest any trend towards monozygosity in OI and ART pregnancies.

Perhaps one additional difficulty in clearly demonstrating any increase in monozygotic twinning with ART is that any potential insult attributable to these techniques should occur so early that only dichorionic twins result. This would certainly be the case if early fracture of the zona is the cause. Thus without careful zygosity studies, and with the pervasive assumption that ART twins should always be dizygotic, monozygosity may be overlooked.

TRIPLETS AND HIGHER-ORDER MULTIPLE GESTATIONS

Triplets and higher-order multiple gestations are much less common in OI and ART procedures than twins, occurring in 6% and 1.5% of pregnancies, respectively.[3] Although national statistics for OI are not centrally maintained, separately published data from a number of programs suggests similar rates of twin, triplet, and higher-order multiple pregnancies.[16,23,54]

It might be supposed that OI is responsible for the majority of quadruplet and higher-order multiple pregnancies, since considerably more cycles are performed annually than ART and since many ART programs are now beginning to limit the maximum number of oocytes or embryos transferred per cycle.

Although less common than twins, triplets and higher-order multiple infants produced by OI and ART represent a high proportion of the total number of these types of pregnancies. For example, they represent 83% of all triplets,[114] 95% of all quadruplets,[28,38] and virtually all infants resulting from higher-order multiple gestations. These types of gestations also account for a disproportionate amount of morbidity and mortality, since gestational age at delivery becomes progressively shorter (less than 32 weeks for quadruplets).

An interesting report from the International Organization for Triplets and Higher Multiples reported trends in German-speaking Europe.[52] Data from 1950 through 1989 were analyzed, showing a tripling of the incidence of triplets from 1/9547 births to 1/3409 over that period. Quadruplet and greater pregnancies increased enormously from about 1/year in Germany to an average of over 20. From 1984 to 1989, two thirds of all triplets and 47/48 higher-order multiple pregnancies were the result of fertility therapies. Most interestingly, and perhaps because of greater recognition and intervention, the average gestational age and birth weights of both triplets and higher-order infants declined over the time of the study, whereas death rates and morbidity increased slightly. The author makes the important point that triplet and higher-order multiple pregnancies should not be considered as wonderful successes in fertility therapy but rather as failures of medical management.

Although cases have rarely been reported for twins, selective reduction or termination, with its attendant risk and costs (and benefit in these cases), is much more commonly utilized in triplet gestations and especially in quadruplet or higher-order multiple gestations. This important topic is addressed more fully in later chapters of this book.

UNUSUAL TWIN GESTATIONS

Yet another effect of the increasing use of ART and OI is an increasing incidence of unusual multiple pregnancies, including combined intrauterine and extrauterine (heterotopic) pregnancies, bilateral ectopic pregnancies, and other combinations. Ectopic pregnancy is clearly more common in ART procedures than normal conceptions, with an average rate of 1/20 intrauterine pregnancies.[3] Since multiple pregnancies are also more common, it is expected that combinations of the two phenomena will be encountered. Although many such combination pregnancies (particularly intrauterine plus extrauterine) may not be recognized, an early report from Britain found 5 extrauterine twin pregnancies out of a total of 124 extrauterine and 1648 intrauterine pregnancies, for an incidence of 1/354 pregnancies.[94] Two other programs reported 4 heterotopic (intrauterine plus tubal ectopic) pregnancies in 428 total pregnancies[35] and 10 heterotopic in 1001 total pregnancies,[78] with the usual background rate of 5% ectopic pregnancies. This seems to suggest a rate of 1/100 for heterotopic pregnancy in ART conceptions, compared with the historic rate of 1/30,000 natural conceptions. Other case reports include a combined triplet intrauterine and bilateral ectopic tubal pregnancy,[33] a bilateral tubal pregnancy after unilateral zygote tubal transfer,[24] and twin pregnancies with one normal fetus and one hydatidiform mole after both

OI[2] and gamete intrafallopian transfer.[112]

Perinatal Risks

An important question in this discussion of risk from OI and ART is whether the spectrum of morbidity and mortality seen in multiple gestations resulting from these techniques is the same as that from naturally conceived multiple gestations. Although the true answer to this question must await the careful tabulation of real data, some appreciation for the likely increase in national perinatal morbidity resulting from ART and OI can be gained by examining the differences in risk between monozygotic and dizygotic gestations, remembering that most ART multiple gestations are probably polyzygotic. More extensive discussions of these issues can be found in later chapters of this book.

RISKS OF MONOZYGOTIC GESTATIONS

Monozygotic gestations have uniquely higher risks than even dizygotic twin gestations. This occurs for the following two reasons: complications may result from monochorionic or monoamniotic placental configurations, and there is a higher incidence of genetic and developmental congenital anomalies (about 7 times the rate in dizygotic or singleton pregnancies).[51] Complications unique to monochorionic pregnancies include placental vascular anastomoses leading to twin-twin transfusion syndrome (TTS).[62] This serious danger is discussed in Chapter 2 of this text. Although it is not common, the demise of a single twin can lead to complications for the survivor that include neurologic compromise and other organ damage. In several series reporting on this problem, nearly all affected surviving infants were part of a monochorionic (and thus generally monozygotic) pregnancy.[5,22,69]

Monochorionic-diamniotic pregnancies have a high incidence of amniotic band syndrome, which can lead to limb deletions, cleft lip and palate, cord accidents, and fetal demise.[48] Monoamniotic gestations have all of the above risks, plus a risk of cord entanglement, and they experience a 50% to 60% fetal mortality rate, compared with a 25% rate in monochorionic-diamniotic pregnancies and a rate of 8.9% in dichorionic pregnancies.[9] Monoamniotic twins include conjoined twins, who have high mortality rates, with universal morbidity for survivors. Monozygotic twins in general have twice the perinatal mortality rate of dizygotic twins.[51,72]

As previously discussed, genetic and developmental abnormalities may in fact be a triggering mechanism for monozygotic twinning. It is not surprising to find an increased incidence of chromosomal anomalies,[42,111] anterior neural tube defects,[115] sirenomelia,[117] caudal duplication,[97] esophageal atresia,[46] and Duhamel anomalad,[106] among other anomalies in monozygotic twins. A subset of data from the National Collaborative Perinatal Project in the United States noted higher rates of macrocephaly, encephalocele, cleft lip and palate, diaphragmatic hernias, tracheoesophageal fistula, intestinal malrotation, hernias, and cystic kidneys.[81] Although exact distributions of these anomalies are not noted, the increase in occurrence was found to be almost entirely attributed to monozygotic twins, who were noted to have a 16% incidence of both major and minor anomalies. These associations certainly add to both morbid and fatal outcomes of twin pregnancies.

In natural conceptions, monozygotic twins constitute approximately one third of all twins. The morbidity and mortality attributable to this type of twinning therefore have a substantial effect on the perinatal risk of all twins. ART- and OI-induced multiple gestations may have a different ratio of polyzygosity to monozygosity and therefore may have a different (and probably lower) risk profile.

RISKS COMMON TO ALL TWIN GESTATIONS

The argument of the previous section certainly should not be used to suggest that there is no increased perinatal risk from ART and OI. Dizygotic twins (and dichorionic-monozygotic twins) should never experience placental vascular anastomoses. Dizygotic twins have no higher individual risk of genetic or developmental anomalies than singletons, but they have exactly twice the risk per pregnancy, which may lead to more intervention (sometimes at relatively early stages of gestation).

The most substantial risk to all twins (up to 70% of all mortality) stems from prematurity.[53] This can be the result of spontaneous labor, or it can be caused by iatrogenic intervention for discordant growth, preeclampsia, or other maternal indications. These risks and their management are discussed in subsequent chapters, but it is important to remember that the median gestational age at delivery for twins is 38 weeks and that 42% to 74% of mothers with twin pregnancies experience preterm labor.[102,107]

Although multiple gestations conceived with ART do not experience premature la-

bor more often than naturally occurring multiple gestations, premature delivery and its associated morbidity is the single greatest risk and cost imposed by the increasing use of OI and ART. In the previously mentioned study of 78 pregnancies from OI,[54] 23 twins, 5 triplets, 2 quadruplets and 1 sextuplet resulted. Because of complications associated with prematurity, 22% of the twin infants, 54% of the triplets, 75% of the quadruplets, and 100% of the sextuplet infants died in the perinatal period. Although this report dates from the late 1960s and many of these deliveries, which occurred between 25 and 32 weeks, might now be salvaged, this still illustrates the great potential for morbidity presented by this problem.

In a more recent study that took place in Australia and New Zealand, a perinatal death rate of 47.5/1000 births was reported, about twice the normal national rate.[6] As in other reports, prematurity played a large role, with 60% of the perinatal deaths being in fetuses and infants of multiple gestations. An expected number (2.3%) of major congenital malformations also contributed morbidity and mortality. Cesarean section occurred in 44% of ART deliveries in the Australian report, 3 times the national rate. Multiple gestations contributed substantially to these numbers as well, although the rate in singleton pregnancies was also high at 39%.

Although many multiple gestations are delivered early, concern is not entirely removed if 38 weeks' gestation is reached. Numerous studies point to the onset of increasing differences in average birth weights of singletons and twins, beginning at 35 to 38 weeks.[51,71] Average birth weights in twins actually decline after 38 weeks, suggesting an increasing imbalance between fetal needs and uteroplacental capacity. Multiple gestations extending beyond 38 weeks may therefore begin to face an increasing risk for growth retardation and perhaps fetal distress or stillbirth. This is probably because of placental crowding. Blecker, Oosting, and Hemrika[13] noted in a study of 3000 singleton and 1500 twin gestations that the ratios of placental to neonate weight are similar in singletons, twins, and triplets, but that placental weights in twin and triplet pregnancies begin to fall behind singletons at 24 weeks. Additional placental problems in twins include a high incidence of marginal and velamentous cord insertions (up to 45%), as well as single umbilical arteries and placental abruption.[68]

Twin gestations, particularly they are if not recognized, are at greater risk for folic acid deficiency. Apart from megaloblastic anemia, which occurs in up to 50% of twin pregnancies in some series,[1] folic acid deficiency has also been linked to abruptio placentae, pregnancy-induced hypertension, premature labor, and stillbirth.[95] Whether this implies a greater risk of these problems in twin pregnancies because of folic acid deficiency, or whether twin gestation is the cause of both folic acid deficiency and these other complications is not clear. In recognized twin pregnancies (as all ART- or OI-caused multiple pregnancies should be) folic acid supplementation should reduce these risks to normal levels.

Many women in ART or OI programs are approaching age 35 or older. In one of the largest British programs, Bourn Hall, the average maternal age was almost 6 years over the national average, and 42% of women who conceived with the program were over 35 years of age, compared with 4% nationally.[107] Chorionic villi sampling (CVS) or amniocentesis is often used in this age group to detect chromosomal anomalies. Such procedures in a twin pregnancy may increase the risk of loss of the pregnancy to some extent over that for singleton pregnancies. One early study of 47 twin pregnancies, 18 of which were not recognized, found loss rates of 17% when both sacs were punctured.[87] A more recent study of 98 twin pregnancies, all with two viable fetuses noted at the time of amniocentesis, found a loss rate of 8.1% by 28 weeks' gestation, compared with a historical control rate for miscarriages of 4.5% in a comparable population of twins.[93] A careful case-control study comparing 101 twin gestations undergoing amniocentesis to 108 control twin pregnancies undergoing ultrasound at the same gestational age but no amniocentesis (monoamniotic twins, discordant growth, and anatomic and genetic anomalies were all excluded) found loss rates of 3.5% versus 3.2%, which is not a significant difference.[47] Another large series of 339 patients undergoing amniocentesis (and a control group of singleton pregnancies undergoing amniocentesis) found gestational mortality rates of 12.6/1000 and 12.1/1000, respectively, which is also not a clear difference.[4] In 128 multiple pregnancies undergoing CVS between 9 and 12 weeks, a 5% loss rate was experienced, which is comparable to the 4% rate found in singleton pregnancies.[88] Accuracy in detecting cytogenetic abnormalities seemed to be as good as it was in singleton pregnancies. In summary, multiple gestations clearly double the risk of at least one infant having a chromosomal abnormality, may or may not increase the risk of diagnostic techniques, and certainly raise the difficult issue of selective termination (with associated risk) if one fetus is found to be aneuploid.

RISKS OF HIGH-ORDER MULTIPLE GESTATIONS

Multiple gestations of three or more infants normally demonstrate a mixture of the risks found in monozygotic twins and dizygotic twins. Prematurity is still the greatest concern, with triplets averaging 33 weeks at delivery and 92% to 100% of triplet gestations experiencing preterm labor.[102,107] As previously mentioned, quadruplets average a gestational age of 30 weeks at delivery,[38] and infants from higher-order multiple gestations are fortunate merely to continue to viability. Placentation is a greater problem than with twins, and even trichorionic triplet gestations show a high incidence (46%) of abnormal chord insertions caused by placental crowding.[7] Since many natural triplet and higher-order multiple gestations have some component of monozygosity, concerns about genetic and developmental abnormalities remain high, although they may not be as high in ART-derived pregnancies.

MATERNAL RISK

The mother of twins or a higher-order multiple gestation assumes obstetric risks beyond the obvious increase in risk of operative delivery. Preeclampsia, anemia, polyhydramnios, hyperemesis, pruritus gravidarum, peripartum cardiac failure, uterine rupture, uterine atony, postpartum hemorrhage, hypertension, and abruptio placentae are all more common in these patients.[70,99,107] Polyhydramnios was studied in one small series (86 twin gestations over 2 years in San Francisco), with the interesting finding that in 9/10 cases of persistent polyhydramnios, fetal anomalies were present.[58] Although zygosity was not noted, the anomalies mentioned (twin-twin transfusion, acephalia, acardia, conjoined twins) strongly suggested monozygosity. This particular risk may therefore not apply to gestations generated by OI or ART.

Most follow-up studies of pregnancies resulting from OI or ART suggest a higher rate of operative delivery than in routine cases. Although this is in part because of the intrinsic difficulty completing vaginal deliveries of multiple gestations, it may also be attributable to the delivering obstetrician's bias toward quick intervention in what is perceived as a "premium" pregnancy. Even singleton pregnancies from OI and ART have higher rates of cesarean sections.[54,107]

Estimated Increase in Perinatal Morbidity and Mortality in the US Related to ART

In the United States, OI (including clomiphene citrate) and ART could be estimated to cause 20,000 to 40,000 pregnancies per year, including 4000 to 6000 twin pregnancies, 800 triplet pregnancies, and about 75 higher-order multiple gestations. These are only approximate numbers. Although good data are available for ART programs, similar national data for OI are not available. As mentioned, these multiple gestations constitute an increase in twin gestations of about 40% to 50% over the natural background incidence but up to a 500% increase in triplet gestations and a 2000% increase in quadruplet gestations. With the prematurity rates given in previous paragraphs, these multiple pregnancies should constitute 3500 to 4500 cases of premature delivery per year, as well as a similar number with threatened preterm labor. The cost of this should be obvious, but it needs to be balanced with the hope and happiness of the new families who were previously infertile.

In addition to the maternal and neonatal medical risks, there is a high economic toll caused by multiple gestations (and consequently OI and ART). A study at the Brigham Womens Hospital examined cost and other factors in multiple pregnancies.[20] They found that 35% of all twins during the study time frame were derived from ART, as were 77% of all gestations of three or more in number. In this study, 24% of singletons were delivered before 38 weeks, versus 67% of twins and 93% of higher-order multiple gestations. The rate of cesarean sections increased from 24% in singletons to 59% in twins and 86% in triplets. Neonatal intensive care unit (NICU) admissions increased from 15% in singletons to 48% in twins and 78% in triplets. Accordingly, the cost per infant (total charges to the family, including maternal, divided by the number of infants) increased from $9845 for singletons to $18,974 for twins and $36,588 for triplets. Although the cesarean section rate and NICU admission rate for singletons certainly indicate that this hospital is a tertiary care referral institution and therefore not particularly representative of most hospitals, it is valid illustration of the rapid escalation in cost as gestational number increases.

The risk of multiple gestation from OI and ART is inversely correlated with age, with a much lower (but not absent) risk of multiple gestation for women over age 40 unless they are using donor oocytes. Ovulatory status is also important; women with chronic anovulation have a moderately higher risk than those with normal ovulation.

Since most pregnancies initiated by ART and OI are polyzygotic and since the majority are singleton or twin pregnancies (95%), it is clear that many of the complications discussed in the previous sections do not apply. There should not be a higher incidence of birth defects (genetic and developmental) than there is for natural conceptions in a comparable group of women (many infertility programs have a higher median maternal age), and this is confirmed by a consistent finding in published reports of birth defect rates of 1% to 2%.[3] Because of the dichorionic (or trichorionic, quadrichorionic, or higher) nature of ART related placentations, TTS should not be a concern.

A variety of factors have been shown to impart increased risk to twin pregnancies, including monozygosity, late detection, low socioeconomic status, labor outside a major medical center, malpresentation, delay of more than 30 minutes between deliveries, early placental separation, and nonrecognition of second twin.[72] Most of these factors, with the exception of malpresentation and early placental separation, do not apply to ART- and OI-generated pregnancies. Factors in labor can be managed to some extent by operative intervention. Some factors affecting twin pregnancy, such as intrauterine growth retardation (IUGR) and low birth weight (LBW), may affect pregnancies conceived with ART more so than matched controls.[107]

The major concern in ART- and OI-generated multiple gestations remains premature delivery. Although early recognition of multiple pregnancies may allow timely intervention with some reduced risk,[89] this risk cannot yet be entirely prevented by medical management. Several studies have documented perinatal morbidity and mortality resulting from infertility therapies.[107] It is important to compare these results with those of a normal population of spontaneous conceptions, which experience a baseline rate of perinatal complications. ART- and OI-generated gestations will probably never do better than this baseline.

Inseparable from the discussion of the risk of ART and OI therapies is consideration of their benefits. For most of the couples participating in such programs, pregnancy is a strongly desired state for which they are willing to take considerable risk. On one hand, it is important to attempt to reduce the risk to the minimal necessary level from the dual perspectives of doing as little harm as possible to patients and minimizing the cost to society. However, the argument that avoiding infertility therapies altogether will avoid all perinatal morbidity is no more ingenious than stating that if only all couples used contraception all the time, there would be no complications attributable to pregnancy.

Reducing the Risk of Multiple Gestation in ART

In spite of the fact that many of the risks found in natural twin and triplet gestations do not apply to ART- and OI-induced conceptions, the major factor of prematurity clearly does. It is most critical in trip-let and higher-order multiple gestations. With current pharmacologic alternatives, prevention of preterm labor is clearly better than treatment. It is important for programs specializing in fertility treatment to develop protocols, if possible, to reduce the risk of these larger multiple gestations. A variety of strategies have been advocated to accomplish this, each with some benefit and cost.

THERAPIES OTHER THAN OVULATION INDUCTION

The single greatest factor in fertility therapy that causes multiple gestation is polyovulation. Therefore treatment alternatives that do not utilize OI reduce this risk. These alternatives may be appropriate in come cases. In situations of unexplained infertility, trials of low cost, low risk, and (unfortunately) lower success rate such as intrauterine inseminations, which pose no higher risk than baseline for multiple gestation, are almost always recommended before more aggressive therapy is started. Clomiphene citrate may also be used although clomiphene therapy includes a risk of about 5% for twin conceptions and perhaps 1% for triplet conceptions. Unfortunately, only about 20% to 30% of couples with unexplained infertility conceive within six cycles with these two alternatives, beyond which efficacy and cost effectiveness are questionable. In older couples (women over age 40), these methods may be attempted, but they are usually used for a shorter time.

In women with mild to moderate endometriosis or tubal disease, or in cases of prior tubal sterilization, surgical management is usually attempted before ART is used. Surgical management in these cases may have several advantages, including lower cost per procedure, better insurance coverage, an opportunity for several conceptions if the procedure is successful, and no more than the normal population risk of multiple pregnancy. Most of these surgical treatments should be accomplished laparoscopically in an outpatient setting, but microreanastomosis is still primarily performed through a laparotomy incision and involves greater pain, disability, and surgical risk than ART procedures. In severe tubal disease of endometriosis or pelvic inflammatory disease, although optimal management is still the subject of considerable debate, ART is generally felt to be a reasonable first therapeutic alternative because of the low rate of success of other surgical interventions. In women age 40 or older, surgical management of even mild or moderate pelvic disease should be considered only rarely, since decreased fecundity renders success rates too low to justify the cost or morbidity. These women also should consider ART as first-line therapy. The choice of treatment, surgery, or ART is complicated and dependent on many technical and socioeconomic factors.[49]

BROMOCRIPTINE AND CLOMIPHENE CITRATE

For couples in whom the primary diagnosis is oligo-ovulation or anovulation, careful consideration should always be given to OI protocols with less risk of polyovulation. In women with galactorrhea or hyperprolactinemia, bromocriptine should always be the first-line choice to establish normal ovulation, since it does not increase the risk of multiple gestation.[110] It can be considered in cases when only mild elevations of prolactin exist (25 to 40 pg/ml), particularly if oligo-ovulation is coexistent. However, it is probably ineffective in normoprolactinemic chronic anovulation or empirically in women with normal menses.

Because of its low cost, ease of administration, and lower risk of multiple gestation, clomiphene citrate remains the first choice for women with eugonadotropic chronic anovulation (World Health Organization [WHO] type-two anovulation). Twins occur in only 5% to 10% of clomiphene citrate conceptions, and triplets are uncommon.[1,29,55] Up to 250 mg/day of clomiphene citrate can be used before concluding that ovulation cannot be achieved with this drug. Once a patient is ovulatory, up to six cycles should be attempted.

PULSATILE GONADOTROPIN-RELEASING HORMONE THERAPY

A second choice for type-two anovulation may be pulsatile administration of gonadotropin-releasing hormone (GnRH). Although it is not always effective in initiating ovulation in this group of women and it often approaches menopausal gonadotropins in cost and difficulty of administration, pulsatile GnRH seems to offer somewhat less risk of polyovulation and multiple gestation. Several large reports (434 and 118 cycles) of this treatment method found good pregnancy rates (23% and 29% per cycle) and relatively low (8%) multiple pregnancy rates.[59,74] This certainly represents a lower multiple gestation rate than is normally expected with gonadotropin therapy and maintains a respectable pregnancy rate. Another series found a higher risk from this type of stimulation, with 24/157 (15%) pregnancies being multiple, including two triplet pregnancies and one quadruplet gestation.[15] The suggestion was made that low pulse frequencies might help alleviate this problem. GnRH should certainly be considered in cases of hypogonadotropic (hypothalamic) amenorrhea (WHO type-one anovulation), where it is usually successful in initiating unifollicular development.

MENOPAUSAL GONADOTROPINS

Human menopausal gonadotropins (HMGs) should only be used when the previously discussed methods are inappropriate. Only 10% to 20% of patients with type-two anovulation should require progression to HMG because of failure of clomiphene therapy.[39] Careful monitoring of estradiol levels and follicular diameters is an important standard of care. Monitoring primarily affects the rate of ovarian hyperstimulation syndrome and not multiple pregnancy.[99] There are several reasons why even the most careful observation does not completely prevent multiple gestations. Estradiol levels and patterns do not correlate well with conception, successful pregnancy, or multiple pregnancy.[11,64,91,118] Cycles can be canceled if ultrasound reveals more than 4 or 5 large follicles, but the risk of multiple gestation is still present.[119] With current methods of administration, a unifollicular response is rare and usually not intentional. A variety of stimulation protocols have been proposed to moderate the response to HMG, including clomiphene-HMG combinations,[65] GnRh agonists in combination with HMG,[43] the use of follicle-stimulating hormone (FSH) rather than HMG, beginning HMG administration later in cycles, using lower doses of HMG over longer times, administering HMG or FSH in pul-

satile subcutaneous fashion,[82] and administering smaller releasing doses of human chorionic gonadotropin (hCG).[99] None of these approaches have yet proven to be consistently successful at removing or even substantially modifying the risks of multiple gestation. Many multiple gestations result from cycles that would be considered completely average. These could not have been prevented unless HMG or FSH were not used at all.

Patients with chronic anovulation most commonly respond to HMG stimulation with the growth of a large number of relatively small follicles and high estradiol levels. Although this response can be slightly modified by application of the techniques listed above, the basic pattern remains the same. To have a chance at ovulation and pregnancy at all (if other types of treatment have failed), these couples must currently endure the risk of possible multiple gestation. Occasionally when there are extreme responses, the clinician should recommend abandoning a stimulation cycle. In some instances, patients then self-administer their own hCG against medical advice. This might be prevented by requiring all patients to return to the office for administration of hCG-releasing injections. Even if hCG is withheld, a spontaneous luteinizing hormone (LH) surge may occur, although it is less likely. Another strategy that has validity, but is expensive, is to convert OI cycles with a vigorous response (large numbers of follicles) to gamete interfallopian transfer (GIFT) or IVF cycles, where control can be exercised over the number of oocytes or embryos returned to the fallopian tubes or endometrial cavity.

Although intrauterine insemination (IUI) when used alone is not associated with an increased risk of multiple gestation, a correlation has been drawn between higher sperm concentrations and an increased risk of multiple gestation when inseminations are used in conjunction with HMG OI.[105] There is also a loose correlation between sperm concentrations and the likelihood of conception in unstimulated (unifollicular) cycles. It is predictable that in the presence of a polyovular cycle, higher sperm counts will increase the chance of any one oocyte being fertilized or of more than one fertilization. A reduction in sperm concentrations would probably lower (but not completely remove) the risk of multiple gestation, but would simultaneously reduce the success rate of HMG with IUI. Whether this approach is reasonable given the high cost of HMG superovulation cycles is not clear. It might make sense in those cycles in which higher-than-average numbers of follicles are present.

ASSISTED REPRODUCTIVE TECHNIQUES

In ART procedures there is a correlation between the number of oocytes or embryos replaced and the risk of both pregnancy and multiple pregnancy. Whereas reducing the number of embryos transferred reduces the number of multiple gestations, it also reduces the success rate of a program. An example from an early Australian program demonstrates this correlation, as well as the fact that multiple gestation remains a risk even with low numbers of embryos being returned. Of 423 embryo transfers in 1983, Wood et al.[116] reported 74 (17%) ongoing pregnancies, a good rate at that time. There were 90 embryo transfers with just one embryo, resulting in 5 pregnancies (6%), including one twin pregnancy (20%). From 140

transfers of two embryos, 18 pregnancies (13%) were obtained, including 3 twin pregnancies (17%). When three embryos were transferred, 45 pregnancies resulted from 174 returns (26% success rate), but the multiple gestation rate jumped to 27% (9 twin pregnancies and 3 triplet pregnancies). The 23 cycles with four embryos transferred led to 6 pregnancies (26%, no improvement over three embryos) with 1 set of triplets (17%). These numbers, though reasonably representative, differ from program to program. Another report of 48 pregnancies in 250 embryo transfers described 10 multiple pregnancies, all of which occurred when three embryos were transferred.[37] They also noted a significantly lower average age (by 3 years) of the women experiencing multiple gestation. Others have also reported this inverse correlation of age and multiple gestation.[30] One of the largest British programs, in reporting obstetric outcomes of ART pregnancies did not detect an effect of maternal age on multiple pregnancy, but it also did not examine the number of women in each age group undergoing embryo transfer. Instead, it only noted the number of pregnant women in each age group.[107] They did note a distinct correlation between number of embryos returned and multiplicity of the pregnancy (the average number of babies per delivery was 1.36 when 4 embryos returned).

Each ART program must determine in an individual fashion the point at which pregnancy rates do not improve with additional embryos transferred and at which multiple gestations begin to increase too greatly. This is generally two or three embryos per return, but varies with patient age and other factors. Even at low numbers (one or two embryos), the risk of multiple gestation may remain well above the usual population risk.

The temptation to improve a clinic's statistics by returning high numbers of embryos must be resisted. Although information on the average number of embryos returned during ART procedures is not readily available, it is interesting to note that of the 10 ART programs with the highest success rates (ongoing pregnancies per oocyte retrieval), six had multiple pregnancy rates over 40%.[17] Although this could be the result of returning higher numbers of embryos, it could simply reflect good laboratory quality with a high implantation rate per embryo.

Striking the appropriate balance between costs, success, and risk is difficult. Cryopreservation of embryos makes the decision somewhat easier, but the implantation rate per cryopreserved embryo is only about half that per fresh embryo. Performing additional procedures (cryopreserved embryo transfer) after the failure of an initial ART procedure adds to costs, leaving this approach less than ideal.

A factor that should be strongly considered is the age of the female patient. This has a strong influence on the likelihood of any pregnancy, as well as multiple gestation. ART programs should examine their success rates by age category and number of embryos transferred to establish individual guidelines for reasonable numbers of embryos to transfer for different age groups. For example, one group of clinicians feels that the optimal number of embryos for women 30 years of age and younger is two. For ages 31 to 35, two to three embryos are generally recommended, and for 36- to 40-year-old patients, three to four embryos are considered appropriate. Women over 40 years old generally do not have a large number of embryos to choose from, but they could consider five or six embryos if that many are available. Other programs have embraced the stricter guideline of only two embryos (rarely three of poor quality), with no substantial decrease in pregnancy rates, and no decrease in twin pregnancy rates, but elimination of triplet and quadruplet pregnancies.[85]

Embryo quality must be considered, but it still involves an imprecise evaluation and cannot be relied on for accuracy. As new techniques such as assisted hatching become more commonly utilized, such protocols will have to be revised. One study of assisted hatching that returned an average of only 3.5 embryos per patient nevertheless reported multiple pregnancy rates of 55% to 60%.[27]

Limiting the number of embryos transferred does not completely remove the risk of twins or triplets, but it should nearly eliminate the risk of quadruplets or higher multiples. It is sometimes difficult to avoid being swayed by an individual patient's situation. It is tempting to increase the number of embryos returned in patients who have been through a number of cycles unsuccessfully. Although this may be appropriate in some instances, decisions made on the basis of only a few data points can easily be wrong. For example, one patient completed her seventh cycle in a program without a successful conception (she had one prior miscarriage), in spite of good quality embryos being returned. To compensate for her apparent poor implantation rate, the clinicians returned five embryos. The result was a triplet pregnancy.

SELECTIVE REDUCTION

With the current need to maintain a reasonable expectation of success for ART in the face of high expenses and the desire to support both the financial and emotional well being of patients, there is no perfect method of preventing multiple pregnancies. Another approach to the problem is correction after the fact. Selective reduction, covered in other chapters in this book, remains a method of reducing risk in more extreme cases (rarely triplets and more often in quadruplets and higher-order multiple gestations) to a manageable level. Selective reduction contributes its own cost and risk to the overall equation. The main risk is total pregnancy loss, which ranges from 10% to 26%. This is balanced by the benefit of increasing the length of gestation of surviving fetuses, which is most clearly evident in quadruplet and higher gestations.[14,34,40,41,109]

Conclusions

It is clear that the increasing utilization of fertility therapies is altering the general understanding of multiple gestation in many ways. The technologies themselves and associated infertility programs act as a laboratory to enhance knowledge of the normal and abnormal processes of early pregnancy and twinning processes. Multiple gestations produced by the therapies not only contribute to national statistics of morbidity and mortality, but they also change the historic incidence of the different classifications of multiple pregnancy, thereby altering the risk patterns that have previously been understood.

Although ART and OI can challenge existing notions of what constitutes twinning and introduce new concepts in human reproduction, technology cannot yet alter many of the fundamental risks of multiple gestation. The human uterus appears designed to best accommodate a single fetus at a time, and multiple fetuses whether natural or iatrogenic, are at considerable increased risk of prematurity, abnormal placentation, IUGR, and a number of maternal obstetric risks. This risks are real, serious, and costly in both a medical and economic sense.

Although a variety of methods have been discussed to minimize the risk of multiple gestation associated with fertility therapy, none are perfect. If current fertility therapies are utilized, a substantial risk of at least twins (and usually triplets) remains. Programs involved in such therapies remain obligated to monitor the success and failures of their therapies and to choose methods that present the least risk. This includes using less successful but less risky techniques (such as insemination or clomiphene citrate) whenever appropriate. OI with bromocriptine and GnRH should be strongly considered. When HMG and ART are used, controlling the number of embryos transferred is critical, even if overall success rates are slightly diminished.

There is certainly a need to aid patients in the pursuit of their goal of parenthood, but extreme care must be taken with these therapies to avoid harming patients more than they are helped. Continued research in embryo culture, implantation, and mechanisms of ovulation offer some hope of improving clinicians' ability to better regulate reproduction in the future.

References

1. Adashi E et al: Gestational outcome of clomiphene-related conceptions, *Fertil Steril* 31:620-626, 1979.

2. Altaras MM et al: Hydatidiform mole coexisting with a fetus in twin gestation following gonadotropin induction of ovulation, *Hum Reprod* 7:429-431, 1992.

3. American Fertility Society, Society for Assisted Reproductive Technology: Assisted reproductive technology in the United States and Canada: 1992 results generated from the American Fertility Society/Society for Assisted Reproductive Technology registry, *Fertil Steril* 62:1121-1128, 1994.

4. Anderson RL, Goldberg JD, Golbus MS: Prenatal diagnosis in multiple gestation: 20 years experience with amniocentesis, *Prenat Diagn* 11:263-270, 1991.

5. Anderson RL et al: Central nervous system damage and other anomalies in surviving fetus following second trimester antenatal death of co-twin, *Prenat Diagn* 10:513-518, 1990.

6. Australian In-Vitro Fertilization Collaborative Group: In-vitro fertilization pregnancies in Australia and New Zealand, 1979-1985, *Med J Aust* 148:429-436, 1988.

7. Baldwin VJ: *Pathology of multiple pregnancy*, New York, 1994, Springer-Verlag.

8. Benirschke K: Origin and significance of twinning, *Clin Obstet Gynecol* 15:220-235, 1972.

9. Benirschke K: *Multiple gestation: incidence, etiology and inheritance.* In Creasy R, Resnik R, editors: *Maternal fetal medicine*, ed 3, Philadelphia, 1994, W.B. Saunders.

10. Benirschke K, Kim CK: Multiple pregnancy, *N Engl J Med* 288:1329-1336, 1973.

11. Bergquist C, Nillius SJ, Wide L: Human gonadotropin therapy. I. Serum estradiol and progesterone patterns during conceptual cycles, *Fertil Steril* 39:761-765, 1983.

12. Bieber FR et al: Genetic studies of an acardiac monster: evidence of polar body twinning in man, *Science* 213:775-777, 1981.

13. Blecker OP, Oosting J, Hemrika DJ: On the cause of the retardation of fetal growth in multiple gestations, *Acta Genet Med Gemellol (Roma)* 37:41-46, 1988.

14. Boulot P et al: Effects of selective reduction in triplet gestation: a comparative study of 80 cases managed with or without this procedure, *Fertil Steril* 60:497-503, 1993.

15. Braat DDM: Multiple follicular growth under pulsatile gonadotrophin releasing hormone stimulation, *Hum Reprod* 8:189-192, 1993.

16. Breckwoldt M et al: Management of multiple conceptions after gonadotropin-releasing hormone analog/human menopausal gonadotropin/human chorionic gonadotropin therapy, *Fertil Steril* 49:713-715, 1988.

17. Brownlee S et al: The baby chase, *U.S. News & World Report*, pp 84-93, Dec 5, 1994.

18. Bsat FA, Seoud MAF: Superfetation secondary to ovulation induction with clomiphene citrate: a case report, *Fertil Steril* 47:516-517, 1987.

19. Bulmer MG: *The biology of twinning in man*, Oxford, 1970, Clarendon Press.

20. Callahan TL et al: The economic impact of multiple-gestation pregnancies and the contribution of assisted-reproduction techniques to their incidence, *N Engl J Med* 331:244-249, 1994.

21. Cameron AH et al: The value of twin surveys in the study of malformations, *Eur J Obstet Gynecol Reprod Biol* 14:347-356, 1983.

22. Carlson NJ, Towers CV: Multiple gestations complicated by the death of one fetus, *Obstet Gynecol* 73:685-689, 1989.

23. Caspi E et al: The outcome of pregnancy after gonadotropin therapy, *Br J Obstet Gynaecol* 83:967-973, 1976.

24. Chan YF, Ho PC: Bilateral tubal pregnancies after pronuclear stage embryo tubal transfer to 1 tube, *Aust N Z J Obstet Gynaecol* 33:315-316, 1993.

25. Chervenak FA et al: Antenatal diagnosis and perinatal outcome in a series of 385 consecutive pregnancies, *J Reprod Med* 29:727-730, 1984.

26. Cohen J et al: Impairment of the hatching process following IVF in the human and improvement of implantation by assisted hatching using micromanipulation, *Hum Reprod* 5:7-13, 1990.

27. Cohen J et al: Implantation enhancement by selective assisted hatching using zona drilling of human embryos with poor prognosis, *Hum Reprod* 7:685-691, 1992.

28. Collins MS, Bleyl JA: Seventy-one quadruplet pregnancies: management and outcome, *Am J Obstet Gynecol* 162:1384-1392, 1990.

29. Correy JF, Marsden DE, Schokman FCM: The outcome of pregnancy resulting from clomiphene-induced ovulation, *Aust N Z J Obstet Gynaecol* 22:18-21, 1982.

30. Corson SL et al: Outcome in 242 in vitro fertilization-embryo replacement or gamete intrafallopian transfer-induced pregnancies, *Fertil Steril* 51:644-650, 1989.

31. Dale B et al: Intercellular communication in

the early human embryo, *Mol Reprod Dev* 29:22-28, 1991.

32. Derom C et al: Increased monozygotic twinning rate after ovulation induction, *Lancet* 8544:1236-1238, 1987.

33. Dietz TU et al: Combined bilateral tubal and multiple intrauterine pregnancy after ovulation induction, *Eur J Obstet Gynecol Reprod Biol* 48:69-71, 1993.

34. Dommergues M et al: Embryo reduction in multifetal pregnancies after infertility therapy: obstetrical risks and perinatal benefits are related to operative strategy, *Fertil Steril* 55:805-811, 1991.

35. Dor J et al: The incidence of combined intrauterine and extrauterine pregnancy after in vitro fertilization and embryo transfer, *Fertil Steril* 55:833-834, 1991.

36. Edwards R, Mettler L, Walters D: Identical twins and in vitro fertilization, *J In Vitro Fertil Embryo Trans* 3:114-117, 1986.

37. El Khazen N et al: A comparison between multiple and single pregnancies obtained by invitro fertilization, *Hum Reprod* 1:251-254, 1986.

38. Elliott JP, Radin TG: Quadruplet pregnancy: contemporary management and outcome, *Obstet Gynecol* 80:421-424, 1992.

39. Evans J, Townsend L: The induction of ovulation, *Am J Obstet Gynecol* 125:321-327, 1976.

40. Evans MI et al: Selective termination: clinical experience and residual risks, *Am J Obstet Gynecol* 162:1568-1575, 1990.

41. Evans MI et al: Efficacy of transabdominal multifetal pregnancy reduction: collaborative experience among the world's largest centers, *Obstet Gynecol* 82:61-66, 1993.

42. Flannery DB et al: Antenatally detected Klinefelter's syndrome in twins, *Acta Genet Med Gemellol (Roma)* 33:51-56, 1984.

43. Gagliardi CL et al: Gonadotropin-releasing hormone agonist improves the efficiency of controlled ovarian hyperstimulation/intrauterine insemination, *Fertil Steril* 55:939-944, 1991.

44. Gemzell CA: Induction of ovulation, *Acta Obstet Gynaecol Scand Suppl* 47:1, 1974.

45. Gemzell CA, Roos P: Pregnancies following treatment with human gonadotropins, *Am J Obstet Gynecol* 94:490-496, 1966.

46. German JC, Mahour GH, Wooley MM: The twin with esophageal atresia, *J Pediatr Surg* 14:432-435, 1979.

47. Ghidini A et al: The risk of second-trimester amniocentesis in twin gestations: a case-control study, *Am J Obstet Gynecol* 169:1013-1016, 1993.

48. Gilbert WM et al: Morbidity associated with prenatal disruption of the dividing membrane in twin gestations, *Obstet Gynecol* 78:623-630, 1991.

49. Gomel V, Taylor PJ: In vitro fertilization versus reconstructive tubal surgery, *J Assist Reprod Genet* 9:306-309, 1992.

50. Gougeon A: Frequent occurrence of multiovular follicles and multinuclear oocytes in the adult human ovary, *Fertil Steril* 35:417-422, 1981.

51. Gruenwald P: Environmental influences on twins apparent at birth, *Biol Neonate* 15:79-93, 1970.

52. Grützner-Könnecke H et al: Higher order multiple births: natural wonder or failure of therapy, *Acta Genet Med Gemellol (Roma)* 39:491-495, 1990.

53. Gunthard HP, Schmid J: Perinatal mortality in twin pregnancies, *Geburtshilfe Frauenheilkd* 38:270, 1978.

54. Hack M et al: Outcome of pregnancy after induced ovulation, *JAMA* 211:791-797, 1970.

55. Hack M et al: Outcome of pregnancy after induction of ovulation: follow-up of pregnancies and children born after clomiphene therapy, *JAMA* 220:1329-1333, 1972.

56. Harris DW: Letter to the editor, *J Reprod Med* 27:39, 1982.

57. Harvey MAS, Huntley RMC, Smith DW: Familial monozygotic twinning, *J Pediatr* 90:246-248, 1977.

58. Hashimoto B et al: Ultrasound evaluation of polyhydramnios and twin pregnancy, *Am J Obstet Gynecol* 154:1069-1072, 1986.

59. Homburg R et al: One hundred pregnancies after treatment with pulsatile luteinising hormone releasing hormone to induce ovulation, *Br Med J* 298:809-812, 1989.

60. Imaizumi Y: Triplets and higher order multiple births in Japan, *Acta Genet Med Gemellol (Roma)* 39:295-306, 1990.

61. James WH: Dizygotic twinning, marital stage and status and coital rates, *Ann Hum Biol* 8:371-378, 1981.

62. Johnson SF, Driscoll SG: Twin placentation and its complications, *Semin Perinatol* 10:9-13, 1986.

63. Kaufman MH, O'Shea KS: Induction of

monozygotic twinning in the mouse, *Nature* 276:707-708, 1978.

64. Kemmann E et al: Induction of ovulation with menotropins in women with polycystic ovary syndrome, *Am J Obstet Gynecol* 141:58-64, 1981.

65. Kistner RW: *Induction of ovulation with clomiphene citrate.* In Behrman SJ, Kistner RW, editors, *Progress in infertility*, Boston, 1968, Little, Brown and Co.

66. Landy HL, Weiner S, Corson S: The "vanishing twin": ultrasonographic assessment of fetal "disappearance" in the first trimester, *Society of Perinatal Obstetrics* sixth annual meeting, San Antonio, Jan 30-Feb 1, 1986.

67. Levi S: Ultrasonic assessment of the high rate of human multiple pregnancy in the first trimester, *J Clin Ultrasound* 4:3-5, 1976.

68. Liban E, Salzberger M: A prospective clinicopathological study of 1108 cases of antenatal fetal death, *Isr J Med Sci* 12:34-44, 1976.

69. Liu S et al: Intrauterine death in multiple gestation, *Acta Genet Med Gemellol (Roma)* 41:5-26, 1992.

70. Long PA, Oats JN: Preeclampsia in twin pregnancy: severity and pathogenesis, *Aust N Z J Obstet Gynaecol* 27:1-5, 1987.

71. Luke B et al: Gestational age-specific birthweights of twins versus singletons, *Acta Genet Med Gemellol (Roma)* 40:69-76, 1991.

72. MacLennan A: *Multiple gestation: clinical characteristics and management.* In Creasy R, Resnik R, editors: *Maternal fetal medicine*, ed 3, Philadelphia, 1994, W.B. Saunders.

73. Macourt DC, Stewart P, Zaki M: Multiple pregnancy and fetal abnormalities in association with oral contraceptive usage, *Aust N Z J Obstet Gynaecol* 22:25-28, 1982.

74. Martin KA et al: Comparison of exogenous gonadotropins and pulsatile gonadotropin-releasing hormone for induction of ovulation in hypogonadotropic amenorrhea, *J Clin Endocrinol Metab* 77:125-129, 1993.

75. Medearis AL et al: Perinatal deaths in twin pregnancy, *Am J Obstet Gynecol* 134:413-421, 1979.

76. Merrell-National Laboratories Product Information Bulletin, 1972.

77. Mettler L et al: Schwangerschaft und Geburt monozygoter weiblicher Zwillinge nach Invitro-fertilization und Embryotransfer (IVF-ET), *Geburtshilfe Frauenheilkd* 44:670-676, 1984.

78. Molloy D et al: Multiple-sited (heterotopic) pregnancy after in vitro fertilization and gamete intrafallopian transfer, *Fertil Steril* 53:1068-1071, 1990.

79. Monga M, Reid RL: Superfoetation in the human: a case report, *J Soc Obstet Gynecol Can* 14:81-84, 1992.

80. Mortimer G: Zygosity and placental structure in monochorionic twins, *Acta Genet Med Gemellol (Roma)* 36:417-420, 1987.

81. Myrianthopoulos NC: Congenital malformations in twins: epidemiologic survey, *Birth Defects* 11:1-39, 1975.

82. Nakamura Y et al: Clinical experience in the induction of ovulation and pregnancy with pulsatile subcutaneous administration of human menopausal gonadotropin: a low incidence of multiple pregnancy, *Fertil Steril* 51:423-429, 1989.

83. Newman HH: *The physiology of twinning*, Chicago, 1923, The University of Chicago Press.

84. Newman RB, Hamar C, Miller MC: Outpatient triplet management: a contemporary review, *Am J Obstet Gynecol* 161:547-555, 1989.

85. Nijs M et al: Prevention of multiple pregnancies in an in vitro fertilization program, *Fertil Steril* 59:1245-1250, 1993.

86. Nylander PPS: *The causation of twinning.* In MacGillivray E, Nylander PPS, Corney G, editors: *Human multiple reproduction*, Philadelphia, 1975, W.B. Saunders.

87. Palle C et al: Increased risk of abortion after genetic amniocentesis in twin pregnancies, *Prenat Diagn* 3:83-89, 1983.

88. Pergament JD et al: The risk and efficacy of chorionic villus sampling in multiple gestation, *Prenat Diagn* 12:377-384, 1992.

89. Persson PH et al: On improved outcome of twin pregnancies, *Acta Obstet Gynaecol Scand* 58:3, 1979.

90. Petrikovsky BM, Vintzileos AM: Management and outcome of multiple pregnancy of high fetal order: literature review, *Obstet Gynecol Surv* 44:578-584, 1989.

91. Pittaway DE, Wentz AC: Evaluation of the exponential rise of serum estradiol concentrations in human menopausal gonadotropin-induced cycles, *Fertil Steril* 40:763-767, 1983.

92. Potter EL, Craig JM: *Pathology of the fetus and the infant*, ed 3, Chicago, 1975, Mosby.

93. Pruggmayer M et al: Incidence of abortion after genetic amniocentesis in twin pregnancies, *Prenat Diagn* 11:637-640, 1991.

94. Rizk B et al: Rare ectopic pregnancies after in-vitro fertilization: one unilateral twin and four bilateral tubal pregnancies, *Hum Reprod* 5:1025-1028, 1990.

95. Rothman D: Folic acid in pregnancy, *Am J Obstet Gynecol* 108:149-175, 1970.

96. Rothman KJ: Fetal loss, twinning and birth weight after oral-contraceptive use, *N Engl J Med* 297:468-471, 1977.

97. Rowe MI, Ravitch MM, Ranninger K: Operative correction of caudal duplication (dipygus), *Surgery* 63:840-848, 1968.

98. Sassoon DA et al: Perinatal outcome in triplet versus twin gestations, *Obstet Gynecol* 75:817-820, 1990.

99. Schenker JG, Yarkoni S, Granat M: Multiple pregnancies following induction of ovulation, *Fertil Steril* 35:105-123, 1981.

100. Schoolcraft WB et al: Assisted hatching in the treatment of poor prognosis in vitro fertilization candidates, *Fertil Steril* 62:551-554, 1994.

101. Segreti WO, Winter PM, Nance WE: *Familial studies in monozygotic twinning*. In Nance WE, editor: Twin research: biology and epidemiology, *Prog Clin Biol Res* 24B:55-60, 1978.

102. Seoud MAF et al: Outcome of twin, triplet, and quadruplet in vitro fertilization pregnancies: the Norfolk experience, *Fertil Steril* 57:825-834, 1992.

103. Shapiro LR, Zemek L, Shulman MJ: Genetic etiology for monozygotic twinning, *Birth Defects* 14:219-222, 1978.

104. Sharav T: Aging gametes in relation to incidence, gender and twinning in Down syndrome, *Am J Med Genet* 39:116-118, 1991.

105. Shelden R et al: Multiple gestation is associated with the use of high sperm numbers in the intrauterine insemination specimen in women undergoing gonadotropin stimulation, *Fertil Steril* 49:607-610, 1988.

106. Smith DW, Bartlett C, Harrah LM: Monozygotic twinning and the Duhamel anomalad (imperforate anus to sirenomelia): a non-random association between two aberrations in morphogenesis, *Birth Defects* 12:53-63, 1976.

107. Tan SL et al: Obstetric outcome of in vitro fertilization pregnancies compared with normally conceived pregnancies, *Am J Obstet Gynecol* 167:778-784, 1992.

108. Terasaki PI et al: Twins with two different fathers identified by HLA, *N Engl J Med* 299:590-592, 1978.

109. Timor-Tritsch IE et al: Multifetal pregnancy reduction by transvaginal puncture: evaluation of the technique used in 134 cases, *Am J Obstet Gynecol* 168:799-804, 1993.

110. Turkalj I, Braun P, Krupp P: Surveillance of bromocriptine in pregnancy, *JAMA* 247:1589-1591, 1982.

111. Uchida IA et al: Twinning rate in spontaneous abortions, *J Hum Genet* 35:987-993, 1983.

112. van de Geijn EJ et al: Hydatidiform mole with coexisting twin pregnancy after gamete intrafallopian transfer, *Human Reprod* 7:568-572, 1992.

113. Vessey M et al: A long-term follow-up study of women using different methods of contraception: an interim report, *J Biosoc Sci* 8:373-427, 1976.

114. Weissman A et al: Management of triplet pregnancies in the 1980s: are we doing better? *Am J Perinatol* 8:333-337, 1991.

115. Windham GC, Sever LE: Neural tube defects among twin births, *Am J Hum Genet* 34:988-998, 1982.

116. Wood C et al: Clinical implications of developments in in vitro fertilization, *Br Med J* 289:978-980, 1984.

117. Wright JCY, Christopher CR: Sirenomelia, Potter's syndrome and their relationship to monozygotic twinning (a case report and discussion), *J Reprod Med* 27:291-294, 1982.

118. Wu CH: Plasma estrogen monitoring of ovulation induction, *Obstet Gynecol* 46:294-298, 1975.

119. Wu CH: Monitoring of ovulation induction, *Fertil Steril* 30:617-630, 1978.

4

Genetics and Genetic Counseling

Arie Drugan, Mark P. Johnson, Eric L. Krivchenia, and Mark I. Evans

The study of twins has been exceptionally important to the understanding of genetic mechanisms and their effects on human reproduction and development of disease. The introduction of the twin method in the evaluation of genetic disease is generally attributed to Galton (1876), who adopted the alternative terms *nature* and *nurture*. Although Galton was probably not aware that there are two types of twins (monozygotic and dizygotic), his basic concept was correct. Monozygotic twins are derived from the division of one zygote and as such, are genetically identical. Phenotypic differences between monozygotic twins could be explained by environmental influences (nurture). Since dizygotic twins have only 50% of their genes in common but are affected by the same environmental influences, they can be used as suitable controls.

Multiple births derived from several oocytes are the rule in most mammals. In humans, only one oocyte per cycle generally matures and is discharged. If two oocytes are ovulated and fertilized by two different sperm, dizygotic twins result. In the same way, polyovulation occasionally leads to multizygotic triplets or quadruplets. Maternal age and genetic predisposition influence the rate of polyovulation (Box 4-1). The incidence of dizygotic twinning increases from puberty to peak between ages 35 and 39, and then gradually declines. Dizygotic twinning rates increase not only with maternal age but also with birth order. Tall, heavy women bear twins 30% more often than small, slender women. Coital frequency also has a positive effect, with a higher rate of twin conceptions within the first 3 months of marriage. Women of Asian descent have lower rates of multiple gestation than white American women. The highest rate of twinning in North America is observed in women of African descent (15/1000 births). These observations are apparently explained by a genetic predisposition for higher follicle-stimulating hormone (FSH) levels in some populations. In recent years, a decrease in naturally occurring multiple gestations has been observed in industrialized countries.[71] However, the total number of multiple pregnancies is increasing in association with the increased use of assisted reproduction techniques (ART) and of agents for ovulation induction (OI).[67]

Box 4-1

Maternal Factors Influencing the Incidence of Multiple Gestations

Age (35 to 39)
Weight (tall, heavy)
Race (black)
Parity (higher)
Coital frequency (increased)
Family history

Familial clustering of dizygotic twins has been observed since the early 1900s. After the birth of spontaneously occurring twins, the subsequent risk of multiple gestation for the mother and her female offspring is approximately 4 times that of the general population. For male dizygotic twins and fathers of dizygotic twins, this risk is not increased. The mode of inheritance seems to be multifactorial, with increased gonadotropin levels most probably being the major genetic determinant.

Monozygotic twinning is the result of the complete division of the embryo at an early cleavage stage, leading to duplication with mirror-image similarity. The rate of monozygotic twinning is fairly constant among different populations (3 to 4/1000 births) and is not influenced by maternal age, parity, or familial predisposition. The factors causing monozygotic twinning to occur are not yet known. Zygosity can be determined by gender difference and by examination of the placenta. Unlike-sex twins are always dizygotic and have dichorionic-diamniotic placentas. About half of all like-sex twins are also dizygotic. Monozygotic twins are always of the same gender.

Depending on the time of separation (days 2 through 15 after fertilization), the placenta in a monozygotic pregnancy can be diamniotic-dichorionic, monochorionic-diamniotic, or monochorionic-monoamniotic. The latter version, which develops when separation of the embryonic disk occurs after development of the amnion (7 to 13 days after fertilization), is observed in only 1% to 2% of monozygotic twin pregnancies and is associated with a high rate of fetal mortality.[59] Although examination of the placenta is feasible only after birth, determination of fetal sex, localization of the placenta, and observation of the dividing membrane and its echogenicity on ultrasound may in some cases help determine zygosity during pregnancy. Technically, this is easier in early gestation. Using a 2-mm thickness of the dividing membrane between the twins as the cutoff, the rates of accuracy for predicting monochorionic and dichorionic twinning have been reported as 82% and 95%, respectively.[75] Other techniques to determine zygosity after birth include blood typing, karyotypic variation, or deoxyribonucleic acid (DNA) restriction fragment-length polymorphisms.

Congenital Anomalies and Pregnancy Loss

Multiple fetuses that are delivered after more than 20 weeks' gestation occur in less than 1% of pregnancies but account for 10% to 12% of perinatal deaths.[43] This can be attributed to maternal complications during pregnancy (such as preeclampsia, anemia, or thromboembolic phenomena), which are more common and appear earlier with multiple pregnancy, and to increased risk of prematurity. These risks increase in direct proportion to the number of live fetuses in utero. However, the main cause of increased perinatal mortality associated with multiple gestation appears to be associated with faulty placentation, competition for intrauterine space, or abnormal insertion of the umbilical cord. Placenta previa, abruptio placentae, and cord prolapse appear to be more common in multiple gestations and contribute to the increased perinatal mortality. Of all intrauterine death in twins, 73.3% are associated with monochorionic placentation.[19] This rate implies that vascular anastomoses with major fluid volume shifts may be the direct cause of death in these cases. Velamentous insertion of the umbilical cord, which makes the fetus more vulnerable to cord compression, fetal distress, and antenatal bleeding from vasa previa, is 6 to 9 times more common in twin pregnancies than in singleton pregnancies.[9] The costs of multiple gestations are known to be substantially increased, averaging in a Boston study to be $9845 for a singleton pregnancy, $37,947 for a twin pregnancy, and $109,765 for a triplet pregnancy.[14]

Congenital anomalies are more common in multiple than in singleton pregnancies and are an important cause of increased pregnancy loss. Monozygotic twins have 2.5 times more structural malformations than dizygotic twins or singletons.[64,65] Dizygotic twins, derived from separate oocytes, have almost 2 times the rate of chromosome anomalies than singletons conceived at identical maternal age, but the rate of nonchromosomal structural malformations is not increased. The increased incidence of some structural malforma-

tions in monozygotic twins (such as anencephaly, holoprosencephaly, and caudal regression syndrome) can be explained by a common insult in early gestation that causes both the twinning and the malformation complex. Disruption complexes are mainly found after the intrauterine death of a twin with a common placenta. Intravascular coagulation and necrosis of the decreased twin and the corresponding area in the placenta with subsequent embolization through placental anastomoses into the circulation of the surviving fetus may lead to microcephaly, porencephalic cysts, and intestinal atresia.[64] Lastly, deformation complexes (such as club foot or craniofacial abnormalities) may arise from crowding in the third trimester. Congenital scoliosis evident in only one of a pair of monozygotic twins underlines the effect of the intrauterine environment on the deformation complex.[54] Since deformation abnormalities are commonly caused by the intrauterine environment with minor genetic contribution, they affect monozygotic and dizygotic fetuses equally, and the risk of recurrence of such abnormalities in sibs is relatively small. Although it has been reported that the amniotic band disruption complex occasionally affects both twins in a monozygotic sibship,[29] twins are most commonly discordant for this disorder; this is also apparently the case for acquired intrauterine lesion.[57]

An increased risk for neural tube defects,[20,36,73,74] congenital heart defects,[13,42] and some craniofacial malformations[21] have been documented in twin surveys. Anencephaly and encephalocele are apparently more common in twins (especially in girls), but meningomyelocele is not. Some rare heart defects (for example, truncus arteriosus) are also exceedingly more common in twins; the excess is specifically documented in twins of like sex, even if they are dizygotic.[39] However, it should be noted that even monozygotic twins are only rarely concordant to the existence, the type, or the severity of an anomaly. In a combined series of 445 monozygotic twins, anomalies were found in 26 pairs (6%); concordant malformations were found in 6 pairs, and discordant malformations were found in 20 pairs.[15] Twins discordant for congenital cardiovascular anomalies,[42] neural tube defects,[36] craniofacial abnormalities,[37] Müllerian agenesis,[60] and skeletal abnormalities[6] have all been reported.

A different phenotype that is discordant for major structural anomalies has been reported in some aneuploid monozygotic twin gestations.[41,46] The difference in phenotypic expression of some anomalies in monozygotic twins can be explained by postzygotic mitotic crossing over (sister chromatid exchange), a phenomenon that occurs in humans and is much more common and more important than generally assumed. Its occurrence before an embryo differentiates into twins is theoretically predicted to have disrupting effects on genomic imprinting and cys-acting sequences, leading to consequences that may range from early lethality to monozygotic twin discordance.[18] The close association of twinning, midline malformations, and disorders of brain asymmetry further suggest a major role of mitotic crossing over in the organization of the oocyte and embryogenesis, as well as in the induction of the twinning process itself.[10,18]

Acardia is a malformation specific to monozygotic twinning in which the normal twin maintains the acardiac twin through arterial and venous anastomoses. The incidence of this abnormality is approximately 1/34,000 pregnancies.[48] Arrest of normal cardiac development secondary to circulatory reversal in the affected twin is the most commonly accepted cause.[9,76] Chromosomal abnormalities have also been documented in some of these cases, the latter being always confined to the abnormal twin. The circulatory abnormality leads to absence or abnormal development of the thorax, upper limbs, and head, and it is always lethal. Anencephaly in the twin of an acardiac fetus has also been reported.[51] The perinatal mortality rate of the normal twin has been reported to be as high as 50% and has been attributed to prematurity or congestive heart failure. Surgical occlusion of the umbilical artery of the acardiac fetus has been tried successfully in an attempt to avoid complications for the normal twin.[55]

Conjoined twins, a rare complication of monozygotic twinning that occurs at a rate of about 1/1500 twin pregnancies, are apparently the result of incomplete embryonic cleavage during the monozygotic twinning process. The most common type of conjoined twins is the thoracophagous variety. Prognosis depends on the potential for surgical correction after birth and is usually grim. Ultrasound diagnosis of conjoined twins before birth has been achieved and most commonly leads to interruption of the abnormal gestation. If conjoined twins are diagnosed during labor, delivery by cesarean section is indicated for maternal causes.

The value of serial ultrasonography in the clinical management of multiple gestations is already well established. Determination of chorionicity and amnionicity in multiple gestations is an important surrogate to zygosity and may be achieved through evaluation of placental locations and the thickness of the membrane between the sacs.[49] Monochorionic pregnancies carry a higher risk of fetal anomalies and of obstetric complications such as twin-twin transfusion. Polyhydramnios, oligohydramnios, differences in growth patterns, and some fetal anomalies are also readily diagnosable on ultrasound.[17]

The diagnosis of congenital anomalies in multiple gestations may be hampered by fetal positioning and crowding, oligohydramnios, and increased distance between the ultrasound transducer and the target organ. Despite these limitations, prenatal ultrasonography for fetal congenital anomalies with cardiac screening (limited to the four-chamber view) in 157 twin pairs provided a detection rate of 39% of all major anomalies and 55% of the noncardiac major anomalies but none of the cardiac lesions.[2] More importantly, ultrasonography detected 69% of the major anomalies for which routine prenatal management should be altered. It is apparent from these results that ultrasound screening for fetal anomalies in twin gestations is at least as effective as it is in singleton pregnancies.

Genetic Counseling: Problems Relevant to Multiple Gestations

The most comprehensive description of modern genetic counseling is provided by Harper, who states, "Genetic counseling is the process by which patients or relatives at risk of a disorder that may be hereditary are advised of the consequences of the disorder, the probability of developing or transmitting it, and the ways in which this may be prevented or ameliorated."[31] This definition includes the following three aspects of genetic counseling: (1) the diagnostic aspect, without which all other aspects of genetic counseling are unfounded; (2) the estimation of risks; and (3) the supportive role of the counselor. Thus the purpose of genetic counseling is to "develop effective modes of communication between counselors and families in order to achieve informed decisions and psychological adjustment regarding the human problems related to the burden of genetic disease."[31]

The most common indication for prenatal genetic counseling and diagnosis is advanced maternal age. Other indications include an abnormal ultrasound scan or abnormal results of biochemical maternal serum screening (that is, alpha-fetoprotein [AFP]). The birth of a child with a known or suspected genetic defect, a positive family history for a genetic disorder, consanguinity, or carrier identification through genetic screening (for example, Tay-Sachs disease, cystic fibrosis, or sickle cell anemia carriers) are indications for prenatal genetic counseling in less than 20% of cases.

The causes of fetal malformations are summarized in Table 4-1. Zygosity affects the risk of twins for sharing a genetic problem. Monogyzotic twins have the same genotype and are almost always concordant for mendelian disorders or for chromosome anomalies, although the phenotype may differ considerably. Genetically, dizygotic twins are essentially no more alike than any other siblings, and their

TABLE 4-1

Causes of Fetal Malformations	
SUSPECTED CAUSE	% OF TOTAL
Polygenic or multifactorial	20
Environmental	5
Single gene mutations	5
Chromosomal	10
Unknown	60

TABLE 4-2

Modification of Genetic Risk in Twin Gestations		
GENETIC DISORDER	SINGLETON	TWINS
Chromosomal (maternal age)	X	X* 5/3
Single gene (mendelian)		
Recessive	1/4	3/8
X-linked†	1/4*	1/3‡
Dominant	1/2	5/6
Multifactorial (/1000 births)		
Congenital heart defects	0.74	1.65
Anencephaly	0.92	1.24
Hydrocephaly	0.61	0.72

*Assuming a 1/2 rate of males and that 1/2 of them will be affected; †A priori risk can be modified by ultrasound diagnosis of fetal sex; ‡Assuming a 2/3 chance that at least one of the twins is male and there is a 1/2 risk for males to be affected

risk of sharing a genetic disorder is not increased above that of other children in the family. For multifactorial disorders, concordance is higher in monozygotic twins than in dizygotic twins and varies with the predominance of genetic factors in the causation of the disease. The risk of sharing a nonmendelian disorder in dizygotic twins is higher than in it is for other siblings, since the twins develop in the same intrauterine environment. The possibilities that both twins are normal, that one twin is normal and the other is abnormal, and finally that both twins are abnormal should all be considered in the calculation of genetic risks.[34] Thus to calculate the risk of chromosome anomalies affecting at least one twin, the risk associated with maternal age should be multiplied by a factor of 5/3. The risk of mendelian and multifactorial disorders affecting at least one twin in a pair is summarized in Table 4-2. It is obvious that the increased risk of anomalies and the ethical problems that may be associated with prenatal diagnosis of an affected fetus should be part of the genetic counseling session before amniocentesis in twin gestations.[21] If after prenatal diagnosis, twins are found to be discordant for congenital anomalies, the op-

tions available to parents are to continue the pregnancy (and deliver a malformed twin), to abort the pregnancy (and thus lose the normal twin as well), or to consider selective termination of the abnormal twin. The ethical considerations associated with selective termination are beyond the scope of this review and have been detailed in other writings.[26] The international experience with selective fetal reduction for one abnormal twin has been recently presented by Evans et al.[28] The procedure was performed in 183 cases, most of them twins who were indicated in 98 pregnancies for chromosome anomalies, in 76 pregnancies for fetal structural anomalies, and in 11 pregnancies for one twin affected with a mendelian disorder. Intracardiac potassium chloride (KCl) injection was the preferred method for selective fetal termination and was successful in all cases. The KCl method was associated with a significantly lower loss rate than other methods (8.3% versus 41.7%, respectively). In all cases with monochorionic placentation, the procedure caused loss of the entire pregnancy. The overall rate of pregnancy loss before 24 weeks of gestation was 12.6%, and another 3.8% delivered between 24 and 28 weeks. The authors of the study conclude that selective termination for an abnormal twin is a safe procedure when performed by experienced clinicians, provided placentation is dichorionic. In monochorionic pregnancies, selective termination should not be performed by KCl injection. Recently, Quintero et al.,[58] at the same institution, have shown that ligation of the umbilical cord under endoscopic visualization can be used in the management of an acardiac twin. Such an approach appears more reasonable, although the experience is still too small for precise risk estimates.

Prenatal Genetic Screening

Prenatal screening to detect heterozygote carriers of genetic disorders is feasible when the following three conditions are met:

1. The disorder occurs mainly in a specific, defined population
2. A test suitable for carrier detection through mass screening is available
3. Prenatal diagnosis is possible in pregnancies of carrier couples

Some disorders that meet these conditions are Tay-Sachs disease (in Ashkenazi Jews), cystic fibrosis (in American populations of Northern European ancestry), sickle cell anemia (in African-Americans), and β-thalassemia (in couples of Mediter-

ranean descent). It is the standard of care to offer all Jewish couples carrier testing for Tay-Sachs disease by determining the hexosaminidase A level in peripheral blood.[1] When both parents carry the Tay-Sachs gene, prenatal diagnosis of affected fetuses is possible through the determination of enzyme activity in cultured amniocytes or chorionic villi.[8]

Multiple gestation is associated with an earlier and more significant increase in maternal plasma volume, which may cause an erroneous diagnosis of some gravidas as carriers through its dilution effect on the enzyme level in peripheral blood. In some cases, this may lead to performing unnecessary procedures for prenatal diagnosis, which are in themselves problematic in multiple pregnancies, as is discussed in the next section of this chapter. However, changes in maternal plasma volume do not affect carrier detection through the assessment of enzyme activity in peripheral lymphocytes or through molecular methods (for example, the detection of delta F508 mutation in cystic fibrosis). Hemoglobin electrophoresis and peripheral blood smears (for detection of sickle cell trait or thalassemia carriers) are also not affected by maternal plasma volume.

A common indication for genetic counseling is an abnormal result of a screening for maternal serum alpha-fetoprotein (MSAFP) and other markers (such as human chorionic gonadotropin [hCG] and estriol). The high acceptance of MSAFP screening as standard of care in pregnancy results from its proven efficacy for the detection of a wide array of fetal malformations (such as neural tube defects or abdominal wall defects) and from adverse pregnancy outcomes after abnormally elevated MSAFP results.[47,63] When the MSAFP level is greater than 2.5 multiples of the median (MOM), the risk for a structurally abnormal fetus is 3% to 5%, and ultrasound and amniocentesis are offered. However, this risk may also be modified according to the degree of MSAFP elevation—the higher the MSAFP level, the higher the risk that the fetus is malformed.[63]

Since the mid-1980s, low MSAFP levels have been associated with increased risk for aneuploidy,[44] and tables have been developed to calculate the risk of Down syndrome in a specific gestation based on maternal age and MSAFP levels.[32] About 45% of pregnancies with trisomy 21 are detected by using a maternal age-dependent low MSAFP cutoff level. It has been noted that other chromosome anomalies may also be associated with low MSAFP, and therefore a risk approximately twice the risk for Down syndrome is quoted in these cases. When amniocentesis is performed as a result of this indication, the overall yield of chromosome anomalies is 1.1%.[23] Moreover, the trend of most laboratories is to use triple serum screening (AFP, β-hCG, and ± unconjugated estriol), which together with maternal age may detect up to 65% to 70% of pregnancies affected by trisomy 21. The yield of amniocenteses is about 1/50.[27,72] The effect of multiple gestation on the efficacy of double or triple serum screening has not been reported, but from the previously cited considerations it is expected to be more significant than when MSAFP is used alone. This topic is currently under investigation in several institutions.

Multiple gestations are commonly associated with high MSAFP levels, since each fetus contributes its own AFP production to maternal circulation. Thus the expected median MSAFP level in twins is approximately twice the MOM for singletons of same gestational age. In a study of 136 twin pregnancies, Johnson et al.[35] reported a median MSAFP level for twins that is parallel to the median level of singletons but 2.5 times higher. In a study of 535 twin pairs, after correction for maternal weight, race, and insulin dependent diabetes, the median AFP level for twins was about 2 times (2.1 ± 0.3) the median of singletons.[23] The MSAFP level in blacks was commonly higher than in whites with pregnancies of comparable gestational age. Using a 4.5 multiple of the singleton median cutoff level in twin pregnancies, 3.9% of results were defined as high, similar to the rate observed in singleton pregnancies. Considering the higher rate of fetal congenital anomalies in twins and the possible confounding effect of an increased MSAFP level after the demise of another fetus in multiple gestation or after multiple pregnancy reduction, a higher percentage of abnormally elevated MSAFP results would have been expected in twin gestations.[30]

Biochemical serum screening for fetal aneuploidy in multiple gestation may be confounded by different fetal contributions to the total level of substrate in maternal circulation. Thus the effect of a low AFP secretion from one fetus, which in a singleton pregnancy may have resulted in the prenatal diagnosis of an abnormal gestation, may be confused by a higher AFP contribution from the normal twin, resulting in a mean AFP value in the normal range and obviating the need for amniocentesis. Simplistically defining low MSAFP results in twins to be AFP values lower than 1.0 multiple of the singleton median (in pregnancies of similar gestational age and race) enables the detection of about 7% of twin gestations that need genetic counseling for increased risk of aneuploidy.[24] The actual yield of abnormal fetal karyotypes detected by amniocentesis performed when such criteria are used has not been reported yet.

Procedures for Prenatal Diagnosis: Special Considerations

The incidence of multiple gestation in patients referred for prenatal diagnosis is 1.3% (ranging from 1.2% to 1.6%).[11,25,50,59,60] With the increased use of ultrasonography in pregnancy, especially in the first trimester, it is rare that a multiple pregnancy is discovered only at amniocentesis. Ultrasonography can also give important information regarding placental chorionicity in twin gestations.

Genetic counseling before procedures should include details of the following issues:

1. The risk of fetal anomalies as calculated for twins with consideration of their zygosity and the indication for prenatal diagnosis
2. The need to sample each fetus separately
3. Possible complications from the procedure
4. The ethical and technical implications in case one fetus is found to be affected.

The risk of fetal aneuploidy is higher in twin gestations than in singleton pregnancies of comparable maternal age, and it has been suggested that prenatal diagnosis should be offered to women age 33 or older who are carrying twins.[62]

However, it should be noted that the risk of pregnancy loss after prenatal diagnosis in patients carrying multiple fetuses is also increased above that reported for patients expecting singletons. A summary of studies reporting complications of amniocenteses performed in over 800 twin pairs shows a mean pregnancy loss to 28 weeks of 4.6% (ranging from 2.1% to 8.1%).*

Although cordocentesis has been attempted successfully in twins, amniocentesis is generally the procedure of choice for midtrimester prenatal diagnosis in multiple gestations.[45,66] Before the procedure, the anatomic relationship between the twins and the membrane separating the sacs should be demonstrated on ultrasound and documented. With continuous ultrasound guidance, it is generally easy to sample both sacs separately. Using a curvilinear- or linear-array ultrasound transducer, the first amniocentesis needle can be left in situ while a second needle is introduced into the other sac, so both needles can be observed simultaneously on ultrasound in the same plane with the chorioamniotic membrane between them.[5] When the relationship between the sacs is less evident, injection of a dye such as indigo carmine into the first sac after aspiration of amniotic fluid may be helpful. Aspiration of clear amniotic fluid proves that the second sample is from the previously untapped sac. However, the use of dyes in these situations should be approached cautiously. The use of methylene blue as a dye marker for genetic amniocentesis in twins has been associated with jejunal atresia in 17/89 twin pairs exposed.[70] The use of a membrane-free maternal hemoglobin hemolysate has been suggested as a

*References 3, 4, 7, 11, 50, 53, 56, 59

useful inert and safe biologic dye for this purpose.[7] Another approach is to withdraw an extra syringe full of amniotic fluid and immediately reinject it. The turbulence and particles scatter, making identification of that sac straightforward. The "clean" sac can then be tapped.

In singleton pregnancies, an abnormally elevated amniotic fluid AFP level indicates the need to test for acetylcholinesterase (AChE) in amniotic fluid. An abnormally elevated amniotic fluid AFP level and a positive AChE test are associated in most cases with fetal malformations or with fetal death. In twin pregnancies, clinical interpretation of amniotic fluid AFP and AChE results may be confused by the transfer of these materials across the membranes.[33] Discordant amniotic fluid AFP results are more common in dizygotic twins, perhaps because of the dichorionic membrane between the sacs. AChE diffuses readily across the membranes and cannot be used to determine which twin is abnormal.[22,68]

First trimester prenatal diagnosis offers the advantages of earlier results and more privacy in reproductive decisions. First trimester ultrasound can accurately predict dichorionicity in 96% of cases and monochorionicity in 88% of cases.[38] Dichorionic twins need separate sampling from each fetus, whereas in genetically identical monochorionic twins, one sample suffices for prenatal diagnosis. Whereas sampling accuracy from each twin is high with second trimester amniocentesis,[53] the incidence of "mixed" sampling confusing prenatal diagnosis results is apparently high with either early amniocentesis[16] or chorionic villus sampling (CVS). Two published series of CVS in multiple gestations have shown that mixed sampling occurs in 4% to 6% of patients.[12,52] This is more than double the contamination rate in singleton gestations.

Summary and Conclusions

Multiple gestations are encountered in more than 1% of patients referred for prenatal diagnosis, and they present special problems of genetic counseling, prenatal testing, and interpretation of results. Structural anomalies are more common in monozygotic twins, and ultrasonographic diagnosis may be hampered by fetal crowding and positioning and by increased distance from the transducer. The risk of aneuploidy is increased in dizygotic twins, suggesting that the age at which prenatal diagnosis is offered in multiple gestations should probably be lowered to 33 years. Biochemical serum screening may be confounded by different contributions of substrate from the fetuses and by more acute changes in maternal plasma volume than observed in singleton pregnancies. The procedure of choice for midtrimester prenatal diagnosis is amniocentesis, but patients should be counseled regarding a somewhat higher risk of postprocedure pregnancy loss than that observed for singleton pregnancies. Moreover, diffusion of amniotic fluid AFP and AChE across the membranes may complicate interpretation of results. In the first trimester, prenatal diagnosis in multiple gestations by CVS is feasible, but the risk of twin-to-twin contamination is relatively high (about 5%). This risk has also been reported for early amniocentesis. The ethical and practical problems associated with one abnormal fetus should also be discussed with patients. Selective fetal reduction of the abnormal fetus is a relatively safe procedure in experienced hands, but it should generally not be attempted in monochorionic gestations except by cord ligation.

References

1. ACOG: Antenatal diagnosis of genetic disorders, *ACOG Technical Bulletin* No 107, Sept 1987.
2. Allen SR et al: Ultrasonographic diagnosis of congenital anomalies in twins, *Am J Obstet Gynecol* 165:1056-1060, 1991.
3. Anderson RL, Goldberg JD, Golbus MS: Prenatal diagnosis in multiple gestations: 20 years' experience with amniocentesis, *Prenat Diagn* 11:263-270, 1991.
4. Antsaklis A et al: Invasive techniques for fetal diagnosis in multiple pregnancy, *Int J Gynaecol Obstet* 34:309-314, 1991.
5. Bahado SR, Schmitt R, Hobbins JC: New technique for genetic amniocentesis in twins, *Obstet Gynecol* 79:304-307, 1992.
6. Beck RB, Brudno DS, Rosenbaum KN: Bilateral absence of the ulna in twins as a manifestation of the split hand-split foot deformity, *Am J Perinatol* 6:1-3, 1989.
7. Beekhuis JR et al: Second trimester amniocentesis in twin pregnancies: maternal hemoglobin as a dye marker to differentiate diamniotic twins, *Br J Obstet Gynaecol* 99:126-127, 1992.
8. Ben-Yoseph Y et al: Diagnosis and carrier detection of Tay Sachs disease: direct determination of hexoseaminidase A using 4 methylumbelliferyl derivatives of beta-N-acetylglucoseamine 6 sulphate and beta-N-acetylgalactoseamine 6 sulphate, *Am J Hum Genet* 37:733-748, 1985.
9. Bernishke K: *Maternal-fetal medicine* ed 2, Philadelphia, 1989, W.B. Saunders.
10. Boklage CE: The organization of the oocyte and embryogenesis in twinning and fusion malformations, *Acta Genet Med Gemellol (Roma)* 36:421-431, 1987.
11. Bovicelli L et al: Genetic amniocentesis in twin pregnancies, *Prenat Diagn* 3:101-106, 1983.
12. Brambati B et al: First trimester prenatal diagnosis in multiple pregnancies: principles and potential pitfalls, *Prenat Diagn* 11:58-60, 1991.
13. Burn J, Corney G: Congenital heart defects and twinning, *Acta Genet Med Gemellol (Roma)* 33:61-69, 1984.
14. Callahan TL et al: The economic impact of multiple-gestation pregnancies and the contribution of assisted-reproduction techniques to their incidence, *N Engl J Med* 331:244-249, 1994.
15. Cameron AH et al: The value of twin surveys in the study of malformations, *Eur J Obstet Gynecol Reprod Biol* 14:347-356, 1983.
16. Christiaens GCML et al: First trimester prenatal diagnosis in twin pregnancies, *Prenat Diagn* 14:51-55, 1994.
17. Coleman BG et al: Twin gestations: monitoring the complications and anomalies with ultrasound, *Radiology* 165:449-453, 1987.
18. Cote GB, Gyftodimou J: Twinning and mitotic crossing over: some possibilities and their implications, *Am J Hum Genet* 49:120-130, 1991.
19. D'Alton ME, Newton ER, Cetrulo CI: Intrauterine fetal demise in multiple gestation, *Acta Genet Med Gemellol (Roma)* 34:43, 1984.
20. Doyle PE et al: Congenital malformations in twins in England and Wales, *J Epidemiol Community Health* 45:43-48, 1991.
21. Drugan A, Johnson MP, Evans MI: Genetic counseling, *Clinical Consultations in Obstet Gynecol* 2:225-231, 1990.
22. Drugan A et al: Clinical implications of amniotic fluid AFP in twin pregnancies, *J Reprod Med* 34:977-981, 1989.
23. Drugan A et al: Counseling for low maternal serum alpha-fetoprotein should emphasize all chromosome anomalies, not just Down syndrome, *Obstet Gynecol* 73:271-274, 1989.
24. Drugan A et al: Similarity of twins to singleton MSAFP ratio by race: no need to establish specific multifetal tables, *Fetal Diagn Ther* 8:84-88, 1993.
25. Elias S et al: Genetic amniocentesis in twin gestations, *Am J Obstet Gynecol* 138:169-174, 1980.
26. Evans MI et al: Selective termination: evolution of clinical experience and residual risks, *Am J Obstet Gynecol* 162:1568-1575, 1990.
27. Evans MI et al: MOMs and DADs: improved specificity and cost effectiveness of biochemical screening for aneuploidy with DADs, *Am J Obstet Gynecol* 1994 (in press).
28. Evans MI et al: Efficacy of second trimester selective termination for fetal abnormalities: international collaborative experience among the world's largest centers, *Am J Obstet Gynecol* 171: 90-94, 1994.
29. Fiedler JM, Phelan JP. The amniotic band syndrome in monozygotic twins, *Am J Obstet Gynecol* 146:864-865, 1983.
30. Grau P et al: Elevated maternal serum alpha-fetoprotein and amniotic fluid alpha-fetoprotein after multifetal pregnancy reduction, *Obstet Gynecol* 76:1042, 1990.
31. Harper PS: *Practical genetic counseling*, ed 3, Wright, Bristol, 1988, Butterworth and Co.

32. Hershey DW, Crandall BF, Purdue S: Combining maternal age and serum alpha-fetoprotein to predict the risk of Down syndrome, *Obstet Gynecol* 68:177-181, 1986.

33. Huber J, Wagenbichler P, Bartsch F: Biamnial alpha-fetoprotein concentration in twins, one with multiple malformations, *J Med Genet* 212:377-379, 1984.

34. Hunter AGW, Cox DM: Counseling problems when twins are discovered at genetic amniocentesis, *Clin Genet* 16:34-42, 1979.

35. Johnson JM et al: Maternal serum alpha-fetoprotein in twin pregnancy, *Am J Obstet Gynecol* 162:1020-1025, 1990.

36. Journel H et al: Neural tube malformations in twins, *J Gynecol Obstet Biol Reprod* 14:819-827, 1985.

37. Keusch CF, Mulliken JB, Kaplan LC: Craniofacial anomalies in twins, *Plast Reconst Surg* 87:16-23, 1991.

38. Kurtz AB et al: Twin pregnancies: accuracy of first trimester abdominal ultrasound in predicting chorionicity and amnionicity, *Radiology* 185:759-762, 1992.

39. Lang MG et al: Dizygotic twins concordant for truncus arteriosus, *Clin Genet* 39:75-79, 1991.

40. Librach CL et al: Genetic amniocentesis in seventy twin pregnancies, *Am J Obstet Gynecol* 148:585-590, 1984.

41. Lin AE, Garver KL: Monozygotic Turner syndrome twins—correlation of phenotype severity and heart defect, *Am J Med Genet* 29:529-531, 1988.

42. Little J, Nevin NC: Congenital anomalies in twins in Northern Ireland. III. Anomalies of the cardiovascular system 1974-1979, *Acta Genet Med Gemellol (Roma)* 38:27-35, 1989.

43. Manlan G, Scott KE: Contribution of twin pregnancy to perinatal mortality and fetal growth retardation: reversal growth retardation after birth, *Can Med Assoc J* 118:365, 1978.

44. Merkatz IR et al: An association between low maternal serum alpha-fetoprotein and fetal chromosome anomalies, *Am J Obstet Gynecol* 148:886-891, 1984.

45. Moise KJ Jr, Cotton DB: Discordant fetal platelet counts in a twin gestation complicated by idiopathic thrombocytopenic purpura, *Am J Obstet Gynecol* 156:1141-1142, 1987.

46. Mulder AFP et al: Trisomy 18 in monozygotic twins, *Hum Genet* 83:300-301, 1989.

47. Nelson LW, Bensen J, Burton BK: Outcomes in patients with unusually high maternal serum alpha-fetoprotein levels, *Am J Obstet Gynecol* 157:572-576, 1987.

48. Nicolaidis P, Nasrat H, Tannirandorin Y: Review: fetal acardia: aetiology, pathology, and management, *J Obstet Gynecol* 10:518-525, 1990.

49. Nyberg DA, Callen PW: *Ultrasound evaluation of the placenta*. In Callen PW, editor: *Ultrasound evaluation in obstetrics and gynecology*, ed 2, Philadelphia, 1988, W.B. Saunders.

50. Palle C et al: Increased risk of abortion after genetic amniocentesis in twin pregnancies, *Prenat Diagn* 3:83-89, 1983.

51. Pavone L et al: Twins with acardia and anencephaly, *Acta Genet Med Gemellol (Roma)* 34:89-93, 1985.

52. Pergament E et al: The risk and efficacy of chorionic villus sampling in multiple gestations, *Prenat Diagn* 12:377-384, 1992.

53. Pijpers L et al: Genetic amniocentesis in twin pregnancies, *Br J Obstet Gynaecol* 95:323-326, 1988.

54. Pool RD: Congenital scoliosis in monozygous twins: genetically determined or acquired in utero? *J Bone Joint Surg* 68:194-196, 1985.

55. Porreco RP, Barton GM, Haverkamp AD: Occlusion of umbilical artery in acardiac acephalic twin, *Lancet* 337:326-327, 1991.

56. Pruggmayer M et al: Incidence of abortion after genetic amniocentesis in twin pregnancies, *Prenat Diagn* 11:637-640, 1991.

57. Pysher TJ: Discordant congenital malformations in monozygous twins: the amniotic band disruption complex, *Diagn Gynecol Obstet* 2:221-225, 1980.

58. Quintero RA et al: Brief report: umbilical-cord ligation of an acardiac twin by fetoscopy at 19 weeks of gestation, *N Engl J Med* 330:469-471, 1994.

59. Redwine FO, Cruikshank DP, Brown J: Antenatal genetic studies in twin gestations, *Acta Genet Med Gemellol (Roma)* 33:39-41, 1984.

60. Regenstein AC, Berkeley AS: Discordance of mullerian agenesis in monozygotic twins: a case report, *J Reprod Med Obstet Gynecol* 36:386-387, 1991.

61. Revenis ME, Johnson LA: *Multiple gestations*. In Avery GB, Fletcher MA, MacDonald MG, editors: *Neonatology: pathophysiology and management of the newborn*, ed 4, Philadelphia, 1994, J.B. Lippincott.

62. Rodis JF et al: Calculated risk of chromosomal abnormalities in twin gestations, *Obstet Gynecol* 76:1037-1041, 1990.

63. Schell DI et al: Counseling patients with elevated maternal serum alpha-fetoprotein: alteration of risk by alpha-fetoprotein level and ultrasound findings, *J Reprod Med* 35:543-546, 1990.

64. Schinzel A: Congenital developmental defects in twins: spectrum, etiology, genetic counseling, *Schweiz Rundsch Med Prax* 74:351, 1985.

65. Schinzel AAGL, Smith DW, Miller JR: Monozygotic twinning and structural defects, *J Pediatr* 95:921, 1979.

66. Shah DM et al: Diagnosis of trisomy 18 in monozygotic twins by cordocentesis, *Am J Obstet Gynecol* 160:214-215, 1989.

67. Shenker JG, Yarkoni S, Granat M: Multiple pregnancy following induction of ovulation, *Fertil Steril* 35:105, 1981.

68. Stiller RJ et al: Amniotic fluid alpha-fetoprotein in twin gestations: dependence on placental membrane anatomy, *Am J Obstet Gynecol* 158:1088-1092, 1988.

69. Tabsh KMA et al: Genetic amniocentesis in twin pregnancy, *Obstet Gynecol* 65:843-845, 1985.

70. Van Der Pol JG et al: Jejunal atresia related to the use of methylene blue in genetic amniocentesis in twins, *Br J Obstet Gynaecol* 99:141-143, 1992.

71. Vogel F, Motulsky AG: *Human genetics*, Heidelberg, 1986, Springer-Verlag.

72. Wald NJ et al: Maternal serum screening for Down syndrome in early pregnancy, *B M J* 297:883-887, 1988.

73. Windham GC, Bjerkedal T: Malformations in twins and their siblings: norway, 1967-1979, *Acta Genet Med Gemellol (Roma)* 33:87-95, 1984.

74. Windham GC, Bjerkedal T, Sever LE: The association of twinning and neural tube defects: studies in Los Angeles, California and Norway, *Acta Genet Med Gemellol (Roma)* 31:165-172, 1982.

75. Winn HN et al: Ultrasonographic criteria for the prenatal diagnosis of placental chorionicity in twin gestations, *Am J Obstet Gynecol* 161:1540, 1989.

76. Wolf HK et al: Acardius anceps with evidence of intrauterine vascular occlusion: report of a case and discussion of the pathogenesis, *Pediatr Pathol* 11:143-152, 1991.

5 Maternal Adaptation

Michael O. Gardner and Katharine D. Wenstrom

Pregnancy causes many physiologic and anatomic changes in the expectant mother that begin soon after conception.[27] The maternal adaptation to twin and higher-order multiple pregnancies can be characterized as an exaggeration of the normal pregnancy response and involves nearly all maternal organ systems.[22] Understanding the unique physiologic demands placed on the mother of a multiple pregnancy is essential for the patient and her physician.

Cardiovascular System

Some of the earliest physiologic adaptations in pregnant women involve changes in the cardiovascular system. In singleton pregnancies, the mean arterial blood pressure decreases from early in the pregnancy until late in the second trimester. The arterial blood pressure then rises until term, returning approximately to the woman's prepregnancy blood pressure. In twin gestations, diastolic blood pressures are even lower in the second trimester and exhibit a greater increase near term. Systolic blood pressures in twin gestations are similar to those of singleton gestations throughout pregnancy. Blood pressure is dependent on maternal position and is highest when the patient is sitting, lowest when she is lying on her side, and in be-

tween when she is standing. These positional changes in blood pressure can lead to postural hypotension. Since women with multiple pregnancies have a greater decrease in mean arterial pressure in the second trimester than women with singleton pregnancies, they may be at greater risk for significant postural hypotension (Figure 5-1).

Another cardiovascular change in pregnancy is an increase in the maternal heart rate of about 15%. This is similar in both twin and singleton gestations.[33] The decrease of 14% in mean circulation time is also similar in single and multiple gestations. In twin pregnancies, the mean total peripheral resistance decreases by 30%, compared with the 20% decrease in singleton pregnancies of similar gestational ages.

The incidence of preeclampsia is increased in multiple pregnancies. It is higher in twin pregnancies than it is in singleton pregnancies, and it is even higher in triplet and quadruplet pregnancies. Campbell[4] reported an incidence of preeclampsia in twin pregnancies of 29% versus 5.8% in singleton pregnancies. The increased incidence of preeclampsia may be the result of the increased placental mass that is associated with multifetal gestation.[5]

Cardiac output is increased in a normal

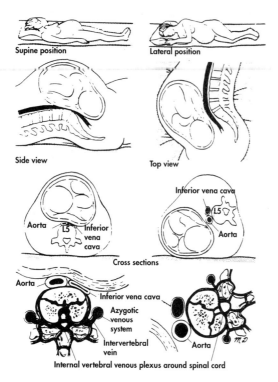

Supine position

Lateral position

Side view

Top view

Inferior vena cava

Aorta   L5   Inferior vena cava

L5

Aorta

Cross sections

Aorta

Inferior vena cava

Azygotic venous system

Intervertebral vein

Aorta

Internal vertebral venous plexus around spinal cord

FIGURE 5-1 Lateral and cross-sectional views of uterine aortocaval compression in the supine position and its resolution by lateral positioning of the pregnant woman. *(From Bonica JJ: Obstetric analgesia and anesthesia, Amsterdam, 1980, World Federation of Societies of Anesthesiologist.)*

singleton pregnancy by 30% to 50%. The majority of this change occurs by the end of the first trimester, but the increase continues until the gestation reaches 32 weeks. The greater cardiac output in early pregnancy is predominately the result of an increase in stroke volume, whereas an increase in the maternal heart rate accounts for the change in cardiac output during the last half of pregnancy. By the third trimester, maternal position also has a significant effect on maternal cardiac output. Because compression of the vena cava by the gravid uterus results in de-

creased venous return, the maternal cardiac output when the woman is supine is 20% less than when she is in the lateral recumbent position. This problem may be potentiated in multiple gestations because the uterus is proportionately larger. Rovinsky and Jaffin[32] determined cardiac output using the Evans blue dye technique in both singleton and multiple gestations.[32] They found that women with twin and triplet pregnancies had higher cardiac outputs than women with singleton pregnancies. Nonpregnant women had an average cardiac output of 5.9 L/min. Women with singleton pregnancies peaked at 8.6 L/min by 25 to 28 weeks, and women with twin and triplet pregnancies peaked at 9.0 L/min by 21 to 24 weeks. The cardiac output in women with twin pregnancies is reported to be even higher during labor or when the mother is treated with beta mimetics (Figure 5-2). However, not all researchers agree with these findings. Campbell et al.[8] were unable to demonstrate a difference in cardiac output between women with normal twin and singleton pregnancies. Using Doppler techniques, they found that cardiac outputs and stroke volumes were similar in mothers with twin gestations and mothers with singleton gestations. In mothers with twin pregnancies complicated by preeclampsia, there was a decrease in cardiac output compared with women who had normal twin pregnancies.

Blood volume increases significantly in pregnancy; this increase in volume directly correlates with the size of the fetal mass.[31] Plasma volume of women with singleton pregnancies increases by 48% to 4.0 L. In women with twin pregnancies the plasma volume increases by 67% (to

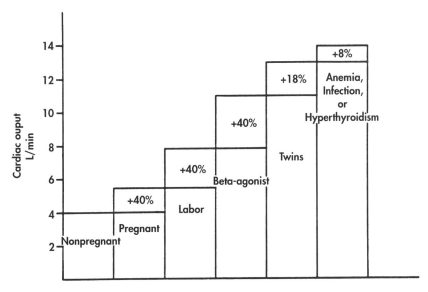

FIGURE 5-2   Cumulative effects of pregnancy and various pregnancy complications on cardiac output. *(From Clark SL et al, editors: Critical care obstetrics, ed 2, Cambridge, Mass., 1991, Blackwell Scientific Publications.)*

4.7L), and in women with triplet pregnancies it increases to 96% above the plasma volume of nonpregnant controls. Fullerton et al.[12] described a quadruplet pregnancy with an increase of the plasma volume to nearly 6L. In contrast, the total maternal red cell volume only increases by approximately 25% in pregnancy. This increase begins early in pregnancy and continues until term (Table 5-1). Because of the disproportionate increase in plasma volume compared with red cell volume, the hematocrit of the expectant mother drops.

The large plasma volume increase in women with multiple pregnancies compared with women pregnant with singletons may thus lead to a dilutional anemia. Hall, Campbell, and Davidson[15] found that in pregnant women who were not receiving routine iron or folic acid supplementation, iron deficiency and folic acid deficiency was more common in women

pregnant with twins than with singletons. However, they did not find evidence of a higher incidence of clinically significant anemia; macrocytosis was evident on peripheral blood smears of only 2.4% of mothers of twins.

Levels of components of the coagulation system are altered during pregnancy. These altered levels cause the pregnant woman to be in a hypercoagulable state until several days postpartum. Fibrinogen levels increase by 50% during pregnancy to about 450 mg/dl near term. The coagulation factors VII, VIII, IX, and X all increase during pregnancy, whereas plasma fibrinolytic activity decreases. These alterations are similar in twin and singleton pregnancies.[9] The levels of plasminogen, fibrin split products, antithrombin III, and α_2-macroglobulin are also similar in singleton and twin pregnancies. However, twin gestations are typically characterized

TABLE 5-1

Blood and Red Cell Volumes in Normal Women Late in Pregnancy and Again When Not Pregnant

	LATE PREGNANT	NONPREGNANT	INCREASE (ml)	INCREASE (%)
SINGLE FETUS (n = 50)				
Blood volume	4820	3250	1570	48
RBC volume	1790	1355	430	32
Hematocrit	37.0	41.7		
TWINS (n = 30)				
Blood volume	5820	3865	1960	51
RBC volume	2065	1580	485	31
Hematocrit	35.5	41		

From Pritchard JA: Anesthesiology 26:393, 1965.

by a greater increase in plasma fibrinogen levels than is seen in singleton pregnancies.

Uterine Changes

Uterine growth begins early in pregnancy. In multiple pregnancies the total intrauterine volume is approximately equal to that of singleton pregnancies until the end of the first trimester. However, by 18 weeks of gestation the intrauterine volume of twin pregnancies is 2 times that of singleton pregnancies (Figure 5-3).[28] This difference continues until term. In fact, by 25 weeks the intrauterine volume in a twin pregnancy is equal to that of a full-term singleton pregnancy. Women with triplet and higher-order multiple pregnancies have an even greater increase in intrauterine volume.

Blood flow to the gravid uterus increases to 500 to 700 ml/min at term in singleton pregnancies. This increase in blood flow is proportional to the increase in uterine size, with most of the excess flow directed toward the placenta. The increase in uterine blood flow in a twin pregnancy is greater than in a singleton pregnancy. The increase results from an increase in cardiac output and may be related to the lower uterine vascular resistance in twin pregnancies compared with singleton pregnancies. Rizzo, Arduini, and Romanini[30] used Doppler velocimetry to show that the resistance index of the uterine arteries (resistance index = [systolic velocity − diastolic velocity]/systolic velocity) was significantly lower in twin pregnancies than in singleton pregnancies. The two placentas in twin gestations may act as parallel low-resistance circuits, thus causing a fall in systemic vascular resistance. However, the increase in uterine blood flow may not be proportional to the increase in uterine volume

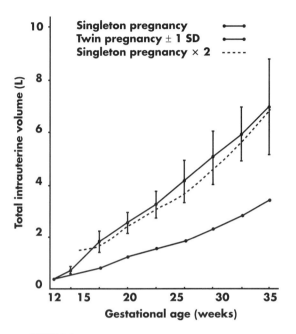

FIGURE 5-3 Total intrauterine volume in singleton and twin pregnancies. *(From Redford DHA: Acta Genet Med Gemellol (Roma) 31:145-148, 1982.)*

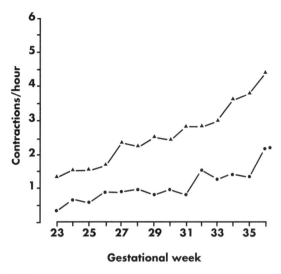

FIGURE 5-4 Uterine activity during pregnancy in ambulatory patients: comparison of singleton and twin gestations. *(From Newman RB et al: Am J Obstet Gynecol 154:530, 1986.)*

when compared with that in singleton pregnancies. In 1955, Morris, Osborne, and Wright[24] injected the isotope ^{24}NaCl into the uterine walls of normal singleton and twin pregnancies after 34 weeks' gestation. The mean clearance time of the ^{24}NaCl from the uterine muscle of twin pregnancies was 50% longer than in singleton pregnancies.

Uterine activity is increased in multiple gestations (Figure 5-4). From 23 weeks until term, women with twin pregnancies have more frequent uterine contractions than women with singleton pregnancies.[26] This may be because of uterine overdistension or other factors such as placental insufficiency or the increased activity of the two fetuses. The frequency of contractions increases until term. Whether this increase in uterine activity results in increased prematurity is not clear.

Endocrine Changes

Multiple pregnancies, like singleton pregnancies, are associated with increases in maternal serum cortisol, aldosterone, and free thyroxine.[22] The hormones made by the placenta are increased in multiple pregnancies compared with singleton pregnancies. Thiery, Dhont, and Vandekerckhove[36] demonstrated that maternal serum human chorionic gonadotropin (hCG) levels in multiple pregnancies were 2.5 times higher than in singleton pregnancies and remained so throughout gestation. The human placental lactogen (hPL) level is also higher in twin gestations than in singleton pregnancies.[34] Although in the 1970s there existed some enthusiasm for using hCG and hPL levels as a screening test for twins, the wide range of normal hormone values made the sensitivity too low to be a clinically useful screening tool.[14,37]

The maternal serum progesterone level in twin pregnancies is double that of singleton pregnancies.[38] Serum estradiol is also elevated in multiple gestations. Jandial et al.[17] found that the level of pregnancy-specific β_1-glycoprotein (SP_1) is higher in twin gestations than in singleton gestations.

Urinary excretion of estriol is increased in multiple gestations. Beischer, Brown, and Smith[2] reported that in twin pregnancies, the urinary estriol level is usually above the ninetieth percentile of that in singleton pregnancies. Likewise, maternal serum estriol levels are higher in twin pregnancies compared with singleton pregnancies of similar gestational ages.[23] Since estriol is produced by the fetoplacental unit, this increase is not surprising. However, plasma estriol levels do not correlate with the combined birthweight of infants from multiple gestations.

The maternal serum alpha-fetoprotein (MSAFP) level is elevated in multiple pregnancies compared with singleton pregnancies. The mean MSAFP value in twin pregnancies is 2.0 to 2.5 multiples of the singleton median (MOM). Ghosh et al.[13] demonstrated that in 11 twin pregnancies complicated by a neural tube defect, the MSAFP value was above 5 MOM. Redford and Whitfield[29] suggested that the MSAFP value be measured in all twin gestations between 16 and 20 weeks. Their study showed that in twin pregnancies with an MSAFP value greater than or equal to 4 MOM but uncomplicated by a neural tube defect, the perinatal mortality rate was 400/1000. In twins without birth defects, the relative risk for perinatal death was 4.8 if the MSAFP value was at least 4 MOM, compared with the gestations of structurally normal twins where the MSAFP values were 2 and 3 MOM. Those twin pregnancies with MSAFP values greater than 4 MOM need evaluation similar to singleton pregnancies with elevated MSAFP values. Specifically, a targeted ultrasound of both fetuses is necessary, and amniocentesis of both amniotic sacs is also possibly required to measure MSAFP and acetylcholinesterase (AChE) levels.

Respiratory Function

The volume of air breathed per minute is increased by 40% in pregnancy. This is accomplished by a similar increase in tidal volume but no increase in respiratory rate.[22] In twin pregnancies, the increase in tidal volume has been reported to be greater than in singleton pregnancies.[22] These changes occur early in pregnancy and continue until delivery. The increase in tidal volume is accompanied by a 20% decrease in the residual volume in both twin and singleton pregnancies. The vital capacity is not significantly changed. The overall increase in ventilation is necessary to compensate for the 20% increase in oxygen consumption in the normal pregnant woman.

Gastrointestinal Function

Several of the physiologic changes in pregnancy involve the gastrointestinal system. Many women experience nausea and vomiting, particularly in early pregnancy. The cause of "morning sickness" is unknown, but it may be related to hCG, since the symptoms mirror the rise and fall of hCG. By the end of the first trimester, most women have relief from their symptoms and an increase in appetite.

Because of decreased lower esophageal sphincter tone and increased intragastric pressure, many patients have symptoms of gastric reflux in pregnancy. Pregnant women also have delayed gastric emptying, which increases the risk of aspiration during general anesthesia. The normal changes in the alimentary system that occur in singleton pregnancies may be exaggerated in multiple pregnancies.[22]

The size of the liver is unaltered in pregnancy. Because of increased estrogen levels in pregnancy and the placental production of an alkaline phosphate isoenzyme, there is a large increase in serum alkaline phosphatase concentration.[22] The rate of elimination of sulfobromophthalein (Bromsulphalein) from liver cells to bile is decreased in pregnancy. The rate of excretion is even lower in a multiple pregnancy.[1] However, the rate of the transfer of sulfobromophthalein from plasma to the liver cells is increased in twins, probably because of increased hepatic blood flow. In normal pregnancy, serum albumin levels and total protein decrease, but there is a substantial increase in serum cholesterol.

Constipation is a common complaint during pregnancy. This is because of decreased muscle tone in the colon, as well as increased water absorption.

Renal Functions

The kidneys increase in size during pregnancy, probably because of an increase in renal blood volume. The renal pelvis and the ureter are dilated. This dilation is thought to be secondary to both obstruction caused by the gravid uterus and the relaxation effect of progesterone. These physiologic changes also occur in multiple gestations.

The glomerular filtration rate increases in pregnancy, starting in the first trimester. Creatinine clearance increases by 50% to about 150 ml/min by 20 weeks. In multiple pregnancies, the glomerular filtration rate is higher than it is in singleton pregnancies.[22]

Carbohydrate Metabolism

In singleton pregnancies there is normally a decrease in the maternal fasting blood glucose level. Dwyer et al.[10] showed that fasting blood glucose levels were significantly lower in mothers with twin pregnancies than in mothers with singleton pregnancies. However, the plasma glucose levels after 1, 2, or 3 hours of the glucose tolerance test in mothers with twin pregnancies were not significantly different from mothers with singleton pregnancies. Dwyer also reported that the incidences of hyperglycemia and hypoglycemia were higher in mothers pregnant with twins (Table 5-2). Spellacy, Buhi, and Burk[35] compared the blood glucose and insulin levels of 24 mothers with twin pregnancies with those of 24 mothers who had singleton pregnancies. Blood glucose and insulin levels were lower in mothers pregnant with twins. This suggests that twin gestations do not place the mother at a higher risk for gestational diabetes than singleton gestations.

Nutrition and Weight Gain

A wide range of maternal weight gain is found in singleton pregnancies. Mothers of multiple fetuses gain more weight during

TABLE 5-2

Incidence of Abnormal Glucose Tolerance in Twin and Singleton Pregnancies

| | INCIDENCE | | | | |
| | TWIN | | SINGLETON | | |
	NO.	(%)	NO.	(%)	SIGNIFICANCE
Gestational diabetes	16	(5.6)	462	(2.47)	(p < 0.01)
Gestational hypoglycaemia	11	(3.9)	316	(1.69)	(p < 0.01)

From Dwyer PL et al: Aust N Z J Obstet Gynaecol 22:131, 1982.

TABLE 5-3

Weight Gain in Twin and Singleton Pregnancies

| PERIOD OF GESTATION, WK | WEIGHT GAIN (kg/wk) BY TYPE OF PREGNANCY | |
	SINGLE	TWIN
13-20	0.42	0.60
20-30	0.47	0.54
30-36	0.40	0.64
0-36	11.1 kg Total gain	14.6 kg Total gain

From National Academy of Sciences: Nutrition during pregnancy. I. Weight gain. II. Nutrient supplements, Washington, D.C., 1990, National Academy Press.

pregnancy than mothers of singletons (Table 5-3). This increased rate of weight gain is evident from early in pregnancy until 36 weeks.[6] Luke et al.[20] described an "ideal" twin pregnancy that had a weight gain of greater than 8/10 lb/wk until 24 weeks' gestation and then a weight gain of 1 lb/wk or more until term. This pattern of weight gain was associated with improved intrauterine growth in twins, which was particularly evident with good weight gain before 24 weeks. This model was designed for twins and has not been tested on higher-order multiple pregnan-

cies. The birthweight of the infant is related to the maternal weight gain. In fact, birthweight in twin gestations is better correlated with maternal weight gain than maternal height or pregravid weight.[19]

The Institute of Medicine recommends that mothers with twin pregnancies gain about 1½ lb/wk during the second and third trimesters for a total weight gain of 35 to 45 lb.[25] Others have recommended weight gains of 45 to 50 lb by 34 weeks in triplets[18] and a weight gain of over 50 lb in quadruplet pregnancies.[11]

The ideal caloric intake for pregnancy is not clear. Some authorities recommend that women pregnant with singletons consume 2400 kcal/day.[25] Although others have recommended 2800 kcal/day for women pregnant with twins, there is no generally agreed upon standard. Likewise, suggestions for caloric intake in high-order multiple gestations are based on anecdotal experience from small case series.[1]

In the face of increased weight gain, one might suspect that mothers with twins would tend to eat more than mothers expecting singletons. In a study by Campbell, MacGillivray, and Tuttle,[7] no significant difference in the dietary caloric intake between mothers with twins and those with singletons was found.[8] Likewise, the dietary consumption of zinc, copper, and iron was similar in women with twin and singleton pregnancies.

Total body water is not significantly different in mothers with twin or singleton pregnancies, in spite of the greater weight gain in twin gestations.[21] Women with twin pregnancies may have more fat storage than those with singleton pregnancies. Maternal serum levels of sodium, chloride, and potassium, as well as maternal serum osmolality, are similar in twin and singleton gestations. Serum folate levels are higher in women with twin pregnancies compared with those in women with singleton pregnancies.[16]

Preconception Counseling

Initially, one might think that preconception counseling is not applicable to multiple pregnancies. By definition, the counseling must occur before the expected pregnancy, and traditionally the conception of twins and higher-order multiple gestations is unanticipated. However, Luke[18] has showed that the incidence of multiple births has increased substantially in the United States between 1973 and 1990. Much of this increase results from use of drugs that cause ovulation induction (OI) and the increase in assisted reproductive techniques (ART) such as in vitro fertilization. This increase in multiple births is not without consequences. The increased rate of prematurity in twins and especially higher-order multiple pregnancies is associated with increased infant morbidity and mortality. Likewise, the cost to society is substantial. A recent economic analysis showed that compared with an average hospital charge of $9800

for singleton births, the charge for a twin delivery was $38,000, and the cost of delivering triplets was approximately $110,000.[3] These and other issues should be discussed with prospective parents before beginning ART.

ART is also associated with an increased risk of monochorionic twinning. Wenstrom et al.[39] reported that the incidence of monochorionicity is at least 3.2% in ART pregnancies, versus 0.4% in the general population. Among ART-induced pregnancies that result in twins or higher-order multiple gestations, the incidence of monochorionicity was approximately 10%. Monozygotic twins have an increased risk of structural anomalies and pregnancy complications, including twin-twin transfusion syndrome (TTS). These complications contribute to the increased perinatal morbidity and mortality found with monochorionic pregnancies. For these reasons, preconceptional counseling may be valuable to the patient and her family before embarking on treatments for infertility.

Conclusion

Mothers with multiple pregnancies have an exaggerated response to the physiologic changes of pregnancy. All the organ systems of the expectant mother are affected, often to a greater degree than they are in singleton pregnancies. Because of the relatively small number of multiple pregnancies and the common occurrence of complications, it is difficult to state with assurance what constitutes the normal maternal response in an uncomplicated multiple pregnancy. In spite of this caution, the clinician caring for mothers with twin and higher-order multiple pregnancies can bear in mind the significant and wide-ranging maternal physiologic responses to multiple gestations.

References

1. Beazley JM, Tindell VR: Changes in liver function during multiple pregnancy using a modified bromsulphthalein test, *J Obstet Gynaecol Br Commonw* 73:658-661, 1966.
2. Beischer NA, Brown JB, Smith MA: The significance of high urinary estriol excretion during pregnancy, *J Obstet Gynaecol Br Commonw* 75:622-628, 1968.
3. Callahan TL et al: The economic impact of multiple gestation pregnancies and the contribution of assisted reproduction techniques to their incidence, *N Engl J Med* 331:244-249, 1994.
4. Campbell DM: Maternal adaption in twin pregnancy, *Semin Perinatol* 10:4-8, 1986.
5. Campbell DM, Campbell AJ: Aterial blood pressure: the pattern of change in twin pregnancies, *Acta Genet Med Gemellol (Roma)* 34:217-233, 1985.
6. Campbell DM, Campbell AJ, MacGillivray I: Maternal characteristics of women having twin pregnancies, *J Biosoc Sci* 6:463-470, 1975.
7. Campbell DM, MacGillivray I, Tuttle S: Maternal nutrition in twin pregnancy, *Acta Genet Med Gemellol (Roma)* 31:221-227, 1982.
8. Campbell DM et al: Cardiac output in twin pregnancy, *Acta Genet Med Gemellol (Roma)* 34:225-228, 1985.
9. Condie R, Campbell D: Components of the hemostatic mechanism in twin pregnancy, *Br J Obstet Gynaecol* 85:37-39, 1978.
10. Dwyer PL et al: Glucose tolerance in twin pregnancy, *Aust N Z J Obstet Gynaecol* 22:131-134, 1982.
11. Elliot JP, Radin TG: Quadruplet pregnancy: contemporary management and outcome, *Obstet Gynecol* 80:421-424, 1992.
12. Fullerton LT et al: A case of quadruplet pregnancy, *J Obstet Gynaecol Br Commonw* 72:791-96, 1965.
13. Ghosh A et al: Prognostic significance of raised serum alpha-fetoprotein levels in twin pregnancies, *Br J Obstet Gynaecol* 89:817-820, 1982.
14. Grennert L et al: Ultrasound and human placental lactogen screening for early detection of twin pregnancies, *Lancet* 307:4-6, 1976.
15. Hall MH, Campbell DM, Davidson RJL: Anemia in twin pregnancy, *Acta Genet Med Gemellol (Roma)* 28:279-282, 1979.
16. Hall MH, Pirani BBK, Campbell D: The course of the fall in serum folate in normal pregnancy, *Br J Obstet Gynaecol* 83:132-136, 1976.
17. Jandial V et al: The value of measurement of pregnancy specific proteins in twin pregnancies, *Acta Genet Med Gemellol (Roma)* 28:319-325, 1979.
18. Luke B: The changing pattern of multiple births in the United States: maternal and infant characteristics, 1973 and 1990, *Obstet Gynecol* 84:101-106, 1994.
19. Luke B, Keith LG, Damewood MD: Maternal characteristics of women delivered of twins natural vs. induced, *Int J Fertil* 38:12-15, 1993.
20. Luke B et al: The ideal twin pregnancy: patterns of weight gain, discordance and length of gestation, *Am J Obstet Gynecol* 169:588-597, 1993.
21. MacGillivray I, Campbell DM, Duffins GM: Maternal metabolic response in twin pregnancy in primigravidae, *J Obstet Gynaecol Br Commonw* 78:530-534, 1971.
22. MacGillivray I, Nylands PPS, Corney G: *Human multiple reproduction*, Philadelphia, 1975, W.B. Saunders.
23. Masson GM: Plasma estriol in normal and preeclamptic multiple pregnancies, *Obstet Gynecol* 42:568-573, 1973.
24. Morris N, Obsborn SB, Wright HP: Effective circulation of the uterine wall in late pregnancy, *Lancet* 265:323-325, 1955.
25. National Academy of Sciences: *Nutrition during pregnancy*, Washington, D.C., 1990, National Academy Press.
26. Newman RB, Gill PJ, Katz M: Uterine activity during pregnancy in ambulatory patients: comparison of singleton and twin gestations, *Am J Obstet Gynecol* 154:530-531, 1986.
27. Parisi UN, Creasy RN: Maternal biologic adaptions to pregnancy. In Reece EA et al, editors: *Medicine of the fetus and mother*, Philadelphia, 1992, J.B. Lippincott.
28. Redford DHA: Uterine growth in twin pregnancy by measurement of total intrauterine volume, *Acta Genet Med Gemellol (Roma)* 32:145-148, 1982.
29. Redford DHA, Whitfield CR: Maternal serum alfa-fetoprotein in twin pregnancies uncomplicated by neural tube defect, *Am J Obstet Gynecol* 152:550-553, 1985.
30. Rizzo G, Arduini D, Romanini C: Uterine artery Doppler velocity waveforms in twin pregnancies, *Obstet Gynecol* 82:978-983, 1993.
31. Rovinsky JJ, Jaffin H: Cardiovascular hemodynamics in pregnancy. I. Blood and plasma volumes in multiple pregnancy, *Am J Obstet Gynecol* 93:1-15, 1965.

32. Rovinsky JJ, Jaffin H: Cardiovascular hemodynamics in pregnancy. II. Cardiac output and left ventricular work in multiple pregnancy, *Am J Obstet Gynecol* 95:781-786, 1966.

33. Rovinsky JJ, Jaffin H: Cardiovascular hemodynamics in pregnancy. III. Cardiac rate, stroke volume, total peripheral resistance, and central blood volume in multiple pregnancy: synthesis of results, *Am J Obstet Gynecol* 95:787-794, 1966.

34. Spellacy WN, Buhi WC, Birk SA: Human placental lactogen levels in multiple pregnancies, *Obstet Gynecol* 52:210-211, 1978.

35. Spellacy WN, Buhi WC, Birk SA: Carbohydrate metabolism in women with a twin pregnancy, *Obstet Gynecol* 55:688-691, 1980.

36. Thiery M, Dhont M, Vandekerckhove F: Serum HCG and HPL in twin pregnancies, *Acta Obstet Gynecol Scand* 56:495-497, 1976.

37. Vandekerckhove F et al: Screening for multiple pregnancy: determination of human chorionic gonadotropin, alpha-fetoprotein and human placental lactogen in blood during the second trimester of pregnancy, *Acta Genet Med Gemellol (Roma)* 33:495-497, 1984.

38. Van Der Molen HJ: Determination of plasma progesterone during pregnancy, *Clin Chim Acta* 8:943-953, 1963.

39. Wenstrom KD et al: Increased risk of monochorionic twinning associated with assisted reproduction, *Fertil Steril* 60:510-514, 1993.

6 Antepartum Management
Laboratory Evaluation and Management

Marcello Pietrantoni

Maternal adaptation to multiple pregnancy has fascinated obstetricians and perinatologists alike. This interest has come about because of the exaggeration of normal pregnancy changes, variable adverse outcomes, and increased perinatal mortality (PNM) and morbidity over a singleton pregnancy. Multiple pregnancies are at increased risk for preeclampsia, gestational diabetes, postpartum hemorrhage, pulmonary edema, operative deliveries, preterm deliveries, and physical and mental handicap in the infants.[108] The gestational age at delivery is often reduced by 2 to 3 weeks for each additional fetus. However, improvement in neonatal resuscitation and care and delivery over the last 20 years is felt to be responsible for a steady decline in mortality rates, particularly in triplets.[38] Nonetheless, the risk of pregnancy loss in a twin pregnancy remains 3 or more times that of a singleton pregnancy, and respiratory distress syndrome (RDS) is the most common cause of death.[88,152]

Despite the inordinate advances in obstetric care, the observed increased PNM in multiple pregnancies is of monumental concern for clinicians caring for pregnant women in today's society. The causes of this concern are the possible complications arising from the expanded applicability of assisted reproductive techniques (ART) such as gonadotropins, gonadotropin-releasing hormones (GnRHs), clomiphene citrate, human menopausal gonadotropin (HMG) (Pergonal), and in vitro fertilization (IVF). Additionally, the incidence of multiple pregnancies has escalated.[96] Women who are healthy, tall, and well nourished are also noted to have higher twin rates.[110]

The physical changes, physiologic alterations, increased placental hormonal response, and biochemical differences are only unique for women with multiple pregnancies. The following discussion explores the physiologic and hormonal adaptations in multiple pregnancies.

Diagnosis

BIOCHEMICAL TESTS

It is well documented that the fetal placental unit of a multiple pregnancy manifests an increase in steroid and protein production.[86] Specifically, plasma estriol, progesterone, maternal serum alpha-fetoprotein (MSAFP), human chorionic gonadotropin (hCG), and human placental lactogen (hPL) are all found to be increased in multiple pregnancies.[68,87,111,181,187] However, the normal values for these hormones range widely and vary by gestational age. This variation, coupled with daily fluctuation, makes biochemical screening for multiple pregnancies disadvantageous. The exception is quantitative hCG and MSAFP screening, which has the additional benefit of detecting fetuses at risk for genetic abnormalities and open neural tube defects.

β-Human chorionic gonadotropin

A glycoprotein hormone with biologic activity, hCG acts on the cell's plasma membrane luteinizing hormone (LH) receptor. The assay for β-hCG is the hallmark for early pregnancy verification. The importance of hCG during pregnancy lies in the maintenance of the corpus luteum, which produces estrogen and progesterone. Both are essential for endometrial implantation and uterine quiescence.

The syncytiotrophoblast is the site of synthesis and secretion of hCG in the placenta. It is speculated that GnRH produced by the cytotrophoblast stimulates hCG production. Nonetheless, the fetal kidney has also been shown to synthesize hCG.[115] In all normal pregnancies, hCG can be detected by 8 to 9 days after the LH peak, 7 to 8 days after fertilization, or 1 day after implantation.[128] The concentration of hCG at the time of the first missed period is 100 to 600 IU/L in a singleton pregnancy.[13] It then rises to a peak of about 100,000 IU/L between 8 and 10 weeks of gestation (dated from the last normal menstrual period), thereafter falling to a stable 10,000 IU/L at 20 weeks through the remainder of the pregnancy. In early singleton pregnancies, the hCG concentration increases exponentially (doubling every 2 to 3 days) until 6 weeks. Therefore the doubling time of hCG in the serum varies with gestational age.[103] It is noted that in second trimester twin gestations, the hCG concentration is approximately double (1.84, 95% CI 1.64-2.07) that in singleton pregnancies.[16,194] However, hCG as a biochemical test leaves an uncertainty for clinical practice because of its daily fluctuations. It also appears to be a less accurate test than either MSAFP or hPL in the diagnosis of a multiple pregnancy.[197]

Additionally, high hCG levels are also found in pregnancies complicated by trophoblastic disease, choriocarcinoma, fetal erythroblastosis, and ectopic endocrine tumors (for example, embryonal carcinomas; teratomas; dysgerminomas; and tumors of the lung, adrenal gland, liver, and bladder). Levels of β-hCG greater than 3.5 ImU/ml are pathologic in origin.[56] Therefore multiple pregnancies may not be easily or clearly differentiated by a single biochemical test like β-hCG.[181]

Human placental lactogen

Maternal serum placental lactogen may also be a biochemical indicator of a multiple pregnancy.[97] The biologic activity of hPL is exerted through the prolactin and human growth hormone (hGH) receptors. A major product of placental secretion, hPL is produced by the syncytiotrophoblast and synthesized from "big-hPL."[162] Three weeks after fertilization, hPL may be found in the maternal serum. Physiologically, hPL is mainly secreted into the maternal compartment to bring about metabolic changes that benefit the fetus. There are several hormonal functions of hPL that are mostly found only in experimental animals. For example, it has a lactogenic and a transient luteotropic effect; it stimulates somatomedin, lipolysis, and glucogenesis; it has an anti-insulin effect; and it is synergistic with hCG in producing estrogen and progesterone. Immunologically, hPL is structurally similar (80% to 94% homology) to hGH; however, it has less than 3% of somatomammotropin activity. Although hPL demonstrates lactogenic properties, it does not appear to be critical for human lactation because it is not present when lactation occurs.[57]

Plasma concentrations of hPL rise from 0.1 to 8 μg/ml between the first and third trimesters.[165] Increased transcription at term accounts for the higher levels of hPL (4 times) than in first-trimester placentas, which varies from placenta to placenta. In multiple, diabetic, or Rh-immunized pregnancies the placentas are usually larger than those of a normal singleton gestation, and higher values of hPL are noted. Therefore hPL levels closely correlate with placental growth, function, and size. Spellacy[171] showed that hPL levels below 5 μg/ml at 30 weeks' gestation reflected the "fetal danger zone," or fetal jeopardy, when either multiple or diabetic pregnancies are involved. However, hPL is clinically not specific or practical in the assessment of normal or abnormal pregnancies. This stems from the fact that both low and

no values have been documented in normal pregnancies.[20,58] Additionally, hPL alone is not sufficiently specific for predicting fetal demise in diabetic pregnancies because of their larger placental size and production. Prolonged starvation during the first trimester may also lead to increased hPL levels. Like hCG, hPL is not confined to the trophoblast. It may be produced by bronchogenic carcinoma, hepatoma, pheochromocytoma, and lymphomas.[195] However, hPL differs from hCG in that it has been found in the sera of men and nonpregnant women.

Sonography and antenatal testing (biophysical profile and nonstress test) have become more popular in assessing high risk pregnancies. However, ultrasound evaluations are costly, and in 1976 Grennert et al.[68] assessed the feasibility of using hPL to select patients suspected of having multiple pregnancies. Thirty-seven of 39 (95%) twin gestations had an hPL value more than 1 standard deviation (SD) above the mean of normal distribution, thereby lowering the proportion of patients requiring ultrasound to 16%. In this study, 70% of twin pregnancies were correctly identified at 16 to 20 weeks, using the ninetieth percentile as a cut-off level. Therefore identifying multiple pregnancies by a biochemical marker may lead to an earlier detection and possibly lower the PNM and morbidity, particularly in areas where ultrasonography is not available.

Early diagnosis of multiple pregnancy is the cornerstone and prerequisite for adequate prenatal care and management of delivery. Knight et al.[98] compared hPL to maternal serum alpha-fetoprotein (MSAFP) and found it to be inferior, identifying only 17/37 (45.9%) versus 29/37 (78.3%) of twins, respectfully. Despite the high sensitivity reported by Grennert et al.,[68] Knight et al.[98] found that hPL screening with one SD as a cut-off level resulted in a high false positive rate.

Maternal serum alpha-fetoprotein

Alpha-fetoprotein (AFP) was first described by Bergstrand and Czar[10] in 1957 in human fetal serum. Seppala, Tallberg, and Ehnholm[166] observed the association between amniotic fluid AFP and Finnish nephrosis, marking the first recognized relationship with a fetal condition. In a non-Finnish population the incidence is 1/40,000.[81]

AFP is an oncofetal protein produced mainly by the fetal liver, with small amounts produced by the gastrointestinal tract and yolk sac. AFP is a major glycoprotein with a function that remains largely unknown. The concentration of AFP is highest in both fetal serum and amniotic fluid around 13 weeks (100-fold dilution). The concentration decreases gradually as pregnancy progresses, whereas maternal serum levels continue to rise until 28 to 32 weeks' gestation. The concentration in the fetal serum (mg) is approximately 150 times that in the amniotic fluid (μg). In the majority of cases, AFP at birth has been demonstrated to correlate with gestational age. The correlation between AFP and birthweight, however, is less distinct.[114,138] There is also a marked difference in AFP concentrations between monozygotic and dizygotic twin pairs. Norqaard-Pedersen[139] demonstrated that the mean intrapair difference in the cord blood of dizygotic twins was significantly greater than in monozygotic twins. They concluded that the concentration of AFP is genetically determined and not solely dependent on gestational age. Both fetuses with a greater birth weight and males tend to have a lower AFP level than fetuses of lower birth weight and females. Other factors that have been noted to affect MSAFP levels are race,[9] maternal weight,[194] and insulin dependent diabetes mellitus.[191] Black women have MSAFP levels that are 10% to 15% higher than white women, and a larger maternal size results in a greater dilutional effect on AFP. Women who are insulin dependent have lower MSAFP. Additionally, cigarette smoking results in a level of MSAFP that is 3% higher than it is in nonsmokers.[14]

Anomalies and raised maternal serum alpha-fetoprotein

All pregnant women are offered MSAFP screening for the detection of neural tube defects between 15 and 20 weeks' gestation from the first day of the last normal menstrual period. However, the optimal time for screening is between 16 and 18 weeks' gestation. MSAFP distribution curves of those who are affected and those who are unaffected generally overlap. Therefore the cut-off point is actually a compromise between the highest detection rate and the lowest false positive rate. Hence women with elevated MSAFP levels at 2 to 2.5 multiples of the singleton median (MOM) are generally referred for genetic and nondirective perinatal counseling, comprehensive obstetric ultrasound evaluation, and possible amniocentesis (4%).[127] The amniocentesis is offered because even in top quality diagnostic ultrasound centers approximately 25% of all defects may not be detected by a comprehensive ultrasound. A patient who is a candidate for genetic amniocentesis must understand the increased risk-to-benefit ratio that is virtually double that of a singleton pregnancy for most clinical situations. The risk of amniocentesis varies with experience and bloody taps. Bloody amniotic fluid is aspirated in 1% to 2% of amniocentesis. In experienced hands, adverse outcomes (spontaneous abortion) occur in only 0.5% of cases. Early amniocentesis (12 to 14 weeks) has the slightly higher risk of spontaneous abortion (approximately 1% to 2%) in singleton pregnancies, again depending on the level of the clinician's experience. Successful sampling of both sacs in a twin pregnancy may be accomplished in the majority of patients (79%).[105] Elias et al.[52] reported a 95% success rate. Tabsh et al.[176] obtained a 98% success rate for ultrasound-guided amniocentesis from both sacs, with a single subsequent pregnancy loss. Indigo carmine dye should be instilled into the first amniotic sac that is entered with approximately 1 to 2 ml of a 0.08% solution. Methylene blue should not be used because of its association with hemolysis, hyperbilirubinemia, and increased risk of respiratory distress.[37]

Elevated MSAFP levels are associated with fetal malformations (5% to 10%),[161] open neural tube defects (NTDs), abdominal wall defects (omphaloceles and gastroschisis), teratomas, cystic hygromas, renal anomalies (Finnish type), placental abnormalities (choriohemangiomas, accreta and percreta, abruption, and placental lakes), hepatitis, preterm delivery, intrauterine growth retardation (IUGR), preeclampsia, stillbirth, fetus papyraceus, chromosomal abnormalities (sex aneuploidies and triploidy), maternal malignancy, and multiple gestation. Iatrogenic causes for elevated MSAFP levels include amniocentesis or chorionic villus sampling (CVS) before obtaining serum for AFP evaluation.

NTDs, including anencephaly, encephalocele, and meningomyelocele (spina bifida occulta), are among the most common major birth defects in the United States (2/1000). There are 2500 to 3000 cases per year that result in infant mortality and serious disabilities. Although genetic disorders may play a role, the bases of most NTDs are unknown. When these defects are not part of a syndrome, 90% are multifactorial or polygenic in origin.

Ghosh et al.[61] was the first to report on a series of 11 twin pregnancies discordant for NTDs. Approximately 10% of pregnancies with MSAFP levels greater than 2.5 multiples of the median (MOM) have multiple gestations. The most common cause for an increased MSAFP level is incorrect estimation of fetal age. However, multiple gestation is the second most common reason for an elevated MSAFP level during the second trimester. In the majority of cases, second trimester MSAFP concentrations are greater in uncomplicated twin pregnancies than in singleton pregnancies. Approximately 20% to 40% of multiple pregnancies have MSAFP levels greater than those of the ninety-fifth percentile for singletons.[93] The basis for the former is that in twin pregnancies, AFP is produced by not one but two fetuses. There is also a greater potential for AFP transfer across a larger area of placenta and membranes; the highest values are usually seen in monoplacentation dichorionic-diamniotic gestations.[190] Levels greater than 4.5 MOM are considered elevated for women with twin pregnancies; in most, the range is 2.5 to 4.5 MOM. The incidence of adverse outcome becomes significant at 4.0 MOM.[61,149] Johnson et al.[90] showed an increased incidence of discordant twins with greater than 4 MOM (72.7%), compared with less than 4 MOM (31.2%). Pretorius et al.[147] reported a lower survival rate in pregnancies with values greater than 4.5 MOM (83% dichorionic-diamniotic and 67% monochorionic-diamniotic) than in twin gestations with normal levels of MSAFP (92% dichorionic-diamniotic, and 96% monochorionic-diamniotic). However, the difference was significant only in the monochorionic-diamniotic group (p = .012). A result greater than 4.5 MOM in a twin gestation should be considered elevated, and a comprehensive ultrasound and possibly amniocentesis should be considered.

In a study of 535 twin pregnancies, Drugan et al.[48] reported that race-specific singleton MOM are sufficient, obviating a specific medium curve for twin gestations. Nevertheless, race-dependent medium values should be used for MSAFP interpretation in twin gestations. This is because MSAFP levels in black women are commonly higher than in white women with similar gestations. Additionally, MSAFP median values vary for some gestational weeks among black women. Therefore separate median curves are advocated for this population.

Chromosome abnormalities are commonly associated with low MSAFP levels (less than 1.0 MOM). Hunter and Cox[83] suggested that the risk of chromosome abnormalities in twins is 1.6 times that observed in singleton pregnancies. However, the risk for structural anomalies is not significantly higher than it is in singleton pregnancies. Pregnancies with monozygotic twins are at higher risk for structural malformations that are typically associated with increased MSAFP levels and uncommon to twins, such as discordant spina bifida and anencephaly.[55] Congenital anomalies typically associated with monozygotic twins are acardia and conjoined twins. The outcome for conjoined twins relates to the site and extent of the union. Xiphopagous, omphalopagous, and pygopagous twins have the potential for a favorable outcome. Identification of a fetus in a multiple pregnancy with a major congenital anomaly necessitates careful perinatal counseling for both parents. A difficult psychologic, ethical, moral, economic, and religious decision is often made by the parents and clinician. Several options are available to the parents: (1) continuation of the pregnancy, (2) termination of the pregnancy, and (3) attempt at selective reduction. In some instances, these discordant anomalous twins or triplets undergo lethal procedures or selective reduction through cardiac puncture and exsanguination,[1] a filtered air-embolus into the umbilical vein with fetoscopy[31] and cardiac puncture with potassium chloride (KCl).[53]

Nevin and Armstrong[137] reported a case of a triplet gestation in which one fetus had an omphalocele and the AFP level was also found to be raised in the amniotic fluid surrounding the normal fetus. This has also been described of a normal fetus from a twin gestation.[19,82] Additionally, an acetylcholinesterase (AChE) test of amniotic fluid is routinely used as a diagnostic marker for fetal NTDs in singleton pregnancies. AChE is a neural enzyme present in high concentration in fetal cerebrospinal fluid, low levels in the fetal serum, and usually absent in the amniotic fluid. However, this large molecule of approximately 300,000 daltons was also found to cross the amniotic-chorionic membrane.[91,164] This is of concern because it could result in termination of a normal fetus from a multiple gestation.

Perinatal centers using the standard cut-off level of 2.5 MOM may expect detection rates in singleton pregnancies of 89% and 75% for open spina bifida and anencephaly, respectively, with a false positive rate of 3.3% or less. Using the same 2.5 MOM level in a twin gestation, detection rates of 99% for anencephaly and 89% for open spina bifida are observed; however, as many as one third of unaffected pregnancies have a positive result. The odds of such a result are not high (1/130 for anencephaly, 1/150 for open spina bifida, if the birth prevalence in singletons is 1/1000 for each defect). To achieve the same false positive rate as in a singleton pregnancy of 3.3% or less, the cut-off level would have to be raised to 5.0 MOM. The corresponding detection rates would then be 83% for anencephaly and 39% for open spina bifida.

In a twin gestation, regardless of the MSAFP screening cut-off level used, a comprehensive ultrasound evaluation is unlikely to be much different from that found in singleton pregnancies (100% for anencephaly and 98% for open spina bifida).[133,198] Sabbagha, Sheikh, and Tamura[160] demonstrated in pregnancies at high risk for birth defects an overall sensitivity of 95% and an overall specificity of 99%, with a 0.6% false positive rate on a prenatal ultrasound. However, difficulties with fetal position, amniotic fluid volume, and maternal habitus make some sonographic evaluations difficult. Nevertheless, a comprehensive ultrasound evaluation should be performed with high resolution equipment and by an experienced perinatologist.

Neural tube defects and preventive measures

In 1965 Hibbard and Smithells[79] first suggested the possible association between NTDs and folic acid. Studies published since then have reported a reduction in recurrence of between 60% to 70% for women taking multivitamins containing folic acid before and during the first 6 weeks of gestation. In 1991, the Medical Research Council of Great Britain reported the results of a randomized, double-blinded study conducted at 33 centers in seven countries. Folic acid supplementation, 4.0 mg/day, produced a 72% reduction in the risk of NTD recurrence in 1817 women at risk (those who had previous NTD-affected pregnancies).[118]

Of eight major epidemiologic studies reported since 1988, seven have suggested that periconceptional intake of vitamin supplements containing folic acid or folic acid alone may have a protective effect against first occurrence of NTD.[123,126,131] The study by Czeizel and Dudas,[40] a placebo-controlled, double-blinded study of women in Hungary, is the best investigation of the preventive effect of folic acid. Women took either a multivitamin supplement containing 0.8 mg of folic acid (n = 2104) or a placebo (n = 2046) during the periconceptional period. The outcome revealed statistically significant results, six NTDs occurred in the placebo group, and there were none in the multivitamin group.

The U.S. Public Health Service has issued two public statements regarding folic acid, one is about folic acid supplementation for high-risk women with previously affected NTD pregnancies, and the other is about folic acid supplementation for the general female population considering pregnancy.[33,34] The Public Health Service recommends that all women of childbearing age who are capable of becoming pregnant should consume at least 0.4 mg of folic acid per day. Women who are at high risk for an NTD-affected pregnancy should be offered a folic acid supplement of 4.0 mg/day during the periconceptional period. Prenatal vitamins contain 0.8 mg or 1 mg of folic acid.

Despite encouraging results from some well-designed studies, we need to remember that folic acid supplementation during the periconceptional period may not eliminate all NTDs.

Multiple pregnancies and triple-marker analysis

Before 1984, Down syndrome screening was limited to offering amniocentesis to pregnant women age 35 or older. However, amniocentesis only identifies 20% to 25% of affected fetuses because of the few women over age 35 having children. Advancement in the detection of in utero Down syndrome was made available with the discovery of its association with low MSAFP levels and maternal age combined (25% to 33% detection rate and a false positive rate of 5%).[45,119] In combination, MSAFP and amniocentesis for genetic analysis may identify up to 45% of affected infants. Since 1988, screening women (with singleton pregnancies) at risk for fetal aneuploidy was further improved by combining low maternal serum unconjugated estriol (uE_3), which is 25% below normal in Down syndrome fetuses), hCG levels that are at least 2 times higher than normal, low MSAFP levels (less than 0.5 MOM), and maternal age. This enabled

the identification of 67% of cases with a false positive rate of 7.2%.[71,193]

In maternal serum screening programs for Down syndrome, uE_3, hCG, and AFP (triple-marker analysis, or AFP-3) values are found to be higher in multiple pregnancies than in singleton pregnancies. However, the small numbers of pregnancies studied thus far leave some uncertainty over the magnitude of the effect. In 1991, Wald et al.[194] studied 200 women with twin pregnancies and showed that using AFP-3 screening for Down syndrome yields a similar false positive rate in twin pregnancies and in singleton pregnancies. Thus they showed that MSAFP values in twin pregnancies are, on average, about as high 2.13 times (95% CI 1.97-2.31) as those of singletons. On the average, uE_3 MOM values are 1.67 times (95% CI 1.56-1.79) as high, and hCG values are 1.84 times as high (95% CI 1.64-2.07).

PHYSIOLOGIC ADAPTATIONS

In general, two maternal physiologic facts are well known and accepted. During a singleton pregnancy, there is a rise in total blood and plasma volumes and in red cell mass, and the relative increase in plasma volume is greater than that of the red cell mass, resulting in a lower hemoglobin and hematocrit concentration. When expressed in terms of body weight, the blood volume near term ranges between 73 and 96 ml/kg.[183] This degree of variation is attributed in part to the different techniques employed in measuring blood volume. However, multiple pregnancies are characterized by impressive changes in renal function (increased glomerular filtration), increased intra- and extravascular fluid volumes, and decreased peripheral resistance. These observed changes in multiple pregnancies are qualitatively similar but quantitatively greater. The total peripheral resistance in multiple pregnancies is likely to be lowered even further than in singleton pregnancies because of the greater production of progesterone and possibly prostaglandins, leading to vasodilation and a lower diastolic blood pressure.[24,84] Current research on peripheral resistance in twin pregnancies has shown a lower absolute value over singleton pregnancies; however, statistical significance was not achieved.[179]

The mechanism behind the changes in volume is multifactorial, with the vasodilation and increased intravascular capacity as essential elements. Recent reports on plasma concentrations and physiologic function of atrial natriuretic peptide (ANP) have demonstrated a highly significant decrease in levels over the nonpregnant state, which may affect the regulation of blood volume and renal function (electrolyte homeostasis) during pregnancy.[17,78] The reports on ANP during pregnancy have been conflicting. The majority of the studies have demonstrated an increased plasma concentration of ANP (p-ANP) during normal pregnancy,[39,125,180] but others found no significant differences from the nonpregnant state.[66,169] Thomsen, Storm, and Thamsborg[180] studied 40 healthy primigravid women prospectively with normal singleton pregnancies and found a significant decrease in p-ANP during the third trimester. The results of the study imply a competitive relationship between ANP and the renin-aldosterone system in regulating sodium balance and maintaining a stable volume of fluid during pregnancy. Therefore if a decrease in p-ANP is paramount

in blood volume and in sodium reabsorption and for the activation of the renin-aldosterone system, then a greater effect is expected with multiple pregnancies. The cause for the paradoxical investigations is not clear. The basis for the contradictory reports could be that the study populations were small and cross sectional. Other causes for these differences may be caused by increased in vitro degradation if too little proteinase inhibitor is used, which leads to false low values. Overall water retention is increased in multiple pregnancies as measured by deuterium oxide.[23] This is particularly increased in primigravid women with twins, whereas it is not true for multiparous women.[25,112] The regarded increased physiologic response has also been associated with a good perinatal outcome in primigravid women but not in multigravid women.[31] At term, it is noted that plasma volume reaches a plateau and increases by 48% in a singleton pregnancy and by 67% in twins.[112,156] Triplet pregnancies show an even further increase in plasma volume, peaking at 96.3% above normal in the third trimester.[156] Plasma volume during pregnancy causes an increased sodium absorption of approximately 4 to 5 mmol/dl (0.03% change), compared with the nonpregnant state. Because of the increase in ANF progesterone, and the glomerular filtration rate, there is an increase in the filtered load of sodium of as much as 15,000 to 20,000 mmol/dl. Therefore sodium balance is maintained by an increase in the tubular sodium reabsorption, which is the most notable renal adaptation during pregnancy.[84]

Digoxin-like immunoreactive factor also has been associated with the regulation of volume expansion and blood pressure during pregnancy.[67] The physiologic properties of digoxin-like immunoreactive factor include the ability to cause a natriuretic effect, peripheral vasoconstriction, and sodium/potassium adenosine triphosphatase inhibition, which are not uncommonly found to be increased in states of volume expansion such as pregnancy, heart failure, and strenuous exercise.[69,167,185] Digoxin-like immunoreactive factor is suspected to originate from both the maternal and fetal adrenal glands.[65,163,168] Digoxin-like immunoreactive factor is mostly protein bound (slow-acting or inactive), whereas the free fraction is the more rapidly acting compound.[185] Jakobi et al.[85] measured maternal total plasma digoxin-like immunoreactive factor levels in 113 third-trimester patients: 51 were normotensive, 23 had twin pregnancies, 20 were preeclamptic, and 19 had latent or chronic hypertension (CHTN). The concentration of digoxin-like immunoreactive factor in patients with twin pregnancies (1143 ± 249 pg/ml) was found to be significantly higher than that in either the normotensive patients (890 ± 161 pg/ml, p < .001) or in the hypertensive group (903 ± 256 pg/ml, p < .01). Although no significant differences were seen between the latter two groups, an increased trend was noted in the patients with CHTN compared with the patients who had preeclampsia (957 ± 212 versus 852 ± 288 pg/ml). The increased digoxin-like immunoreactive factor in multiple pregnancies may suggest a contribution from multifetal origin resulting in an increase in blood volume and cardiac output over singleton pregnancies.[188] In singleton pregnancies an increase in maternal stroke volume is usually mediated by an increase in heart size, whereas multiple pregnancies are affected by increased heart rate and contractility and not by further heart enlargement. Therefore the increased digoxin-like immunoreactive factor might be a physiologic adaptive mechanism in multiple pregnancies that yields a higher cardiac output because of its possible cardiotropic effect.

Like plasma renin (p-renin), serum aldosterone concentrations are found to be markedly increased in twin pregnancies over singleton pregnancies in the twentieth week (834 pmol versus 530 pmol, p < 0.05), twenty-eighth week (3531 pmol versus 1170 pmol, p < 0.01), and thirty-second week (3614 pmol versus 1781 pmol, p < 0.01) of gestation.[178] Thomsen, Fogh-Anderson, and Jaszczak[179] reported a negative correlation between changes in p-AN and changes in aldosterone (r = −0.66, p < 0.0001) and p-renin (r = −0.52, p < 0.01).

Plasma volume and birth weight

There also appears to be a relationship between plasma volume and the combined birth weight of twins. Campbell and MacGillivray[28] studied 117 primigravid twin gestations at greater than or equal to 37 weeks that were divided according to the presence or absence preeclampsia. They demonstrated a significant difference in the combined centile birth weights and plasma volume in normotensive and transient hypertensive women.[28] In both groups the mean plasma volume in those women whose twins were under the 25 percentile birth weight or over the 75 percentile birth weight was decreased and increased, respectively. Additionally, the group identified with proteinuric hypertension demonstrated a slight increase in the plasma volume as the birth weight increased. There is also a relationship between intravascular albumin and protein mass and the infant's birth weight when the baby is small for dates, but not for appropriate gestational age (AGA) and large gestational age (LGA) babies or in twins.[49] In 1977 Campbell and MacGillivray[26] studied the maternal physiologic responses and birth weights of infants from singleton and twin pregnancies by parity. Their observations suggested that in subsequent pregnancies (maximum increase at approximately greater than or equal to 30 weeks) there was a greater volume expansion than during the first pregnancy (maximum increase at greater than or equal to 34 weeks). Such a significant volume expansion was also found in multigravid women with twin pregnancies. Therefore it appears that the greater weight of the neonate in the second pregnancy may be the result of the greater volume expansion and earlier peak when compared with the first pregnancy.

Hemoglobin, iron, and folic acid

A consequence of the augmented plasma volume is an increase in hemodilution, which results in any of the water-soluble substances being markedly decreased in the plasma. The suspected deficiencies in folate concentrations in multiple pregnancies were also thought to be the result of a more rapid renal clearance. However, red-cell folate and total circulating concentrations have been found to remain unchanged.[51,72] Interestingly, the incidence of megaloblastic anemia in twins is found to be increased in multiple pregnancies.[174,203] This is thought to occur because of a decrease in transfer of maternal folate to the twin fetuses compared with that in a singleton pregnancy before term. Additionally, the smaller twin seems

to receive less folate than the larger twin, as noted from their red cell folate concentrations.[51] Nevertheless, folic acid supplementation is recommended in women who are at risk for NTDs.[33] The Centers for Disease Control now recommend that all women of childbearing age who are capable of becoming pregnant be advised to consume at least 400 μg of folate daily.[34] Additionally, both plasma zinc and plasma albumin concentrations are known to be lower in multiple pregnancies than in singleton pregnancies, but the protein mass remains the same.[26,29,111] The rationale for the lower zinc levels is the result of both increased volume expansion and albumin metabolism.[182] Zinc is a component of more than 70 metaloenzymes and is bound to albumin (60% to 70%). However, serum copper levels in twin pregnancies are conflicting.[75,76] At 20 to 22 weeks' gestation, plasma copper concentrations were reported by Campbell, MacGillivray, and Tuttle[29] as unchanged at 31.1 ± 5.6 μmol/L in twins and 29.0 ± 5.4 μmol/L in singletons. At 30 to 32 weeks, it was 33.1 ± 5.8 μmol/L in twins and 30.8 ± 5.6 μmol/L in singletons. More than 90% of elemental copper in maternal serum is found as ceruloplasmin, which is increased because of an estrogenic effect of pregnancy.[159]

It also has been reported that the hemoglobin levels and hematocrit concentrations are lower in multiple gestations. This is apparent because of the greater hemodilution in multiple pregnancies and because of a greater demand for iron and folic acid or for their combination. The mean red blood cell mass in twin pregnancies is increased by 40.2% at term and an even greater amount is seen in triplets.[11,117] Hall et al.[73] reported on 123 twin pregnancies and their hematologic profiles, 24% of which had a hemoglobin value of less than 10 g/dl at any time, 9% had a value of less than 9 g/dl, and only 3% had a value of 8 g/dl. Eighteen (15%) of the subjects demonstrated evidence of hypochromia (iron deficiency), 7% had equivocal changes on a peripheral blood smear, and 40% showed absent or reduced iron storage from a bone marrow aspiration. However, only 2.4% demonstrated macrocytosis (similar incidence in untreated singleton pregnancies is 1.9%), and 8 (6.5%) showed megaloblastic hematopoiesis on bone marrow aspiration. Only one woman with megaloblastic change showed significant anemia. The presence of macrocytosis with hypersegmentation of neutrophils in peripheral blood is usually considered indicative of developing megaloblastic anemia. None of the women in the study by Hall et al.[73] received any iron or folic acid supplements. Assessment of the red cell mass in twin pregnancies has demonstrated a significant increase in mass, which is indicative of a markedly increased oxygen-carrying capacity. Neither the mean hemoglobin concentration nor the mean cell volume is altered in multiple pregnancies.[73] Nevertheless, iron and folic acid supplementations are indicated in multiple pregnancies because of the increased incidence of anemia of approximately 40%.[70,112,153]

Plasma fibrinogen levels in a singleton pregnancy range from 200 to 400 mg/dl during early gestation to 300 to 600 mg/dl in the third trimester. Fibrinogen and fibrin levels were found to be consistent, but they were not significantly elevated in twin pregnancies from 20 weeks to term. MacGillivray[112] showed absolute plasminogen levels in twin pregnancies to have a downward trend, and no significant differences were noted. Antithrombin III, α_1-antitrypsin, and fibrin split products demonstrated no differences. Condie and Campbell[35] suggested that the etiology of the increase was plausible because of the pronounced estrogenic enhancement of fibrinogen synthesis seen in multiple pregnancies.

The polymorphonuclear leukocyte (PMN) count in a singleton pregnancy is manifested by variable levels. Normal values reported in a nonlaboring patient range from 5000 to 12,000/mm^3. In laboring patients without evidence of infection the leukocyte count may rise to as high as 25,000/mm^3. Not uncommonly the circulating PMN cells in patients who smoke have been shown to be elevated above normal values.

Blood pressure

Blood pressure (BP) in singleton pregnancies is normally lower at the beginning of the second trimester and does not begin to rise until about the 30th week of gestation.[113] Campbell and Campbell[24] demonstrated that after adjustments for maternal weight and maternal age, a significantly lower diastolic blood pressure can be observed (during mid-pregnancy) in twin pregnancies than in singleton pregnancies. They also showed that there was a greater increase in the diastolic BP by delivery. Nevertheless, the incidence of pregnancy-induced hypertension (PIH) is still elevated over singleton pregnancies.[24]

Cardiac output

Cardiac output was observed to be significantly higher in multiple pregnancies than in singleton pregnancies, but only in the twentieth week.[157,179] When stroke volume and cardiac output are measured when the patient is in the left lateral position, they are both found to be higher than when the patient is in the supine position. Campbell et al.,[30] using a noninvasive technique (transcutaneous aortic velography, [TAV])[157] reported that only in normotensive women is there a tendency for cardiac output to decrease as arterial BP increases like it does in nonpregnant women, but they also found that this is not the case not for women who developed PIH. TAV uses the Doppler shift effect from a continuous ultrasound that is transmitted and received from the transducer at the suprasternal notch.[148] This technique is independent of weight and height.

Nutrition

Food intake is known not to be increased or different in women with multiple pregnancies, despite greater fetal growth (by weight). Campbell, MacGillivray, and Tuttle[29] found that the energy and protein intake as measured by 24-hour urinary nitrogen tests were similar in twin and singleton pregnancies. Despite the fact that no differences were found, the energy intake was 300 to 400 kcal, which is less than the 240 kcal recommended by the United Kingdom Department of Health and Social Security.[42] However, MacGillivray[109] demonstrated a lower urinary nitrogen output in twin pregnancies. These findings of protein and energy intake mean that women with twin pregnancies either have less protein energy intake or are able to more efficiently utilize the food they take in. These data suggest that the physiologic adaptation in multiple pregnancies is exaggerated. Therefore it seems likely that the absorp-

tion and utilization of nutrients is increased to meet the requirements of the greater fetal mass. Woman with twin pregnancies are recommended to have a weight gain of 35 to 45 pounds.[2] Approximately 300 additional calories of energy per day above basal requirements are required during pregnancy.[136]

Glucose tolerance

Diabetes mellitus in pregnancy poses many complications for mother and fetus or neonate.[102,146] The overall prevalence of gestational diabetes is approximately 3.5%, with a relative increase among Hispanics, African Americans, and Asian woman.[47] Of the 3.5% of pregnancies affected by diabetes, 90% of cases are represented by gestational diabetes mellitus (GDM). GDM places women at an increased risk for diabetes in the nonpregnant state, preterm birth, macrosomatia,[41,116] hydramnios,[178] preeclampsia, spontaneous abortion,[124] increased operative deliveries, stillbirths, and neonatal death.[144] When antenatal care is provided, the rates of the latter complications have been reduced and found to be similar to those recorded for uncomplicated pregnancies.[36,122,143]

GDM is defined by glucose intolerance that is first recognized during pregnancy.[175] It is suspected that women with GDM have an underlying and possibly inherited defect in insulin action, which may be masked by insulin resistance of late pregnancy.[15] Insulin resistance is caused in part by increased placental secretion of human chorionic somatomammotropin, increased placental consumption, and decreased sensitivity of the peripheral tissues to insulin.[92] Thus during the second half of pregnancy there is a relative increase in resistance, a compensatory hyperinsulinemia, and an altered renal threshold impairing the disposal of maternal glucose.[21] Diabetes mellitus in multiple pregnancies involves the same complex interaction of genetic predisposition and environmental influences.[89] Johansen et al.[89] showed that in monozygotic twins, concordance for diabetes mellitus was less than 50% before age 40 and almost 100% when diabetes mellitus first manifests after 40 years of age. GDM has been reported by some authors to exist in twin pregnancies at the same rate that it does in singleton pregnancies[99,101] and by others at an increased incidence of 5.6% versus 2.5%, respectively.[50] Interestingly, fasting insulin levels are slightly increased but not significantly higher in twin pregnancies than in singleton pregnancies.[135] Women with twin pregnancies have also been shown to have a lower fasting plasma glucose level but no significant differences in 1-, 2-, and 3-hour glucose levels.[50] Spellacy, Buhi, and Burk[172] evaluated carbohydrate metabolism in 24 singleton pregnancies and 24 twin pregnancies and found significantly lower fasting 5- and 15-minute blood glucose levels in women with twin pregnancies. There was also a significantly lower 15-minute insulin level in the twin group. Campbell and MacGillivray[27] examined intravenous glucose tolerance tests using a glucose load of 25 gm in 54 twin pregnancies. Mean glucose disappearance rates were slower in twin pregnancies than in singleton pregnancies. However, there was a greater tendency toward obesity in the women with twin pregnancies above the seventy-fifth and eighty-fifth percentiles according to Kemsley scales for weight and height.[94] Placental hormones, hPL, estrogen, and progester-

one are theorized as the reasons for the slower rate of glucose disappearance in twins. Naidoo et al.[135] reported on 20 patients with twin pregnancies and 20 with singleton pregnancies who were matched for age, parity, weight, height, and gestational age. Intravenous glucose tolerance tests were performed using a glucose load of 0.5 gm/kg of body weight. They ascertained that all postinfusion insulin levels were significantly higher in twin pregnancies. They also noticed that the glucose disappearance rates (K) were not found to be different between the two groups. Moodley et al.[129] assessed carbohydrate metabolism using the 100-gm oral glucose tolerance test in 21 women with twin pregnancies and in 21 woman with singleton pregnancies. No significant differences in venous plasma glucose were found between them; however, significance in insulin response was lower at 60 minutes in the twin group. Thus women with twin gestations are not at higher metabolic risk for gestational diabetes than women with singleton pregnancies. Therefore it appears that the 50-gm oral glucose challenge test may appear to be an appropriate screening test in multiple pregnancies, as well as in singleton pregnancies. Screening for GDM is performed with a 50-gm oral glucose load with a glucose determination 1 hour later.[120] Screening should be performed between 24 and 28 weeks of gestation. High risk patients (with prior GDM) should be screened earlier, with subsequent screening if normal results are initially obtained. The American College of Obstetrics and Gynecology[5] suggests screening pregnant women who have significant risk factors or universal screening for those with a high background prevalence of Type II diabetes. The recommended screening threshold for the 50-gm glucose test is suggested at greater than or equal to 140 mg/dl. Patients whose plasma glucose levels equal or exceed the screening value should be evaluated with a diagnostic 3-hour glucose tolerance test.

Pulmonary lung maturity

RDS is a major cause of neonatal death in premature infants. Prematurity and RDS occur 4 times more often in infants from multiple pregnancies than in singletons.[18,158] Despite an overall decline in morbidity and mortality, RDS occurs in infants from multiple pregnancies for the same reason it occurs in singletons: that is, prematurity.[100,189] Commonly, both twins are equally affected with RDS, particularly if they are delivered by cesarean section and if they are preterm. Occasionally, only the second twin is affected.[6] Usually, the first twin delivered vaginally has an increased amniotic fluid lecithin to sphingomyelin (L/S) ratio and increased blood cortisol levels compared with the second twin, who is also delivered vaginally.[140,141] It is suspected that head compression during labor serves as the stimulus for the increased cortisol production.[6] Fetal RDS is often associated with immaturity of the lung or insufficient surfactant production. Nonetheless, fetal lung maturity is known to occur at an earlier gestational age (31 to 32 weeks) in multiple pregnancies than in uncomplicated singleton pregnancies when assessed by the L/S ratio.[104,145] This ratio has become the most generally accepted method of assessment of morbidity and mortality in infants threatened with premature delivery.[133]

Pulmonary alveolar stability is dependent on the amount of surfactant produced by the alveolar membranes of the fetus.[64] Premature male newborns are at greater risk for RDS than female infants.[3,121] Fetal lung maturity in male rats has been shown to be delayed compared with female rats.[3] Surfactant decreases surface tension (less than 10 dyne cm^{-1}) at the air-to-liquid interface of the alveoli, thereby increasing oxygenation.[7] The metabolism of pulmonary surfactant is dependent on the maturation of type II pneumonocytes.[186] Surfactant consists of 80% to 90% lipids, 10% to 20% protein, and 2% carbohydrate.[77] In the lipid component of surfactant, up to 90% is comprised of phospholipids (85% lecithin).[95] Almost 50% of the phosphatidylcholine is in the form of disaturated phosphidylcholine, largely dipalmitoyl phosphatidylcholine.[74] Phosphatidylglycerol (6% to 11% of total phospholipid) is the second most abundant phospholipid in mature surfactant.[154]

Fetal lung maturity may be estimated by a ratio of two phospholipids, lecithin (phosphatidylcholine) and sphingomyelin.[63] During the last trimester of pregnancy increasing concentrations of surfactants (lecithin and sphingomyelin) appear in the amniotic fluid and reflect fetal pulmonary maturity. Lecithin and sphingomyelin in a singleton pregnancy are both nearly equal until 35 weeks' gestation (dated from the last normal menstrual period), where lecithin then increases fourfold with advancing fetal maturation.[64] Interestingly, the average gestational age at delivery for twin pregnancies is approximately 35 weeks.[32] Fetal lung maturity is presumed when an L/S ratio of 2:1 is achieved in a nondiabetic pregnancy. Infants born to mothers with insulin dependent diabetes mellitus are at increased risk for RDS in 2% to 3% of cases despite an L/S ratio of 2:0.[46,151] However, the appearance of phosphatidyl-glycerol (greater than or equal to 3% of total phospholipids) in the amniotic fluid of a diabetic pregnancy has a negative predictive value of approximately 100%. A variety of animal research in which diabetes mellitus has been induced into the animals has demonstrated a decrease in the production of phosphatidylcholine.[150] Therefore knowledge of fetal lung maturity is essential in the management of multiple pregnancies. However, some potential errors in L/S ratio determinations have been recognized. Blood and meconium in the amniotic fluid may adversely affect the L/S ratio.[22,80]

In a study of 47 twin pregnancies and 47 control singleton pregnancies, the L/S ratios obtained by amniocentesis were found to be similar and were comparable between Twin A and Twin B for a given gestational age.[199] No patients received corticosteroids before fetal lung maturation determination. Norman et al.[141] found no differences before the onset of labor in 30 African twin pregnancies with a mean of 37.7 weeks' gestation in the lecithin (L), phosphatidylinositol, phosphatidylethanolamine (PE), and phosphatidyl-glycerol to sphingomyelin (S) levels between Twin A and Twin B. However, in the presence of uterine contractions there was a significant increase in L/S and PE/S ratios (L/S ratio: Twin A = 10.8 ± 5.2, Twin B = 7.0 ± 3.8, $p < 0.05$; PE/S ratio: Twin A = 0.7 ± 0.2, Twin B = 0.4 ± 0.1, $p < 002$). These findings are similar to those previously reported by Spellacy et al.,[173] where no differences in the L/S ratio before the onset of labor was found in 14 sets of twins. However, no gestational ages

were noted, and only 7 had L/S ratios less than 2.0. In the study by Norman et al.,[141] it was speculated that glucocorticoids (cortisol and corticosteroids) induced surfactant production in the fetal lung of the leading twin. Additionally, Norman et al.[140] (1983) demonstrated that both free and conjugated steroids were increased in the amniotic fluid from the leading twin after labor had begun; the correlation between glucocorticoid conjugates and the L/S ratio was 0.48 (n = 50, $p < 0.001$). Their results suggest a fetal adrenal origin for the increase in amniotic fluid conjugated steroids from the leading twin, whereas maternally derived glucocorticoids would be expected to be equally increased in both twins.[54,132] Weller et al.[196] found similar results in the L/S ratio of tracheal effluent of the leading infant, which was greater than in the second infant of a multiple pregnancy. Leveno et al.[104] compared the L/S ratios of 42 twin pregnancies and found them to be similar at the time of cesarean section, independent of sex, zygosity, and birth weight with a discordance up to 40%. Sims, Cowan, and Parkinson,[170] in a prospective study, assessed the L/S ratio in 20 twin pregnancies and suggested a ratio of 2.5:1 as the lower limit to predict the functional lung maturity of both twins. This would allow for the differences in L/S ratios of twins and planimetric errors. However, in their investigation, Sims et al.[170] included amniotic fluid collected at the introitus of patients before and during labor. Dhall et al.[44] collected amniotic fluid from 16 pairs of twins soon after amniotomy and demonstrated a high degree of correlation between Twin A and Twin B (r = 0.8768). In the very premature infant the risk of

RDS with an immature L/S ratio (less than 2.0) was predicted in only 30% of cases, indicating its unreliability. Wolf et al.,[200] in a retrospective study of 104 twin infants weighing 500 to 1499 gm and 496 singleton infants born alive after 24 to 31 weeks' gestation demonstrated no differences between twins and singletons in RDS (63% versus 71%), pulmonary interstitial emphysema (14% versus 16%), and bronchopulmonary dysplasia (27% versus 46%) (p = 0.001). Premature rupture of the membranes appeared to reduce the degree of RDS in twins; however, the incidence of chorioamnionitis was not noted.[202]

Thus twin pregnancies do not appear to accelerate fetal lung maturation. Secondly, gestational age is paramount in the determination of fetal lung maturation, since similar rates of maturation occur among fetuses of similar gestational age. Fetal lung maturation in multiple pregnancies is synchronous until labor ensues. Finally, the development of RDS is strongly linked to prematurity and lack of surfactant synthesis.

Corticosteroid use in pregnant women at risk for preterm labor has been shown to reduce RDS and mortality in preterm infants by approximately 40%.[59,62,106] Corticosteroids are most effective between 30 and 34 weeks' gestation; however, the published meta-analysis shows a beneficial but less significant effect at earlier gestational ages. Even though corticosteroid therapy does not completely decrease the incidence of RDS in infants born at 24 to 28 weeks' gestation, it does reduce the severity of RDS and the incidence of intraventricular hemorrhage (IVH). Antenatal corticosteroid therapy may be associated with a small increase in the risk of infection in women with premature rupture of the membranes.[60] However, there is no convincing evidence that neonatal infection or adrenal suppression is increased.[177] Nonetheless, the benefits of corticosteroid therapy in the reduction of RDS and IVH outweigh any small risk of infection.[142] Patients with insulin dependent diabetes treated with corticosteroids manifest an increased blood sugar level. Therefore close monitoring of maternal serum glucose is recommended to avoid such clinical conditions as ketoacidosis. Other agents, such as thyroxine (T_4), triiodothyronine (T_3), and thyrotropin-releasing hormone (TRH), have also been used to accelerate fetal pulmonary maturity.[201] The human fetal lung is known to be enriched with T_3 receptors, compared with other organs.[12] Rooney, Gross, and Warshaw[155] administered TRH to pregnant rabbits and observed an enhanced lung maturation. The mechanism of action of TRH is its enhancement of morphologic indices of lung maturation.[43] Additionally, TRH in combination with corticosteroids has demonstrated a markedly increased lung distensibility (lung compliance) in the fetal lamb.[107] Moraga et al.[130] demonstrated a significant combined effect with glucocorticoid and TRH treatment over betamethasone alone in undisturbed preterm ewes. Betamethasone plus TRH significantly increased fetal lung compliance, which is expressed as milliliter of air per gram of wet weight at 40 cm H_2O and 5 cm (0.82 ± 0.13 and 0.35 ± 0.10 ml/gm, respectively) versus betamethasone (0.37 ± 0.02 and 0.07 ± 0.02). Additionally, total phospholipids and saturated phosphatidyl concentrations were significantly elevated in the combined method ($27.3 \pm$

4.9 and 16.9 ± 4.3 µg/gm wet lung) versus betamethasone alone (10.9 ± 3.5 and 6.7 ± 2.1 µg/gm wet lung). Knight, Liggins, and Wealthall,[97] in a randomized, placebo-controlled, double-blind trial of antepartum TRH and betamethasone that was conducted in 378 pregnant women between 24 and 32.6 weeks' gestation, demonstrated a significant reduction in RDS and fetal death. The incidence of RDS was reduced from 52% to 31% (RR 0.61; 95% CI, 0.41-0.89).

Treatment for the prevention of RDS should consist of either 2 doses of 12 mg of betamethasone, intramuscularly, given 24 hours apart or 4 doses of 6 mg of dexamethasone, intramuscularly, given 12 hours apart. Additionally, TRH in combination with betamethasone in 2 doses of 400 µg each, intravenously, given 12 hours apart is suggested. Optimal pulmonary effect begins 24 hours after initiation of therapy and lasts 7 days.

References

1. Aberg A et al: Cardiac puncture of fetus with Huler's disease avoiding abortion of unaffected co-twin, *Lancet* 2:990-991, 1978.
2. Abrams B: *Maternal nutrition environmental influences on fetal development.* In Creasy RK, Resnick R, editors: *Maternal-fetal medicine, principles and practice*, Philadelphia, 1994, WB Saunders.
3. Adamson IYR, King GM: Sex differences in development of fetal rat lung. I. Autoradiographic and biochemical studies, *Lab Invest* 50:456, 1984.
4. Adamson IYR, King GM: Sex-related differences in cellular composition and surfactant synthesis of developing fetal rat lungs, *Am Rev Respir Dis* 129:130, 1984.
5. American College of Obstetricians and Gynecologists: *Diabetes and pregnancy*, Technical Bulletin No. 200, December 1994.
6. Arnold C et al: Respiratory distress syndrome in second-born versus first-born twins: a matched case-control analysis, *N Engl J Med* 317:1121, 1987.
7. Avery ME, Mead J: Surface properties in relation to atelectasis and hyaline membrane disease, *Am J Dis Child* 97:517, 1959.
8. Ballard PL: Hormonal influences during fetal lung development: metabolic activities of the lung, Ciba Foundation Symposium, Vol. 78, Amsterdam, 1980, Excerpta Medica.
9. Baumgarten A: Racial differences and biological significance of maternal serum alpha fetoprotein. *Lancet* 2:573, 1986.
10. Bergstrand CG, Czar B: Paper electrophoretic study of human fetal serum proteins with demonstration of a new protein fraction, *Scand J Clin Lab Invest* 9:277-286, 1957.
11. Berlin NI et al: The blood volume in pregnancy as determined by P^{32} labeled RBC. *Surg Gynecol Obstet* 97:73, 1953.
12. Bernal J, Pekonen F: Ontogenesis of the nuclear 3,5,3′-triiodothyronine receptor in the human fetal brain, *Endocrinology* 127:278, 1984.
13. Bernaschek G, Rudelstrofer R, Csaicich P: Vaginal sonography versus serum human chorionic gonadotropin in early detection of pregnancy, *Am J Obstet Gynecol* 159:608-612, 1988.
14. Bernstein L et al: Cigarette smoking in pregnancy results in marked decrease in maternal HCG an oestradiol levels, *Br J Obstet Gynaecol* 96:92-96, 1989.
15. Botta RM et al: Evaluation of B-cell secretion and peripheral insulin resistance during pregnancy and after delivery in gestational diabetes mellitus with obesity, *Acta Diabetol Lat* 25:81, 1988.
16. Braunstein GD et al: First-trimester chorionic gonadotropin measurements as an aid in the diagnosis of early pregnancy disorders, *Am J Obstet Gynecol* 131:25-32, 1978.
17. Brenner BM et al: Diverse biological actions of atrial natriuretic peptide, *Physiol Rev* 3:665-699, 1990.
18. Brenner WE, Edelman DA, Hendricks CH: Characteristics of patients with placenta previa and results of "expectant management," *Am J Obstet Gynecol* 132:180-191, 1978.
19. Brock DJH, Scrimgeour RG, Nelson MM: Amniotic fluid alpha-fetoprotein measurements in the early diagnosis of central nervous system disorders, *Clin Genet* 7:163, 1975.
20. Brorody IB, Carlton MA: Isolated defect in human placental lactogen synthesis in a normal pregnancy, *Br J Obstet Gynaecol* 88:447, 1981.
21. Buchanan TA et al: Insulin sensitivity and B-cell responsiveness to glucose during late

pregnancy in lean and moderately obese women with normal glucose tolerance or mild gestational diabetes, *Am J Obstet Gynecol* 162:1008, 1990.

22. Buhi MS, Spellacy WN: Effects of blood or meconium on the determination of the amniotic fluid lecithin-sphingomyelin ratio, *Am J Obstet Gynecol* 121:321, 1975.

23. Campbell DM: Maternal adaptations in twin pregnancy, *Semin Perinatol* 10:14-18, 1986.

24. Campbell DM, Campbell AJ: Arterial blood pressure: the pattern of change in twin pregnancies. *Acta Genet Med Gemellol (Roma)* 34:217-223, 1985.

25. Campbell DM, MacGillivray I: Comparison of maternal response in first and second pregnancies in relation to baby weight, *Br J Obstet Gynaecol Commonw* 79:684, 1972.

26. Campbell DM, MacGillivray I: Maternal physiological responses and birthweight in singleton and twin pregnancies by parity, *Eur J Obstet Gynec Reprod Biol* 1:17-24, 1977.

27. Campbell DM, MacGillivray I: Glucose tolerance in twin pregnancy, *Acta Genet Med Gemellol (Roma)* 28:283-287, 1979.

28. Campbell DM, MacGillivray I: The importance of plasma volume expansion and nutrition in twin pregnancy, *Acta Genet Med Gemellol (Roma)* 33:19-24, 1984.

29. Campbell DM, MacGillivray I, Tuttle S: Maternal nutrition in twin pregnancy, *Acta Genet Med Gemellol (Roma)* 31:221-227, 1982.

30. Campbell DM et al: Cardiac output in twin pregnancy, *Acta Genet Med Gemellol (Roma)* 34:225-228, 1985.

31. Campbell S: Paper presented at British Medical Ultrasound Society Annual Scientific Meeting, London, December 14-15, 1981.

32. Caspi E et al: The outcome of pregnancy after gonadotrophin therapy, *Br J Obstet Gynaecol* 83:967-973, 1976.

33. Centers for Disease Control: Use of folic acid for prevention of spina bifida and other neural tube defects-1983-1991, *MMWR* 40:513-516, 1991.

34. Centers for Disease Control: Recommendations for the use of folic acid to reduce the number of cases of spina bifida and neural tube defects, *MMWR* 41:1, 1992.

35. Condie R, Campbell D: Components of the haemostatic mechanism in twin pregnancy, *Br J Obstet Gynaecol* 85:37-39, 1978.

36. Coustan DR, Imarah J: Prophylactic insulin treatment of gestational diabetes reduces the incidence of macrosomia, operative deliveries,

and birth trauma, *Am J Obstet Gynecol* 50:836-842, 1984.

37. Cowett RM et al: Untoward neonatal effect of intramniotic administration of methylene blue, *Obstet Gynecol* 48(suppl):74S-75S, 1976.

38. Creinin M, Katz M, Laros: Triplet pregnancy: changes in morbidity and mortality, *J Perinatol* 11:207-212, 1991.

39. Cusson JR et al: Plasma concentration of atrial natriuretic factor in normal pregnancy, *N Engl J Med* 19:1230-1231, 1985.

40. Czeizel AE, Dudas I: Prevention of the first occurrence of neural-tube defects by periconceptional vitamin supplementation, [see comments] *N Engl J Med* 327:1832-1835, 1992 and 327:1875-1877, 1992.

41. Dandrow RV, O'Sullivan JB: Obstetrical hazards of gestational diabetes, *Am J Obstet Gynecol* 96:1144-1147, 1966.

42. Department of Health and Social Security: Recommended daily amounts of food energy and nutrients for groups of people in the united kingdom. Her Majesty's Stationary Office, 1979, London.

43. Devaskar U et al: Transplacental stimulation of functional and morphological fetal rabbit lung maturation: effect of thyrotropin-releasing hormone, *Am J Obstet Gynecol* 157:460, 1987.

44. Dhall K, Majumdar S: Fetal lung maturation in twin gestation, *Indian J Med Res* 83:422-425, 1986.

45. DiMaio MS et al: Screening for fetal Down's syndrome in pregnancy by measuring maternal serum alpha fetoprotein levels, *N Engl J Med* 317:342-346, 1987.

46. Donald IR et al: Clinical experience with the amniotic fluid lecithin/sphingomyelin ratio. I. Antenatal prediction of pulmonary maturity, *Am J Obstet Gynecol* 115:547, 1973.

47. Dooley SL et al: The influence of demographic and phenotypic heterogeneity on the prevalence of gestational diabetes mellitus, *Int J Gynaecol Obstet* 35:13-18, 1991.

48. Drugan A et al: Similarity of twins to singleton maternal serum alpha-fetoprotein ratio by race: no need to establish specific multifetal tables, *Fetal Diagn Ther* 8:84-88, 1993.

49. Duffus GM, MacGillivray I, Dennis KI: Maternal metabolic response to twin pregnancy in primigravidae, *J Obstet Gynaec Br Commonw* 78:97, 1971.

50. Dwyer PL et al: Glucose tolerance in twin pregnancy, *Aust N Z J Obstet Gynaecol* 22:131-134, 1982.

51. Ek J: Plasma and red cell folate in newborn twins and their mothers in relation to gestational age, *Acta Obstet Gynecol Scand* 60:379, 1981.

52. Elias S et al: Genetic amniocentesis in twin gestations, *Am J Obstet Gynecol* 138:169-174, 1980.

53. Evans MI et al: Selective first-trimester termination in octuplet and quadruplet pregnancies: clinical and ethical issues, *Obstet Gynecol* 71:289-296, 1988.

54. Fenci M deM, Koos B, Tulchinsky D: Origin of corticosteroids in amniotic fluid, *J Clin Endocrinol Metab* 50:431-436, 1980.

55. Finlay D, Dillon A, Heslip M: Ultrasound screening in a twin pregnancy with high serum alpha-fetoprotein. *J Clin Ultrasound* 9:514-515, 1981.

56. Franchimont P, Renter A: *Evidence of alpha and beta-subunits of hCG in serum and urines of pregnant women.* In Margoulies M, Greenwood FC, editors: *Structure-activity relationship of protein and polypeptide hormones,* 1972, Amsterdam, Excerpta Medica.

57. Friesen HG: Lactation induced by human placental lactogen and cortisone acetate in rabbits, *Endocrinology* 79:224, 1966.

58. Gaede P, Trolle D, Pedersen H: Extremely low placental lactogen hormone (hPL) values in an otherwise uneventful pregnancy preceding delivery of a normal baby, *Acta Obstet Gynecol Scand* 57:203, 1978.

59. Gamsu HR et al: Antenatal administration of betamethasone to prevent respiratory distress syndrome in premature infants: report of a UK multicentre trial, *Br J Obstet Gynaecol* 96:401-410, 1989.

60. Garite TJ et al: Prospective randomized study of corticosteroids in the management of premature rupture of the membranes and the premature gestation, *Am J Obstet Gynecol* 141:508-515, 1981.

61. Ghosh A et al: Prognostic significance of raised serum alpha-fetoprotein levels in twin pregnancies, *Br J Obstet Gynaecol* 89:817-820, 1982.

62. Gilstrap L, Phelan JP: Expert exchange: when and how to give prenatal steroids, *OBG Management* 6:27-28, 1994.

63. Gluck L: Diagnosis of the respiratory distress syndrome by amniocentesis, *Am J Obstet Gynecol* 109:440-445, 1971.

64. Gluck L: Pulmonary surfactant and neonatal respiratory distress, *Hosp Pract* 6:45, 1971.

65. Gonzales AR et al: Digoxin-like immunoreactive substance in pregnancy, *Am J Obstet Gynecol* 157:660-664, 1987.

66. Grace AA: Atrial natriuretic peptide concentrations during pregnancy, *Lancet* II:1267, 1987.

67. Graves SW et al: Endogenous digoxin-immunoreactive substance in human pregnancies, *J Clin Endocrinol Metab* 58:748-751, 1984.

68. Grennert L et al: Ultrasound and human-placental-lactogen screening for early detection of twin pregnancies, *Lancet* 1:4-6, 1976.

69. Gruber KA, Whitaker JM, Buckalew VM Jr: Endogenous digitalis-like substance in plasma of volume expanded dogs, *Nature* 287:743-749, 1980.

70. Guttmacher AF: Analysis of 573 cases of twin pregnancy. II. The hazards of pregnancy itself, *Am J Obstet Gynecol* 38:277, 1939.

71. Haddow JE et al: Prenatal screening for Down's syndrome with use of maternal serum markers, *N Engl J Med* 327:588-593, 1992.

72. Hall MH, Pirani BBK, Campbell DM: The cause of the fall in serum folate in normal pregnancy, *Br J Obstet Gynaecol* 83:132, 1976.

73. Hall MH et al: Anemia in twin pregnancy, *Acta Genet Med Gemellol (Roma)* 28:279-282, 1979.

74. Hallman M et al: Evidence of lung surfactant abnormality in respiratory failure: study of bronchoalveolar lavage phospholipids, surface activity, phospholipase activity, and plasm myoinositol, *J Clin Invest* 70:673, 1982.

75. Halsted JA, Hackley BM, Smith JC: Plasma zinc and copper in pregnancy and after oral contraceptives, *Lancet* 2:278, 1968.

76. Hambridge KM, Droegmuller W: Changes in plasma and hair concentrations of zinc, copper, chromium, and magnanese during pregnancy, *Obstet Gynecol* 44:666, 1974.

77. Harwood JL et al: Characterization of pulmonary surfactant from ox, rabbit, rat and sheep, *Biochem J* 151:707, 1975.

78. Hatjis CG et al: Interrelationship between atrial natriuretic factor concentrations and acute volume expansion in pregnant and nonpregnant women, *Am J Obstet Gynecol* 163:45-50, 1990.

79. Hibbard ED, Smithells RW: Folic acid metabolism and human embryopathy, *Lancet* I:1254, 1965.

80. Hobbins JC et al: L/S ratio in predicting pulmonary maturity in utero, *Obstet Gynecol* 39:660, 1972.

81. Hogge WA et al: Congenital nephrosis: detection of index cases through maternal serum alpha-fetoprotein screening, *Am J Obstet Gynecol* 167:1330-1333, 1992.

82. Huber J, Wagenbichler P, Bartsch F: Biamnial alpha fetoprotein concentration in twins, one with multiple malformations, *J Med Genet* 21:377-395, 1984.

83. Hunter AGW, Cox DM: Counseling problems when twins are discovered at genetic amniocentesis, *Clin Genet* 16:34-42, 1979.

84. DeSwiet M: *The cardiovascular system.* Hytten F, Chamberlain G, editors: *Clinical physiology in obstetrics*, Oxford, 1991, Blackwell Scientific Publications.

85. Jakobi P et al: Digoxin-like immunoreactive factor in twin and pregnancy-associated hypertensive pregnancies, *Obstet Gynecol* 74:29, 1989.

86. Jandial V et al: The value of measurement of pregnancy-specific proteins in twin pregnancies, *Acta Genet Med Gemellol (Roma)* 28:319, 1979.

87. Javanovic L, Landesman R, Saxenna BB: Screening for twin pregnancy, *Science* 19B:738, 1977.

88. Jeffrey RL, Bowes WA, Delany JJ: Role of bed rest in twin gestation, *Obstet Gynecol* 43:822, 1974.

89. Johansen K et al: Serum insulin and growth hormone response patterns in monozygotic twin siblings of patients with juvenile-onset diabetes, *N Engl J Med* 293:57-61, 1975.

90. Johnson JM et al: Maternal serum alpha-fetoprotein in twin pregnancy, *Am J Obstet Gynecol* 162:1020-1025, 1990.

91. Johnson VP et al: Alpha-fetoprotein and acetylcholinesterase in twins discordant for neural tube defect, *Prenat Diagn* 9:831-837, 1989.

92. Karam JH, Salber PR, Forsham PH: *Pancreatic hormones and diabetes mellitus.* In Greenspan FS, Forsham PH, editors: *Basic and clinical endocrinology*, Norwalk, Conn., 1986, Appleton-Century-Crofts.

93. Keilani Z, Clarke PC, Kitau MJ: The significance of raised maternal plasma alpha-fetoprotein in twin pregnancies, *Br J Obstet Gynaecol* 85:510, 1978.

94. Kemsley WFF, Billewicz WZ, Thomson AM: A new weight for height standard based on British anthropometric data, *Br J Prev Med* 16:189-195, 1962.

95. Khosla SS et al: Influence of sex hormones on lung maturation in the fetal rabbit, *Biochim Biophys Acta* 750:112, 1983.

96. Kiely JL, Kleinman JC, Kiely M: Triplet and higher-order multiple births: time trends and infant mortality, *Am J Dis Child* 146:862-868, 1992.

97. Knight DB, Liggins GC, Wealthall SR: A randomized, controlled trial of antepartum thyrotropin-releasing hormone and betamethasone in the prevention of respiratory disease in preterm infants, *Am J Obstet Gynecol* 171:11-16, 1994.

98. Knight GJ et al: Efficiency of human placental lactogen and alpha-fetoprotein measurement in twin pregnancy detection: communications in brief, *Am J Obstet Gynecol* 141:585-586, 1981.

99. Kohl SG, Casey G: Twin gestation, *Mt Sinai J Med* 43:523, 1975.

100. Koivisto M et al: Twin pregnancy neonatal morbidity and mortality, *Acta Obstet Gynecol Scand Suppl* 44:21-29, 1975.

101. Kovacs BW, Kirschbaum TH, Paul RH: Twin gestations. I. Antenatal care and complications, *Obstet Gynecol* 74:313-317, 1989.

102. Kucera J: Rate and type of congenital anomalies among offspring of diabetic women, *J Reprod Med* 7:61, 1971.

103. Lagrew DC, Wilson EA, Jaured MJ: Determination of gestational age by serum concentrations of human chorionic gonadotropin, *Obstet Gynecol* 62:37, 1983.

104. Leveno KJ et al: Fetal lung maturation in twin gestation, *Am J Obstet Gynecol* 148:405-411, 1984.

105. Librarch CL et al: Genetic amniocentesis in seventy twin pregnancies, *Am J Obstet Gynecol* 148:585, 1984.

106. Liggins GC, Howie RN: A controlled trial of antepartum glucocorticoid treatment for prevention of respiratory distress in premature infants, *Pediatrics* 50:515-525, 1972.

107. Liggins GC et al: Synergism of cortisol and thyrotropin-releasing hormone on lung maturation in fetal sheep, *J Appl Physiol* 65:1880, 1988.

108. MacGillivray I: Some observations on the incidence of pre-eclampsia, *J Obstet Gynaecol Br Emp* 65:536-539, 1958.

109. MacGillivray I: Nutrition in twin pregnancy, *Acta Genet Med Gemellol (Roma)* 28:289-291, 1979.

110. MacGillivray I: Presidential address: the Aberdeen contribution to twinning, *Acta Genet Med Gemellol (Roma)* 33:5, 1984.

111. MacGillivray I, Campbell DM, Duffus GM: Maternal metabolic response to twin preg-

nancy in primigravidae, *Br J Obstet Gynaecol* 78:530-534, 1971.

112. MacGillivray I, Nylander PPS, Corney G: *Human multiple reproduction,* Philadelphia, 1975, WB Saunders.

113. MacGillivray I, Rose GA, Rowe D: Blood pressure survey in pregnancy, *Clin Sci* 37:395-407, 1969.

114. Marlein G, Rings M: Quantitative immunologische Bestimmung des Alpha₁-fetoproteins in Serum reifer and unreifer Neugeborener sowie in Serum von Sauglingen und Kindern, *Z Kinderheilk* 113:327-335, 1972.

115. McGregor WG, Kuhn RW, Jaffe RB: Biologically active chorionic gonadotropin synthesis by the human fetus, *Science* 220:306, 1983.

116. Modanlou HD et al: Large-for-gestational-age neonates: anthropometric reasons for shoulder dystocia, *Obstet Gynecol* 60:417-423, 1982.

117. McLennan CE, Thouin LG: Blood volume in pregnancy: a critical review and preliminary report of results with a new technique, *Am J Obstet Gynecol* 55:189, 1948.

118. Medical Research Council Vitamin Study Research Group: Prevention of neural tube defects: results of the Medical Research Council vitamin study, *Lancet* 338:131-137, 1991.

119. Merkatz IR et al: An association between low maternal serum alpha-fetoprotein and fetal chromosomal abnormalities, *Am J Obstet Gynecol* 148:886-894, 1984.

120. Metzger BE: Summary and recommendations of the Third International Workshop-Conference on Gestational Diabetes Mellitus, *Diabetes* 40(Suppl2):197-201, 1991.

121. Miller HC, Futrakul P: Birth weight, gestational age, and sex as determining factors in the incidence of respiratory distress syndrome of premature infants, *J Pediatr* 72:628, 1968.

122. Mills JL, Baker L, Goldman AS: Malformations in infants of diabetic mothers occur before the seventh gestational week: implications for treatment, *Diabetes* 28:292, 1979.

123. Mills JL et al: The absence of a relation between the periconceptional use of vitamins and neural-tube defects. National Institute of Child Health and Human Development Neural Tube Defects Study Group, *N Engl J Med* 321:430-435, 1981.

124. Mills JL et al: NICHD diabetes in early pregnancy study: incidence of spontaneous abortion among diabetic women whose pregnancies were identified within 21 days of conception, *N Engl J Med* 319:1617, 1988.

125. Milson I, Hedner J, Hedner T: Plasma atrial natriuretic peptide (ANP) and maternal hemodynamic changes during normal pregnancy, *Acta Obstet Gynecol Scand* 67:71-??, 1988.

126. Milunsky A et al: Multivitamin/folic acid supplementation in early pregnancy reduces the prevalence of neural tube defects, *JAMA* 262:2847-2852, 1989.

127. Milunsky A et al: Predictive values, relative risks and overall benefits of high and low maternal serum alpha-fetoprotein screening in singleton pregnancies: new epidemiologic data, *Am J Obstet Gynecol* 161:291-297, 1989.

128. Mishel DR Jr et al: Initial detection of human chorionic gonadotropin in serum in normal human gestation, *Am J Obstet Gynecol* 118:990, 1974.

129. Moodley SP et al: Carbohydrate metabolism in African women with twin pregnancy, *Diabetes Care* 7:72-74, 1984.

130. Moraga FA et al: Maternal administration of glucocorticoid and thyrotropin-releasing hormone enhances fetal lung maturation in undisturbed preterm lambs, *Am J Obstet Gynecol* 171:729-734, 1994.

131. Mulinare J et al: Periconceptional use of multivitamins and the occurrence of neural tube defects, *JAMA* 260:3141-3145, 1988.

132. Murphy BEP, Silverman AY: Comparison of glucocorticoid conjugates with other indexes of fetal maturation, *Obstet Gynecol* 54:35-38, 1979.

133. Myers JL, Harrell MJ, Hill FL: Fetal maturity: biochemical analysis of amniotic fluid, *Am J Obstet Gynecol* 121:961-967, 1975.

134. Nadel AS et al: Absence of need for amniocentesis in patients with elevated levels of maternal serum alpha-fetoprotein and normal ultrasonographic examinations, *N Engl J Med* 323:557-561, 1990.

135. Naidoo L et al: Intravenous glucose tolerance tests in women with twin pregnancy, *Obstet Gynecol* 66:500, 1985.

136. National Academy of Sciences, National Research Council Food and Nutrition Board: *Recommended dietary allowances,* ed 10, Washington, D.C., 1989, author.

137. Nevin NC, Armstrong MJ: Raised alpha-fetoprotein levels in amniotic fluid and maternal serum in a triplet pregnancy in which one fetus had an omphalocele, *Br J Obstet Gynaecol* 82:826, 1975.

138. Norgaard-Pedersen B: α₁-Fetoprotein concentration in cord serum as a parameter for gestational age, *Acta Paediatr* 62:167-170, 1970.

139. Norgaard-Pedersen B: α_1-Fetoprotein concentration in cord blood from twins and from a set of quadruplets: a case of superfetatio? *Hum Hered* 26:72-80, 1976.

140. Norman RJ, Joubert SM, Marivate M: Amniotic fluid phospholipids and glucocorticoids in multiple pregnancy, *Br J Obstet Gynaecol* 90:51, 1983.

141. Norman RJ et al: Twin pregnancy as a model for studies in fetal cortisol concentrations in labour: relation to prostaglandins, prolactin and ACTH. *Br J Obstet Gynaecol* 90:1033, 1983.

142. Ohlsson A: Treatments of preterm premature rupture of the membranes: a meta-analysis, *Am J Obstet Gynecol* 160:890-906, 1989.

143. O'Sullivan JB: *Long term follow-up of gestational diabetes*. In Camerini-Davalos RA, Cole HS, editors: *Early diabetes in early life*, Third International Symposium, New York, 1975, Academic Press.

144. O'Sullivan JB et al: Gestational diabetes and perinatal mortality rate, *Am J Obstet Gynecol* 116:901, 1973.

145. Parsons M: Effect of twins: maternal, fetal, and labor, *Clin Perinatol* 15:41-53, 1988.

146. Pedersen J: *The pregnant diabetic and her newborn: problems and management*, ed 2, Baltimore, 1977, Williams & Wilkins.

147. Pretorius DH et al: Twin pregnancies in the second trimester in women in an alpha-fetoprotein screening program: sonographic evaluation and outcome, *Am J Radiol* 161:1007-1013, 1993.

148. Rawles J, Haites N: Doppler ultrasound measurement of cardiac output, *Br J Hosp Med* 31:292-297, 1984.

149. Redford DHA, Whitfield CR: Maternal serum alpha-fetoprotein in twin pregnancies uncomplicated by neural tube defect, *Am J Obstet Gynecol* 152:550-553, 1985.

150. Rhoades RA, Filler DA, Vannata B: Influence of maternal diabetes on lipid metabolism in neonatal rat lung, *Biochim Biophys Acta* 572:132, 1979.

151. Roberts MF et al: Association between maternal diabetes and the respiratory-distress syndrome in the newborn, *N Engl J Med* 294:357-360, 1976.

152. Robertson JG: Twin pregnancy: influence of early admission on fetal survival, *Obstet Gynecol* 23:854, 1964.

153. Robertson JG: Twin pregnancy: morbidity and fetal mortality, *Obstet Gynecol* 23:330, 1964.

154. Rooney SA, Canavan PM, Motoyama EK: The identification of phosphatidylglycerol in the rat, rabbit, monkey and human lung, *Biochim Biophys Acta* 360:56, 1974.

155. Rooney SA, Gross I, Warshaw JB: Thyrotropin releasing hormone stimulates surfactant secretion in the fetal rabbit, *Am Rev Respir Dis* 117:386, 1978.

156. Rovinsky JJ, Jaffin H: Cardiovascular hemodynamics in pregnancy. I. Blood and plasma volumes in multiple pregnancy, *Am J Obstet Gynecol* 93:1-15, 1965.

157. Rovinski JJ, Jaffin H: Cardiovascular hemodynamics in pregnancy, *Am J Obstet Gynecol* 95:781-786, 1966.

158. Rush RW et al: Contribution of preterm delivery to perinatal mortality, *Br Med J* 2:965-968, 1976.

159. Russ EM, Raymunt J: Influence of estrogens on total serum copper and ceruloplasmin, *Soc Exp Biol Med* 92:465, 1956.

160. Sabbagha RE, Sheikh Z, Tamura RK: Predictive value, sensitivity, and specificity of ultrasonic targeted imaging for fetal anomalies in gravid women at high risk for birth defects, *Am J Obstet Gynecol* 152:822-827, 1985.

161. Schell DL et al: Combined ultrasonography and amniocentesis for pregnant women with elevated serum alpha fetoprotein: revising the risk estimate, *J Reprod Med* 35:543-546, 1990.

162. Schneider AB, Kowalski K, Sherwood LM: *Chemical structure and biologic immunologic activity of "big" human placental lactogen*, In Pecile A, Mueller EE, editors: *Growth hormone and related peptides*, Amsterdam, 1976, Excerpta Medica.

163. Schreiber V et al: Digitalis-like biological activity and immunoreactivity in chromatographic fractions of rabbit adrenal extract, *Endocrinol Exp* 15:229-236, 1981.

164. Selbing A, Larsson L: Acetylcholinesterase activity in amniotic fluid of normal and anencephalic fetus in diamniotic twin pregnancy, *Acta Obstet Gynecol Scand* 65:93-94, 1986.

165. Selenkow HA et al: *Measurement and pathophysiologic significance of human placental lactogen*. In Pecile A, Finzi C, editors: *The Foeto-placental unit*, Amsterdam, 1969, Excerpta Medica.

166. Seppala M, Tallberg T, Ehnholm C: Studies on embryo-specific proteins: physiological characteristics of embryo-specific alpha-globulin, *Ann Med Exp Biol Fenn* 45:161-169, 1967.

167. Shilo L et al: Endogenous digoxin-like immu-

noreactivity in congestive heart failure, *Br Med J* 295:415-416, 1987.

168. Shilo L et al: Endogenous digoxin-like material is adrenal origin, *Isr J Med Sci* 23:294-295, 1987.

169. Shrivastav P et al: Secretion of atrial natriuretic peptide and digoxin-like immunoreactive substance during pregnancy, *Clin Chem* 5:977-980, 1988.

170. Sims CD, Cowan DB, Parkinson CE: The lecithin/sphingomyelin (L/S) ratio in twin pregnancies, *Br J Obstet Gynaecol* 83:447-451, 1976.

171. Spellacy WN: Human placental lactogen in high-risk pregnancy, *Clin Obstet Gynecol* 16:298, 1973.

172. Spellacy WN, Buhi WC, Birk SA: Carbohydrate metabolism in women with a twin pregnancy, *Obstet Gynecol* 55:688, 1980.

173. Spellacy WN et al: Amniotic fluid L/S ratio in twin gestation, *Obstet Gynecol* 50:68-70, 1977.

174. Sterling MK, Blackledge DG, Goodall HB: Diagnosis and management of folate deficiency in low birthweight infants, *Arch Dis Child* 54:271, 1979.

175. *Summary and recommendations of the Third International Workshop-Conference on Gestational Diabetes Mellitus*, Diabetes 40(suppl 2):197, 1991.

176. Tabsh KMA et al: Genetic amniocentesis in twin pregnancy, *Obstet Gynecol* 65:843, 1985.

177. Teramo K, Hallman M, Raivio KO: Maternal glucocorticoid in unplanned premature labor: controlled study of the effects of betamethasone phosphate on the phospholipids of the gastric aspirate and on the adrenal cortical function of the newborn infant, *Pediatr Res* 14:326-329, 1980.

178. Thomas RM: *Diabetes in pregnancy (obstetric complications)*. In Creasy RK, Resnick R, editors: *Maternal-fetal medicine, principles and practice*, Philadelphia, 1994, W.B. Saunders.

179. Thomsen JK, Fogh-Anderson N, Jaszczak P: Atrial natriuretic peptide, blood volume, aldosterone, and sodium excreation during twin pregnancy, *Acta Obstet Gynecol Scand* 73:14-20, 1994.

180. Thomsen JK, Storm TL, Thamsborg G: Increased concentration of circulating atrial natriuretic peptide during normal pregnancy, *Eur J Obstet Gynecol Reprod Biol* 27:197-201, 1988.

181. Thiery M, Dhont M, Vandekerckhove D: Serum HCG and HPL in twin pregnancies, *Acta Obstet Gynecol Scand* 56:495, 1976.

182. Tuttle S et al: Zinc and copper nutrition in human pregnancy: a longitudinal study in normal primigravidae and in primigravidae at risk of delivering a growth retarded baby. *Am J Clin Nutr* 5:1032-41, 1985.

183. Ueland K: Maternal cardiovascular dynamics. VII. Intrapartum blood volume changes. *Am J Obstet Gynecol* 126:671, 1976.

184. Valdes R Jr, Graves SW: Protein binding of endogenous digoxin immunoreactive factors in human serum and it's variation with clinical condition, *J Clin Endocrinol Metab* 60:1135-1143, 1985.

185. Valdes R Jr et al: Endogenous digoxin-like immunoreactivity in blood is increased during prolonged strenuous exercise, *Life Sci* 42:103-110, 1988.

186. Van Golde LMG: Metabolism of phospholipids in the lung. *Am Rev Respir Dis* 114:977, 1976.

187. Van der Molen HJ: Determination of plasma progesterone during pregnancy. *Clin Chim Acta* 8:943, 1963.

188. Veille JC, Morton MJ, Burry KJ: Maternal cardiovascular adaptations to twin pregnancy. *Am J Obstet Gynecol* 153:261-3, 1985.

189. Verduzco RT, Rosario R, Rigatto H: Hyaline membrane disease in twins: A 7 year review with a study on zygosity. *Am J Obstet Gynecol* 125:668, 1976.

190. Veress L, Szabo M, Toth Z, Papp Z: Relationship between placentation and maternal serum alpha-fetoprotein in twin pregnancies. *Acta Chirurgica Hungarica* 29:2;183-186, 1988.

191. Wald NJ et al: Maternal serum alpha-fetoprotein and diabetes mellitus, *Br J Obstet Gynaecol* 86:101-105, 1979.

192. Wald NJ et al: The effect of maternal weight on maternal serum alpha-fetoprotein levels, *Br J Obstet Gynaecol* 88:1094-1096, 1981.

193. Wald NJ et al: Maternal serum screening for Down's syndrome in early pregnancy, *Br Med J* 297:883-887, 1988.

194. Wald NJ et al: Maternal serum unconjugated oestriol and human chorionic gonadotrophin levels in twin pregnancies: implications for screening for Down syndrome, *Br J Obstet Gynaecol* 98:905-908, 1991.

195. Weintraub D, Rosen SW: Ectopic production of human chorionic somatomammotropin (HCS) in patients with cancer, *Clin Res* 18:375, 1970.

196. Weller PH et al: Pharyngeal lecithin/sphingo-

myelin ratios in newborn infants, *Lancet* I:12-15, 1976.

197. Wenstrom KD, Gall SA: Incidence, morbidity and mortality, and diagnosis of twin gestations, *Clin Perinatol* 15:1-10, 1988.

198. Whitehead N et al: Follow-up of elevated maternal serum alpha-fetoprotein levels: ultrasonography or amniocentesis [Letter], *Am J Obstet Gynecol* 164:1688-1689, 1991.

199. Winn HN et al: Comparison of fetal lung maturation in preterm singleton and twin pregnancies, *Am J Perinatol* 9:326-328, 1992.

200. Wolf EJ et al: A comparison of pre-discharge survival and morbidity in singleton and twin very low birth weight infants, *Obstet Gynecol* 80:436-439, 1992.

201. Wu B et al: The effect of thyroxine on the maturation of fetal rabbit lungs, *Biol Neonate* 22:161-168, 1973.

202. Yeung CY: Effects of prolonged rupture of membranes on the development of respiratory distress syndrome in twin pregnancy, *Aust Pediatr J* 18:197-199, 1982.

203. Zuelzer WW, Ogden FN: Megaloblastic anemia in infancy, *Am J Dis Infancy* 71:211, 1947.

Sonographic and Doppler Assessment

Joseph A. Spinnato

The widespread availability of diagnostic ultrasound for clinical obstetrics has dramatically altered both the scientific understanding of human twinning and its management. The advantages brought to management include: (1) earlier and more precise diagnoses of fetal number, zygosity, and chorionicity; (2) improved identification of anomalies unique to multiple pregnancy, such as acardiac or conjoined twinning and discordance for anomaly; and (3) improved identification and management of disease states unique to multiple gestation, such as "vanishing twins," discordant growth, twin reversed arterial perfusion (TRAP) syndrome, single twin demise, and twin-twin transfusion syndrome (TTS). The subsequent introduction of Doppler technology to clinical practice has further helped clinicians understand the pathophysiologic mechanisms of various twin disease states, and although its utility requires further definition and fine tuning, Doppler ultrasound may further enhance the care of twin gestations. This chapter explores the use of ultrasound and Doppler technology for the diagnosis and management of twin gestation.

Diagnosis

Up to 14% of twin gestations are undiagnosed before labor and delivery.[25,83] Ultrasound evaluation reduces the failed diagnosis rate to less than 5%.[25,47,83] Ewigman, LeFevre, and Hesser[47] evaluated 915 of 2171 pregnant patients who had no indication for ultrasound at their first prenatal visit and randomly assigned them to receive either a single routine screening ultrasound or usual prenatal care. Both sets of twins were detected in the screened group. In the usual-care group, five of seven pairs of twins (71%) were diagnosed by 24 weeks' gestation. LeFevre et al.,[83] in a randomized clinical trial of 15,530 women that was designed to test the hypothesis that screening ultrasonography in low-risk pregnancies would improve perinatal outcome (RADIUS study), evaluated 68 multiple pregnancies in the routinely screened group and 61 multiple pregnancies in the control group. All but one noncompliant patient in the screened group had the diagnosis of multiple pregnancy established before 26 weeks' gestation. In contrast, 23 women (37%) with multiple gestations in the control group were not identified by ultrasonography until after 26 weeks. Eight women had no scan before the delivery admission. Perrson and Kullander[108] evaluated 43,000 routine ultrasound examinations performed on 22,400 pregnant women over 10 years. There were 249 multiple gestations detected in the screening program. The early examination detected 98% of the twin pregnancies with no false positive results, but multiple pregnancies were overlooked in 2% of the first examinations. The authors speculated that the treatment after early detection of twin pregnancies had a marked effect on perinatal mortality and morbidity, prematurity, and length of newborn stay when compared with the twins managed in the preceding 5 years when routine ultrasound was not employed. This potential for improved twin pregnancy outcomes afforded by earlier detection lends support to routine ultrasound screening.

In clinical practices that do not employ routine obstetric ultrasound screening, a high clinical index of suspicion is necessary to detect multiple gestation. In the well-dated pregnancy, suspicion begins with the history. A history of assisted reproduction, particularly with techniques known to be associated with the ovulation of multiple ova such as clomiphene citrate or gonadotropin stimulation with or without in vitro fertilization (IVF), ultrasound determination of fetal number is recommended. The incidence of multiple gestations after clomiphene therapy is 5% to 10%, and it is even higher when gonadotropins are used. A personal or family history of twinning should prompt ultrasound evaluation, particularly when the history is accompanied by suggestive clinical signs such as size greater than expected for menstrual dates or elevated maternal serum alpha-fetoprotein (MSAFP) levels. In situations where uterine size does not match menstrual dates or when the congruency of size and dates cannot be accurately assessed because of unknown last menses, irregular menses, maternal obesity, uterine leiomyomata, uterine duplication, late prenatal care, or any other factor that interferes with the assessment of uterine size or gestational age, liberal use of ultrasound is urged to both confirm gestational age and exclude multiple gestation.

When MSAFP is used as a clinical screen for incorrect gestational age or multiple gestation, caution is necessary. The *ACOG Technical Bulletin*[2] notes that MSAFP levels are elevated in multiple gestations and comments that with expanded screening programs, more twin gestations will be identified earlier. Johnson et al.[74] measured MSAFP concentration at 14 to

20 weeks' gestation in 138 twin pregnancies. Two pregnancies were discordant for open fetal defects (one anencephaly, one gastroschisis). The median MSAFP value in the remaining 136 twin pregnancies paralleled a curve 2.5 times the median curve for singleton pregnancies over the gestational range studied. Theoretically, MSAFP screening would have detected 56.5% of the twins in this study when a cut-off level of 2.5 multiples of the median (MOM) was used. Clearly, 44% of twin gestations would have been missed if an MSAFP value greater than 2.5 MOM had been relied on for twin diagnosis. Parenthetically, in this study both anomalies associated with an elevated MSAFP level occurred in pregnancies where the MSAFP value was greater than 5 MOM. The threshold for abnormal MSAFP levels in twin gestations is not as well studied as it is in singleton gestations, and a commonly used cut-off of 4 MOM for elevated MSAFP levels in known twin gestations may be associated with a higher false positive rate than is noted for the 2.5 MOM threshold used in singleton gestations.

If multiple gestation is suspected on the basis of clinical examination, an ultrasound evaluation should be performed. Multiple gestational sacs can be visualized by endovaginal imaging as early as 4 to 5 weeks' gestation, with defined fetal poles and cardiac activity as early as 5 to 6 weeks. The gestational sac can be imaged as early as 4 weeks and 2 to 3 days. By 4½ to 5 weeks the yolk sac can be imaged, and by 5 weeks the embryo is seen. The amnion is the last structure to be visualized. The earliest identification of the amnion is at 6 to 6½ weeks' gestation. Before this time the amnion snugly surrounds the embryo and contains a small amount of amniotic fluid. Detection of the amnion is difficult until about 7½ to 8 weeks, when it separates from the fetal body and becomes quite easy to image. If the first ultrasound evaluation of a twin pregnancy is performed before 8 weeks, a repeat evaluation is suggested to clarify the amniotic and chorionic type (see the discussion of chorionicity in Chapter 2).

A note of caution is necessary if a significant difference in size of first-trimester twin fetuses is noted. Weissman et al.[148] identified five twin pairs where the first-trimester difference in gestational age between the two was 5 or more days discordant, representing a 19.5% to 50% difference in the crown-rump lengths (CRLs). In each of the five, the smaller twin had significant congenital anomaly. Unfortunately the predictive values of this finding were not calculated by the authors. It is advisable to reevaluate twins at 15 to 20 weeks' gestation if such discordant CRLs are identified.

Vanishing Twin

Most reports suggest that approximately 1.2% to 1.6% of pregnancies delivered after 20 weeks' gestation are twin gestations. A recent report by Luke,[89] using data from the National Center for Health Statistics, noted a dramatic recent increase in the incidence of twin gestations, which accounted for 2.3% of all births in 1990. However, reports over the last 20 years of clinical ultrasound use have suggested that there is a higher actual incidence of twins that accounts for up to 5% of all pregnancies.[34,81,86,143] These reports also suggest that as many as 75% of these early twin gestations go on to lose one of the fetuses and result in the subsequent delivery of a singleton.* However, of these reported losses, many occurred in early pregnancy before the demonstration of fetal cardiac activity. Often the diagnosis of twins was based solely on sonographic visualization of two sac-like intrauterine fluid collections. Under close scrutiny, it is likely that many of the "second sacs" were fluid collections adjacent to a single gestational sac. The true rate of postconceptional loss in multiple gestations is not known.

Landy et al.[81] reviewed the sonographic findings of 1000 pregnancies with viable gestations in the first trimester and reported a minimum incidence of twinning of 3.29%. Of these, 21.2% demonstrated the vanishing twin phenomenon, often with associated bleeding. The incidence of first-trimester bleeding of the 54 patients in this study was 18.5%, versus only 7.2% among the remaining 946 patients. First-trimester bleeding may be the result of a vanishing twin more often than currently is realized.

The prognosis for the remaining fetus was good and paralleled that expected for singletons. An additional 2.1% of pregnancies possibly had vanishing twins (with less confidence that the second sac represented twinning), with as high as a 5.4% incidence of twins and a vanishing twin rate of 52%. The authors note that false interpretation of either physiologic conditions associated with pregnancy (including the amniotic cavity, chorionic sac, extraembryonic coelom, and yolk sac) or technical ultrasound artifacts can incorrectly imply the presence of an additional

gestational sac on an early sonogram. Other physiologic conditions with the potential for overdiagnosis of multiple gestation include an intrauterine collection of blood at the site of the trophoblast in a singleton pregnancy or in an abnormally progressing pregnancy, hydropic change in chorionic villi, or a decidual reaction in the second horn of a bicornuate uterus.

Kelly et al.[76] described and compared the rate of rise of human chorionic gonadotropin (hCG) in vanishing twin and normal twin pregnancies during the first trimester. Forty patients who conceived after treatment of infertility and who had two gestational sacs on ultrasound examination were included in the study after the following criteria were met: (1) both sacs progressed to exhibit a fetal pole, and (2) the day of LH surge or the day of hCG administration was known. The rate of rise of hCG was slower in vanishing twin pregnancies than in normally progressing twin gestations for the entire period studied. A vanishing twin occurred in one third of the twin pregnancies. Forty-six percent of these losses occurred after fetal heart activity had been established. The lower slope of rise of hCG was already notable in the earliest days of its detection. The authors concluded that in pregnancies destined for vanishing twins, the abnormality is present from the time of implantation and that it is likely that vanishing twin pregnancies represent a part of a spectrum of gestational losses resulting from embryonic causes.

Jauniaux et al.[72] studied the pathologic findings in placentas from 10 multiple gestations complicated by the vanishing twin phenomenon. Postpartum evidence of the vanishing twin phenomenon was found in five cases. Morphologically, the lesions

*References 25, 34, 66, 81, 86, 119, 143

were characterized by well-delineated plaques of perivillous fibrin deposition that occasionally included embryonic remnants. They comment that this focal degenerative change of the placental mass, which also exists in about 25% of placentas from uncomplicated term pregnancies, may be the only clue to the disappearance of one conceptus.

Rudnicki, Vejerslev, and Junge[124] caution that postconceptional nondisjunction, leading to tetraploidy in one twin conceptus, may explain demise in early pregnancy. Tetraploidy observed by chorionic villus sampling (CVS) must be confirmed by amniocentesis before interruption of the pregnancy is considered. The vanishing twin phenomenon may be the explanation for discordance between clinical findings or amniocentesis with CVS for fetal gender or aneuploidy, and it should be considered.

Benson, Doubilet, and Laks[10] conducted a prospective study to assess pregnancy outcome after a first-trimester ultrasound examination demonstrated intrauterine twins with heart beats. The study population included 68 cases of twin gestations, in which a first-trimester scan demonstrated two heart beats. Among all 68 cases, 54 (79%) delivered viable twins, 8 (12%) delivered one infant, and 6 (9%) delivered none. The outcome in dichorionic gestations (83% delivered twins, 12% singletons, and 5% none) was significantly better than in monochorionic gestations (56%, 11%, and 33%, respectively). In this study the vanishing twin phenomenon was not observed if the two fetal hearts were beating after 8 weeks' gestation. By design this study underestimates the true risk of the vanishing twin phenomenon but provides useful information regarding the cardiac positive twin gestation. The strict criteria used by Landy et al.[81] that indicated a 21% rate of vanishing twins might similarly underestimate the true incidence of vanishing twins, which may approach 50%.

Zygosity, Chorionicity, and Amnionicity

Dizygotic twins result from the fertilization of separate ova produced in the same cycle. Monozygotic twins result from the subsequent cleavage of a single fertilized ovum. Among dizygotic conceptions, the incidence of male and female fetuses is random and equal. Using the Hardy-Weinberg rule, (male [M] + female [F]) = 1, $(M + F)^2 = 1$, and $(MM + 2MF + FF) = 1$. Therefore among dizygotic twins, the incidence of like-sex twins (MM plus FF) equals the incidence of unlike-sex twins (MF), approximating 50%. Among all twins, the incidence of monozygotic twins (that are always of like sex) equals the excess of like-sex twins noted above 50%. Since approximately 65% of twins are of like sex, 35% of twins are of unlike sex, approximately 30% of twins are monozygotic (65% minus 35%), and 70% are dizygotic.

Dizygotic twins are always dichorionic-diamniotic—each twin is contained within its own amnion and chorion (outermost layer)—and have placentae that may be entirely separate or fused to varying degrees (Figure 6-1). Whereas fusion may or may not be present, the vascular systems of the two placentae remain separate. Approximately 30% of monozygotic pregnancies are also dichorionic-diamniotic and share with dizygotic twins the unique in-

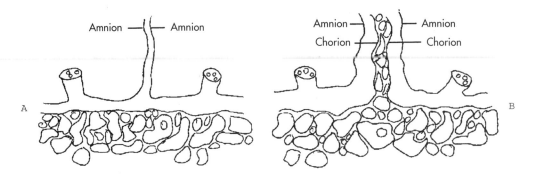

FIGURE 6-1   Artistic rendering of A, monochorionic-diamniotic versus B, dichorionic-diamniotic placentation. Note the trophoblast between the chorion membranes.

tegrity of each fetus' circulation. As a consequence, dichorionic-diamniotic twinning accounts for approximately 79% of twins. Because of the discrete fetal circulations among dichorionic-diamniotic twins, there are two conditions known to uniquely occur in twin gestations (TRAP and TTS) that do not occur in dichorionic-diamniotic twins. If dichorionic-diamniotic twinning can be known with confidence, the pregnancy can be managed without regard for these diagnoses. For example, when a single twin's demise occurs, conservative management schemes need not include a concern for fetal periventricular leukomalacia or dissemination intravascular coagulation in the surviving twin, as seen with TRAP syndrome. Similarly, when discordant fetal growth or the discordant presence of hydramnios or oligohydramnios occurs in a dichorionic-diamniotic gestation, evaluation can focus on discordant fetal genetics, nutrition (placentation), or anomaly without regard for TTS in the differential diagnosis. This determination is also of importance if pregnancy reduction of twins or higher-order multiple fetuses is considered (discussed in Part 4 of this chapter).

Chorionicity is also important when amniotic fluid analysis is performed for elevated MSAFP levels or suspected discordance for fetal anomaly associated with elevated amniotic fluid AFP (AFAFP) or acetylcholinesterase (AChE) in a twin gestation. Stiller et al.[135] evaluated placental membrane anatomy after delivery in 65 twin pregnancies undergoing genetic amniocentesis with AFAFP and AChE determinations when indicated. Each twin in the 57 uncomplicated twin pregnancies was found to have an AFAFP concentration similar to that of singletons at an equivalent gestational age. Eight twin pregnancies were found to be discordant for fetal anomalies associated with an elevated AFAFP and AChE level. The AFAFP concentration in the unaffected fetus in these eight cases was found to be dependent on placental membrane structure. Of the five discordant twin pregnancies with dichorionic-diamniotic placentas, all unaffected twins demonstrated an AFAFP concentration within the normal range for gestational age and a normal

AChE level. In three twin pairs with monochorionic-diamniotic placentas, the unaffected twin member had significantly elevated AFAFP and AChE levels, which suggested diffusion of AFAFP and AChE through the amnion-amnion interface.

Monozygotic twins do have at least twice the risk of fetal anomaly when compared with dizygotic twins. The perinatal mortality risk of monozygotic twins is 2 to 3 times higher; much of this can be explained by the complications of monochorionicity. However, for most clinical concerns the knowledge of chorionicity is of greater importance than is knowledge of zygosity. Therefore it is clinically prudent to attempt to determine the probability of monochorionicity early in a twin gestation. Such determinations begin with the history and an awareness that most gestations are dichorionic. Twinning that is a consequence of assisted reproductive technologies (ART), whether ovulation induction (OI) with clomiphene citrate, gonadotropin, or another technique, is dizygotic in most instances (and therefore dichorionic). However, it should be noted that there is no reason why monozygotic twinning cannot occur after in vitro fertilization. The incidence of this event has not been reported.

Twins that are discordant for gender are always dizygotic and therefore always dichorionic. If fetal gender is determined ultrasonographically in the second or third trimester to be discordant, the pregnancy is assured to be dichorionic. Reece et al.[113] prospectively determined fetal gender by ultrasonography in 115 patients with singleton pregnancies between 16 and 20 weeks of gestation. The rate of visualization of the fetal external genitalia was 83.5%. The accuracy rate for gender de-termination was 90% for males and 100% for females, with an overall rate of prediction of 92.7%. Watson[145] determined the accuracy of fetal gender determination with ultrasound at 13 to 19 weeks' gestation. A determination could be made in 91/100 women. The overall accuracy of gender prediction was 92.3%; for males it was 89.5%, and for females it was 97.1%. Significantly fewer errors were noted as the clinician's experience with gender identification increased. Natsuyama[102] evaluated 1879 pregnant women between 12 and 40 weeks of gestation by obtaining transverse, frontal, and sagittal sections of the fetal lower pelvic region. At 20 weeks' gestation, 96.5% (109/113) of male fetuses and 93.4% (114/122) of female fetuses were correctly identified. The success rate for gender identification among twin gestations has not been specifically reported, but it is reasonable to assume that the accuracy would be similar to that reported for singleton gestations. The success rates in the second trimester reported by these and other investigators suggest that dichorionicity can be assured among the 35% of twins that are discordant for sex.[12,109]

Many authors have used several different ultrasonographic findings in the second and third trimesters to determine the placentation (monochorionic versus dichorionic) present in twin pregnancies. These include the visualization of separate placentae,[93] the thickness of the intervening membranes,[6,68,140,150] the identification of separate layers in the dividing membranes,[36] and the imaging of a triangular projection of placental tissue beyond the chorionic surface at the origin of the dividing membrane as evidence of dichorionicity.[11,48] Finberg[48] referred to this sign as the "twin peak sign" (Figure 6-2) and

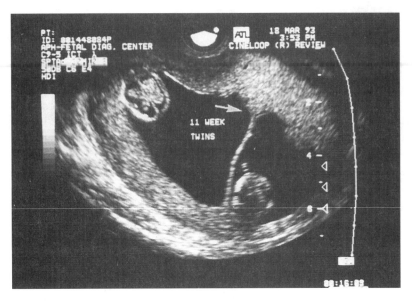

FIGURE 6-2   The "twin peak" sign of a first trimester monochorionic-diamniotic twin gestation.

was able to identify dichorionicity with this sign in the 15 twin pregnancies that he scanned between 14 and 35 weeks. Bessis and Papiernik[11] called this projection the "lambda sign" and correctly predicted 20/24 dichorionic pregnancies. The presence of the lambda sign or the twin peak sign indicates that the gestation is dichorionic, but the absence of this sign does not exclude dichorionicity. Using transabdominal scanning Kurtz et al.[79] examined 105 twin pregnancies in the first trimester. By assessing thickness of the membranes only (greater than 2 mm), they achieved a 92% correct diagnosis of dichorionic-diamniotic pregnancies (Figure 6-3). When determinations of membrane thickness and placental site were combined, the detection rate increased to 96%. However, the lambda sign was not observed often (7% of their cases). Monochorionicity was correctly diagnosed in 88% of the cases. Monteagudo, Timor-Tritsch, and Sharma[100] determined the chorionic and amniotic types in multiple pregnancies with transvaginal ultrasonography at weeks' or earlier gestation. At or before 14 weeks' gestation, 212 multiple pregnancies were scanned transvaginally. In the 43 patients with both ultrasonographic and pathologic assessment, there were 40 twin pregnancies, five of which were the monochorionic-diamniotic type. In all 43 patients, transvaginal ultrasonography correctly predicted the chorionic and amniotic type as determined by the pathologic findings. The authors conclude that transvaginal ultrasonography at 14 weeks or less can easily and accurately determine the chorionic and amniotic type in multiple pregnancies. If they observed a wedge-shaped junction, they considered that to be an indication of the fusion of two chorionic membranes (dichorionic). If a T-shaped junction was seen, it was regarded as the fusion of two amniotic membranes and more likely to be indicative of monochorionicity.

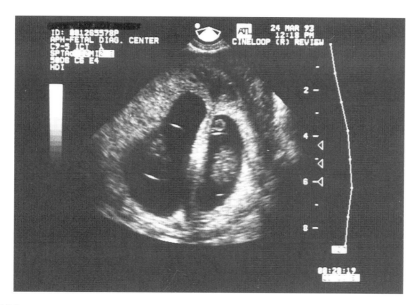

FIGURE 6-3   Thickened dividing membrane of a dichorionic-diamniotic twin gestation. Note the small amount of fluid in the amniotic space.

Later in gestation, a subjectively thin wisp-like membrane is again associated with monochorionicity (Figures 6-4 and 6-5). With optimal transducer resolution, the intervening membrane can occasionally be identified to contain three or four separate layers, which identifies dichorionicity reliably (Figure 6-6).

Monoamniotic Twinning

Monochorionic-monoamniotic twins—in which both fetuses are in the same amniotic sac—account for 1% to 2% of all twins. They are always monozygotic. Conjoined twins are of this type. Sonographic diagnosis of monoamniotic twinning is less certain in most cases than for diamniotic twins. Identification of a membrane separating the fetuses excludes this diagnosis reliably. Unfortunately, failing to observe a membrane does not reliably establish the diagnosis. It is important to exclude mono-

amnionicity before the third trimester, when fetal crowding might obscure the membrane. As a consequence of fetal movement, entanglement of the umbilical cords is a common occurrence and has been associated with as much as a 50% to 71% risk of perinatal death. McLeod and McCoy[96] reported an unusual cord complication at the time of delivery of monoamniotic twins. The cord of the second twin presented as a nuchal cord to the first twin and was unknowingly divided at the time of delivery of the first twin. An awareness of monoamnionicity and the potential for this occurrence could prevent mishaps.

Several studies have shown that lack of sonographic visualization of a membrane is not predictive of monoamnionicity on its own.[6,13,68,93,140] Rodis et al.[121] note that before the diagnosis of monoamniotic twins can be entertained, the following criteria must be fulfilled: (1) no dividing am-

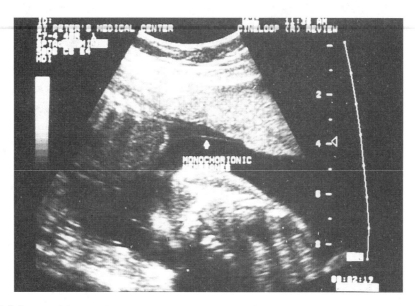

FIGURE 6-4   Wisp-like membrane noted in the second trimester of a monochorionic-diamniotic gestation.

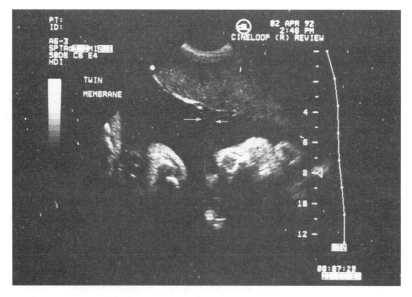

FIGURE 6-5   Separation of each amnion is noted at the placental surface of a monochorionic-diamniotic twin gestation where the twin peak sign is not identified.

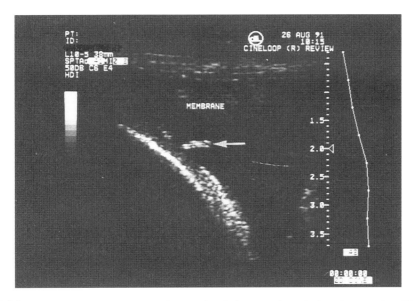

FIGURE 6-6   Section of a trilaminar membrane of a dichorionic-diamniotic twin gestation. The two layers of the chorion appear fused.

nionic membrane should be visualized, (2) only one placenta should be seen, (3) both fetuses must have the same sex, (4) the fetuses must have adequate amniotic fluid surrounding them, and (5) both fetuses must move freely within the uterine cavity. They emphasize this last point to avoid the pitfall encountered in some diamniotic pregnancies in which oligohydramnios in one sac causes the membrane to be plastered against the fetus, thus making it difficult to visualize. This twin is usually pressed against the uterine wall because of hydramnios or oligohydramnios induced by TTS or fetal anomaly causing hydramnios in one sac with compression of the other sac. They recommend three consecutive ultrasound examinations to confirm the diagnosis when monoamniotic twinning is suspected. It should be noted that because of the rarity of monochorionic-monoamniotic twins, none of the reported techniques have been as-

sessed for their accuracy (positive and negative predictive values). Whether Rodis' criteria alone suffice to reliably diagnose monochorionic-monoamniotic twins is unknown, but the attractiveness lies in the lack of an invasive and potentially morbid component.

Beyond the minimal criteria set by Rodis et al., documentation that both umbilical cords extend from the fetuses into a common tangled set of looped cords provides definite evidence of monoamnionicity, but the rate of detecting this finding has not been prospectively studied.[103,139] Fetal crowding may obscure segments of the cords, preventing continuous visualization of the cords from each fetus into the clump of cord loops. Belfort et al.[7] used color-flow Doppler to study the umbilical cords in three cases suspected to be monoamniotic because of apparent cord entanglement. In each case, they described "branching" of the umbilical artery within the entanglement and evidence of two different heart rates in the two segments of the branch. Kofinas, Penry, and Hatjis[77] noted an unusual flow velocity waveform pattern in a case of cord entanglement. The umbilical artery systolic to diastolic (S/D) ratio was abnormally high (greater than the ninety-fifth percentile for gestation), and diastolic notching was present. The umbilical vein flow velocity waveform was pulsatile, and the flow was absent during the diastolic phase of the cardiac cycle.

Although monoamniotic twinning has been diagnosed in the first trimester by visualizing both fetuses in the same sac, the reliability of this sign has not been studied and false positive diagnoses may occur before 7 to 8 weeks' gestation, when the amnion may not be visualized because of its close proximity to the fetus.[95]

Sequential amniocentesis with dye has been employed when monochorionic-monoamniotic twins were suspected, with failure to obtain dye-free amniotic fluid when sampling near the opposite fetus, thus implying monoamnionicity.[138] Carlson and Nageotte[23] used a technique of bubble dispersion (amniocentesis with withdrawal of 5 to 7 ml of amniotic fluid that is agitated with 2 to 3 cc of air and reinjected) to visualize an intervening membrane between twins. This technique allows the clinician to avoid a second amniocentesis and ionizing radiation.

Amniography with plain radiography has been used to detect swallowed contrast agent in the intestines of both twins, successfully diagnosing monoamniotic twins.[82] Finberg and Clewell[49] suggested that if a contrast-enhanced radiographic study is to be used, computerized tomography (CT) has several advantages over plain radiography for this task. With CT, a lower dose of contrast agent is needed. The selected CT planes reduce overall fetal radiation dose. They note that 1 ml of methylglucamine diatrizoate (or an equivalent water-soluble iodinated contrast agent) per 100 ml of anticipated amniotic volume provides diagnostic levels of amniotic fluid opacification. The normal fetus swallows often, and contrast medium can be seen in the stomach within 30 minutes by the 16th gestational week. Finberg and Clewell caution that visualization of a fluid-containing stomach before the test in each twin is necessary to exclude a false negative diagnosis from esophageal obstruction or swallowing dysfunction.

Pseudomonoamniotic Twins

Pseudomonoamniotic twins have been described, wherein the dividing membrane in diamniotic twins has been disrupted either spontaneously or by amniocentesis or funipuncture.[55,97] Its incidence is unknown. Megory et al.[97] described a single case following-up amniocentesis and funipuncture that traversed the dividing membrane. At delivery, cord entanglement was noted. They suggested that whenever possible, clinicians using techniques of amniocentesis and funipuncture should avoid traversing the dividing membrane. Gilbert et al.[55] reported eight cases of intrauterine rupture of the dividing membranes in diamniotic twin gestations. In only one case was iatrogenic trauma the cause. Possible alternative causes include fetal trauma to the dividing membranes, infection, and developmental disturbances. They suggest that intrauterine rupture of diamniotic twin membranes carries a perinatal mortality consistent with that of true monoamniotic gestations and that this entity may in fact be more common than previously thought. They note that a suspected monoamniotic gestation cannot be ruled out by the historic presence of a dividing membrane on previous ultrasound examination. Pseudo-monoamniotic twins may have a similar risk of cord entanglement, as do true monoamniotic twins. Prenatal disruption of the dividing membrane of a diamniotic twin gestation may be associated with amniotic band syndrome.[87]

FETOPLACENTAL ANOMALIES ASSOCIATED WITH TWINNING

The scope of this chapter does not include a discussion of all of the fetoplacental anomalies that could plague a twin gestation. Clearly, the full range of anomalies noted antenatally in singleton gestations may occur in one or both twins. Readers are encouraged to consult other texts for this information. Allen et al.[1] evaluated whether serial ultrasonographic examinations with basic anatomic surveys provide an adequate screen for congenital abnormalities that are more common in twins. Prenatal sonograms and neonatal examinations for 314 twins (157 pairs) were compared. Of those, 33 twins (9.5%) had 40 anomalies; 28 (9%) were major, and 12 (4%) were minor. Thirty-nine percent of all major anomalies, 55% of noncardiac major anomalies, but none of the cardiac lesions were identified. They concluded that serial prenatal ultrasonographic examinations are useful in detecting noncardiac anomalies for which twins are at increased risk, but the four-chamber view was not an adequate screen for the cardiac malformations of twins. Clearly, prenatal

ultrasound assessment of twin gestations for anomalies, although far from perfect, is commonly performed.

There are several fetoplacental abnormalities that occur more often or exclusively in multiple gestations. These include conjoined twins, acardiac twin, velamentous insertion of the umbilical cord (occurs more often), TRAP, and TTS. The latter two conditions are included to permit a discussion of the ultrasound findings resulting from them.

Conjoined Twins

Conjoined twins are a variant form of monozygotic, monoamniotic twins that are the result of incomplete division of the embryonic disk occurring 13 to 15 days after conception. This rare condition occurs in approximately 1/100,000 pregnancies and approximately 1/1500 twin gestations. A wide range and type of abnormalities have been described (Figure 6-7), each with varying location, severity of attachment, and amount of organ sharing. At the extreme of organ sharing, the "parasitic" twin is only partially developed and may appear, for example, as excess extruded lower extremities from the complete twin. The more commonly reported types are those joined at the chest (thoracopagus), head (craniopagus), and between the xiphoid and umbilicus (omphalopagus) (Figures 6-8 and 6-9).

The prenatal diagnosis of conjoined twins requires a high index of suspicion. In late gestation, when fetal crowding and a decreased relative amount of amniotic fluid is present, the diagnosis is more difficult. Recently, the first trimester identification of conjoined twins was reported.[92] More commonly, second trimester identi-

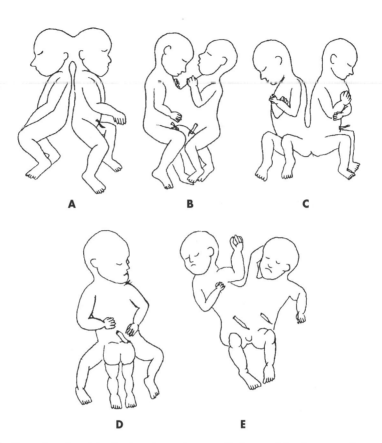

FIGURE 6-7   Examples of conjoined twins: A, craniopagus, B, thoracoabdominopagus, C, pygopagus, D, dipygus, E, dicephalus.

fication occurs.[141] Because of the nature of the attachment of most conjoined twins, both are likely to assume the same position (for example, vertex-vertex, breech-breech, or transverse-transverse). Exceptions to this are more likely when the point of attachment is close to the fetal poles (caudally or cranially). However, several years ago the possibility of thoracopagus twins first presenting with ruptured membranes, in labor in a vertex-breech presentation with 180-degree torsion at the site of attachment, was considered but not diagnosed.

When evaluating conjoined twins, the

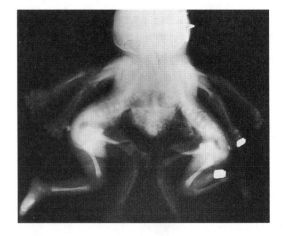

FIGURE 6-8   Radiographic image of conjoined twins.

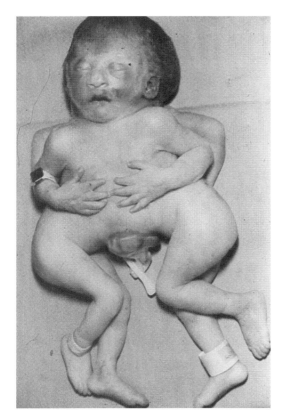

FIGURE 6-9   Postmortem appearance of conjoined twins from Figure 6-8.

process for determining chorionicity leads to a failure to identify an intervening amniotic membrane. When monoamniotic twins are suspected, careful scanning along the longitudinal plane of proximity of the two fetuses is necessary to ensure separation. With fetal crowding in late gestation or after amniorrhexis, this determination can be difficult.

Once conjoined twins are identified, it is important to identify the point and extent of attachment and the degree, if any, of organ sharing. The classification of conjoined twins ranges from hopeless sharing of anomalous vital organs (particularly the heart and great vessels) to twins that are simply attached and have an excellent prognosis for dual intact survival. Both twins should have a complete anatomic survey. As monozygotic twins, the general incidence of anomalies not limited to the point of attachment is increased. Careful sonographic evaluation at the point of attachment may be enhanced by magnetic resonance imaging (MRI) that provides additional anatomically precise clinical data.[141] This may be particularly true for thoracopagus or omphalopagus, where the degree of organ sharing may be difficult to determine. Echocardiographic evaluation is extremely important when sharing of the heart and great vessels is suspected. Both the hearts and great vessels may be completely duplicated, incompletely duplicated, completely shared, or anomalous. Saunders et al.[126] reported four cases of thoracoabdominally conjoined twins where careful echocardiography was performed. The presence and extent of cardiac conjunction was correctly determined in each case, but the major associated cardiac defects with important features that tended to worsen prognosis were inconsistently detected and missed in three cases. They nonetheless conclude that the ability to determine the status of the cardiovascular system prenatally in most cases of conjoined twins should facilitate management. Color Doppler evaluation of the cardiac chambers and particularly the great vessels is important to establish the degree of anomaly and sharing. The integrity of each fetal diaphragm is an important confounder to survival and should be carefully assessed. The general prognosis for thoracopagus is poor, and accurate antenatal determination of the extent of disease assists difficult management decisions.

Acardiac Twinning and the TRAP Sequence

An acardiac twin is a monozygotic twin whose development is sustained, despite the absence of a cranium, thorax, or heart (Figure 6-10), by arterial perfusion from its normal twin. This is possible because of the TRAP sequence that occurs via artery-to-artery anastomoses within the monochorionic placenta that nourishes the acardiac twin. Umbilical Doppler evaluation has identified reversed arterial blood flow within the umbilical artery as early as the first trimester.[129,136,154] Crade, Nageotte, and MacKenzie[33] used color Doppler sonography to demonstrate retrograde arterial flow toward each iliac artery of an acardiac fetus. Pulsed Doppler sampling demonstrated an arterial waveform but failed to identify a fetal abdominal aorta, inferior vena cava, or umbilical vein within the abdomen that could carry blood back toward the umbilical cord insertion. The authors suggested that a more direct pelvic-to-umbilical vein route exists for venous return within an acardiac fetus. Although this blood flow is adequate to promote and sustain the development and growth of the abdomen and lower extremities of the acardiac twin, it is apparently inadequate, or for whatever unknown reasons, unable to promote further growth.

Moore, Gale, and Benirschke[101] reported the perinatal outcomes of 49 pregnancies complicated by acardiac twinning. Invasive therapy was limited to therapeutic amniocentesis in four pregnancies. The overall perinatal mortality rate was 55% and was primarily associated with prematurity. Mean (±standard deviation [SD])

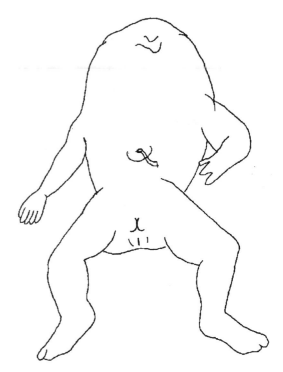

FIGURE 6-10   Artistic rendering of an acardiac twin.

gestational age at delivery was 29 ± 7.3 weeks, with a mean (±SD) normal twin weight of 1378 ± 1047 gm. The weight of acardiac twins averaged 651 ± 571 gm. Of the pregnancies with potentially viable fetuses, 12% ended in stillbirth of the normal (pump) twin. Five pump twins died in the neonatal period, resulting in the survival of only 24 infants (50%). Hydramnios was a major maternal complication (40%) and often associated with preterm labor and congestive heart failure of the pump twin. The authors suggested that pharmacologic treatment of the pump twin or surgical interruption of acardiac umbilical flow may alter the prognosis in selective cases. Clearly, the excess demand on the pump twin's heart caused by maintaining blood flow to the acardiac twin threatens its survival.

Occlusion of the umbilical arterial circulation to an acardiac fetus has been successfully achieved through the use of a thrombogenic coil inserted either around or into the umbilical artery under direct ultrasonic guidance.[64,110] Successful endoscopic laser coagulation of the umbilical cord in two of four acardiac twins has been reported.[144] Operative surgical ligation of the umbilical cord has also been described.[50] Cox et al.[32] described a case of spontaneous cessation of blood flow to an acardiac fetus that occurred gradually over time in the late second and early third trimester with eventual cessation of flow at 34 weeks' gestation. The surviving twin was delivered at 39 weeks without signs of cardiac decompensation. Torsion of the umbilical cord secondary to movement of the acardiac twin was identified as the cause. The authors suggested that whereas attempts to occlude reverse arterial flow to an acardiac fetus may be justified in the preterm pregnancy that shows clear evidence of cardiac decompensation in the pump twin, cases with reduced or absent flow to the acardiac twin and no evidence of cardiac decompensation in the pump twin, do not need in utero surgical intervention.

Chitkara et al.[29] reported the selective termination of an anomalous fetus during the second trimester in 17 pregnancies in which one twin in each pregnancy was diagnosed to be anomalous. The affected twin had a chromosomal aneuploidy in 14 cases, a neural tube defect (NTD) in two cases, and an inborn error of metabolism in one case. However, their primary technique was intracardiac injection of potassium chloride (KCl). This technique is not applicable to the acardiac twin. Most of the perinatal deaths reported for normal twins appear avoidable by interrupting blood flow to acardiac twins by techniques to occlude their umbilical cords. Continued experience with such techniques is needed. Although TRAP complicated by hydramnios has been treated by maternal administration of indomethacin, this management awaits decompensation of the pump twin.[3]

Although the TRAP sequence has been reported as a unique occurrence of acardiac twinning, a condition similar to it may occur with the demise of one monochorionic twin in cases of TTS. Jou et al.[75] reported sudden development of fetal distress in the recipient twin following the spontaneous demise of the pump twin. Despite absent cardiac activity in the donor twin, reverse arterial pulsation was detected in its umbilical cord. Fetal distress may have been the result of sudden hypotension and hypoperfusion induced by the acute reversal of blood flow in its placental artery-to-artery anastomoses. Pathologic evidence to support the possibility of acute reversed twin-twin transfusion had been previously reported by Bendon and Siddiqi.[8] It appears likely that should the cardiac activity of either twin be interrupted spontaneously or by pharmacologic intervention, sudden hypotension may occur in the other twin because of the loss of arterial resistance provided by the opposing cardiac activity.

TTS and the "Stuck Twin"

TTS is a well-described condition that occurs only in monochorionic monozygotic twins, wherein blood is exchanged between fetuses via vascular anastomoses within the placenta that result in a net blood flow from one twin to the other, creating a donor twin and a recipient twin.* Approximately 15% of monochorionic twins are afflicted, representing 4% to 5% of all twins. Its occurrence may be underreported because of the minimal abnormalities present in milder cases. At its extreme, the donor twin is anemic (at least a 5-gm difference in hemoglobin from its twin), hypovolemic, growth retarded, 20% or more discordant in weight to the recipient twin, oliguric, and virtually devoid of amniotic fluid. The recipient is plethoric and hypervolemic, can be hydropic, and produces large quantities of amniotic fluid secondary to polyuria. This subset of TTS with oligohydramnios or hydramnios gives rise to the "stuck twin" appearance, wherein the donor twin appears plastered to the uterine wall. This often creates an inability to visualize its amniotic membrane and is in stark contrast to the recipient twin, who moves freely in a large amniotic fluid space. Without cautious examination and an awareness of the condition, these pregnancies can be mistaken for monoamniotic twins. A key to the differentiation is the fixed position against the uterine wall of the stuck donor twin. In monoamniotic twinning, both fetuses' movements are largely unimpeded. Less extreme cases of TTS do exist,[22] and in all probability represent cases of vascular anastomoses with lower net blood transfer. In these cases the pronounced differences between twins (hemoglobin, discordant weight, and amniotic fluid volume) may

not be observed, and outcomes may be more favorable than with more severe cases.

Vascular anastomoses between the placental circulations of both twins occur in most, if not all, monochorionic gestations. These can be vein-to-vein or artery-to-artery anastomoses. If blood exchange occurs in such cases, it is relatively balanced and is not be expected to show a net change of the individual twins' blood volume or hemoglobin concentration. However, if the anastomoses that occur are artery-to-vein anastomoses, a unidirectional transfer of blood occurs. DeLia and Cruikshank,[38] who have pursued a surgical solution to TTS involving fetoscopically directed laser ablation of the anastomoses, studied the chorion vasculature of fresh monochorionic twin placentas and compared their observations with existing artistic renditions of the pathology of artery-to-vein anastomoses. In each of these prior drawings, a rather substantial degree of separation was depicted between the supplying artery and draining vein of a common (shared) villus (Figure 6-11). DeLia and Cruikshank note that such anatomic findings do not exist in the placenta. In contrast, they note that the deep vascular communications emerge as prominent vessels on the chorion surface at the equator of the placenta (Figure 6-12). This appearance facilitates fetoscopic identification of the culprit vessels.

The stuck twin usually first appears between 16 and 26 weeks' gestation.[9,44] However, Bromley et al.[18] reported three patients diagnosed with mild oligohydramnios or hydramnios that underwent late worsening with a stuck twin seen only after 26 weeks. Indeed, the diagnosis has

*References 18, 21, 27, 52, 56, 65, 94, 112, 117, 142, 151

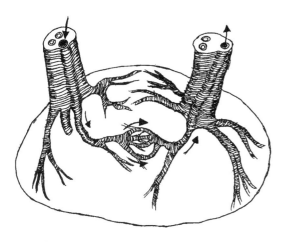

FIGURE 6-11   Artistic rendering of artery-to-vein anastomosis in TTS. *(Redrawn from Gabbe SG, Niebyl JR, Simpson JL, editors: Obstetrics: normal and problem pregnancies, New York, 1991, Churchill Livingston.)*

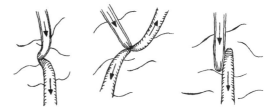

FIGURE 6-12   Fetoscopic appearance of variable types of artery-to-vein anastomoses seen on surface of monochorionic placentas affected by TTS. *(Redrawn from DeLia JE, Cruikshank DP: Am J Obstet Gyn 170:1480, 1994.)*

been first made as late as 34 weeks' gestation.[21]

Most authors have suggested that approximately 95% of pregnancies with stuck twin syndrome are structurally normal twins.[27,93,106,147] Conditions simulating the stuck twin syndrome include fetal anomalies, placental insufficiency, and perhaps abnormal cord insertion (see the discussion of velamentous insertion of the cord). Mahoney et al.,[94] in a series of 17 cases with stuck twins identified two additional hydramniotic twin sets that had sonographically detectable structural abnormalities (one case of esophageal atresia and one case of congenital heart disease). Obviously, careful evaluation for anomaly-causing polyhydramnios must be made before TTS can be assumed. Uteroplacental insufficiency that produces discordance and oligohydramnios in one sac usually is a later occurrence in the third trimester when compared with the earlier occurrence of TTS. However, late-

presenting TTS may be difficult to distinguish from severe discordance because of uteroplacental insufficiency. However, TTS generally occurs earlier in gestation than does discordance caused by uteroplacental insufficiency.

The value of Doppler ultrasound in the identification and management of TTS is uncertain. Yamada et al.[151] evaluated 31 pairs of twins: 6 pairs with TTS, 4 discordant pairs, and 21 concordant pairs. Seven cases had intertwin differences in the pulsatility index (PI) above 0.5, and six of those had TTS. The difference in PI, noted before the appearance of hydrops fetalis, seemed to predict the risk of TTS, whereas the difference in PI from discordant twin cases (except for those with the syndrome) was low. Giles et al.[56] reported 11 patients with TTS who were diagnosed on the basis of their having like-sex twins with monochorionic placentation and umbilical venous blood hemoglobin differences exceeding 50 g/L at delivery. Umbilical artery velocity-time waveform studies were performed in these pregnancies as part of a large series of 456 twin pregnancies. In all 11 cases, the S/D ratio differences between the twins were less than 1 unit (mean 0.4 ± 0.2). The authors suggested that in TTS, umbilical artery S/D ratios are concordant even in the presence of discordancy in fetal size. The pulsatility indexes of these pregnancies were not reported, but minimal differences could be expected, in contrast to the previous study. Whereas Doppler ultrasound may enhance clinicians' understanding of TTS, it would seem unlikely to improve its diagnosis beyond the capabilities of the standard ultrasound biometry. Management options that are facilitated by Doppler are not readily identified in the literature.

Velamentous Insertion of the Umbilical Cord and TTS

Velamentous insertion of the umbilical cord occurs with 4 to 9 times higher incidence in twins than it does in singletons.[131] The cause of velamentous insertions is not known. However, Robinson, Jones, and Benirschke[120] suggest that its higher incidence in twin gestations and particularly in monochorionic twin gestations occurs when embryos implanted in close proximity of each other compete for the same placental territory. Jauniaux et al.[72] noted that marginal and velamentous insertions of the umbilical cord were observed more often in the vanishing twin syndrome, both for the surviving twin and for the fetus papyraceus. Marginal insertion of the cord occurs in 5.6% of singletons[51] and in 15.9% of singletons conceived through IVF,[45] suggesting a possible excess of vanishing twins in IVF pregnancies. This rate is increased to 10.6% and 22.1% in dichorionic and monochorionic twins, respectively and strongly suggests an intrauterine environmental origin for this anomaly.[14]

Velamentous cord insertions are more common in TTS pregnancies and are theorized by some authors to contribute to the development of discordant fetal growth and to the disparity in amniotic fluid volume that is sometimes seen. Fries et al.[52] reported on 38 cases of monochorionic-diamniotic twins, 11 of which showed TTS. The prevalence of velamentous cord insertion in the TTS subset was 63.6%, compared with 18.5% in those without (p < .01). The authors speculate that the membranously inserted cord can be easily compressed, reducing blood flow to one twin and note that large-volume amniocenteses may reduce this compressive force on the cord insertion. They offer this as a mechanism explaining the reported success of this mode of intervention in the treatment of TTS. Whether serial large-volume amniocenteses would less successfully treat TTS if velamentous insertion of the cord were not present is unknown. Eddleman et al.[42] noted an incidence of velamentous cord insertion in singleton and twin gestations of 0.48% and 2%, respectively and noted that the mean birth weight was significantly lower in the velamentous cord insertion group than in the control group. Whether velamentous insertion of the cord is a critical part of the pathophysiology of discordant growth and TTS and particularly the cause of the hydramnios or oligohydramnios of the stuck twin, or is merely an associated phenomena but largely unrelated to the observed physiology is unknown. However, Sherer et al.[131] suggest that in cases of marked growth discordancy in twins, velamentous insertion should be considered a possible cause, and sonographic inspection of the placental insertion of the umbilical cord, particularly the cord of the smaller twin, should be performed.

Velamentous insertion of the umbilical cord is a necessary prerequisite to vasa praevia. Vasa praevia is a phenomena wherein the naked vessels of a velamentously inserted umbilical cord, unprotected by Wharton's jelly or cord structure, course over the cervical os within the chorioamnionic membranes. This condition can result in spontaneous or iatrogenic (at time of amniotomy) laceration of the vessels with resultant catastrophic fetal hemorrhage. Given the increased incidence of velamentous insertion of the cord in twin gestations, an increased index of suspicion for vasa praevia is warranted. During ultrasound evaluation of twin pregnancies (or perhaps all pregnancies) when a funic presentation is noted with coils of umbilical cord presenting at or near the cervical os, careful tracing of the umbilical cord towards its placental insertion may identify a velamentous insertion of the cord and an increased risk for vasa praevia. Gianopoulos et al.[54] first reported the antenatal identification of vasa praevia using real-time ultrasound without M-mode or color Doppler enhancement. It is expected that both of these techniques could more easily facilitate the diagnosis. It should be noted that a vasa praevia may first occur after delivery of the first twin, with velamentous insertion of the second twin's cord. Bleeding at amniotomy to deliver the second twin may likewise be the result of the rupture of a fetal vessel.

Intrauterine Growth Retardation

Intrauterine growth retardation (IUGR) is substantially increased in multiple gestations (12% to 47%) compared with singleton pregnancies (5% to 7%).[28] Fetal growth restriction is a major factor in the neonatal morbidity of twins.[90] The perinatal mortality rate for twins with IUGR is 2.5 times higher than it is for twins without IUGR.[60] The reduced growth rate usually affects only one twin of a pair, and discordant fetal growth has been reported to occur in up to 29% of twin pregnancies.[5,46,60,85]

Attempts to identify IUGR accurately and to increase surveillance so as to improve outcome are an important part of twin management. Some degree of controversy exists as to the appropriate growth tables to use in the evaluation of growth adequacy. The current ACOG Technical Bulletin[2] states that it is important to use growth tables derived from multiple pregnancies when assessing the growth of twins. Such tables do exist and largely demonstrate a flattening of growth in the late third trimester in twin gestations. Thus at or near term, the tenth percentile of growth is lower for twins and fewer fetuses are classified as small for gestational age (SGA).

It is reasonable to argue that there is no intrinsic genetic reason for twin growth to be less than singleton growth, and the differences observed are probably the consequence of environmental factors such as crowding or an increased likelihood of uteroplacental insufficiency (UPI) when there is more than one fetus to be grown. Support for an increased risk of UPI in twin pregnancies is found in a study by Ohel et al.,[104] who sonographically determined placental gradings of 158 twin pregnancies and 474 singleton pregnancies and noted the distributions of placental grades. Grades I to III were significantly different throughout the third trimester, with a preponderance of Grade III placentas in the twin group. The growth curves of the fetal biparietal diameter (BPD),[115] long bones (femur length [FL]),[116] and transverse cerebellar diameter[84,132] in twin gestations have recently been demonstrated to be similar to those of singleton gestations. Although twin growth curves for the abdominal circumference are not available, it is reasonable to conclude that most of the flattening of twin growth curves is the result of a similar flattening of the rate of growth of the abdominal circumference (AC) caused by UPI.

In 1994, Luke, Minogue, and Witter[89] reported a retrospective survey of over 19,600 normal twin and singleton infants and noted a lack of significant differences between twin and singleton growth until late in the third trimester. Between 24 and 36 weeks, the mean birth weights of twins and singletons were comparable. However, between 36 weeks and delivery, the twins' birth weights were reduced when compared with singletons. Twin growth is expected to parallel normal singleton growth through 36 weeks' gestation. After that, ultrasound evaluation is important to detect abnormal growth beyond the mild degree that is expected in near-term, normal twins.

Thus to avoid diminished sensitivity for the detection of abnormal fetal growth, it seems prudent to use the percentiles of weight for gestational age established for singleton pregnancies when evaluating twin growth. It is this author's opinion that twin growth charts offer little to twin management and may decrease the sensitivity of IUGR detection, and therefore they are not be presented in this chapter. Whereas mild slowing of twin growth might be expected, especially at term, some caution is advised when it occurs.

Although the use of fundal height measurements as a screening tool for IUGR enjoys wide acceptance for the management of singleton gestations, the use of fundal height measurements as a technique to detect IUGR or discordant twins is not advised. In an attempt to establish such nomograms, Egan et al.[43] evaluated 160 women with twin pregnancies between 16 and 36 weeks who were to undergo ultrasound examinations. The sensitivity of fundal height to detect discordant growth in twins was 23.5%, the specificity was 82.5%, the positive predictive value was 13.8%, and the negative predictive value was 90.1%. Clearly fundal height is inadequate to assess for abnormalities of growth or amniotic fluid volume. However, sudden fundal height increases may be related to TTS or fetal anomaly, and fundal height measurements should be routinely performed.

After the diagnosis of a twin gestation is established, its chorionicity determined, and an anatomic survey performed, serial ultrasound biometry is advised (beginning at 24 to 26 weeks' gestation) to evaluate the appropriateness of fetal growth and evaluate for growth discordance. If the twins are thought to be dichorionic (two placentas, unlike sex, or thick dividing membranes), sonograms are recommended at least every 4 weeks.[123] If they are thought to be monochorionic (like sex, one placenta, or thin dividing membrane), serial sonograms should be performed at 2- to 3-week intervals. If a growth disturbance is identified, ultrasound examinations should be performed at 1- to 2-week intervals, depending on the clinical situation. In gestations diagnosed to be monochorionic, a greater early concern is present because of the risk of TTS. When gestations are diagnosed to be dichorionic (with no risk of TTS), serial surveillance might begin somewhat later.

As implied in the previous discussion, the identification of IUGR in twin gestations is substantially the same as for singleton gestations. Deviations of estimated fetal weight (EFW) for one or both twins (using singleton charts) that approach or fall below the tenth percentile for gestational age, particularly when they are associated with an abnormal head circumference (HC) to AC ratio (HC/AC) or worrisome Doppler studies, should prompt testing for fetal well-being and a consideration for early delivery. Rodis et al.[122] noted among 60 pairs of concordant twins that the mean FL/AC ratio is 22.4 ± 1.5 in twin gestations and appears to be independent of gestational age between 20 and 40 weeks. Stefos et al.[134] demonstrated the utility of fetal assessment in twin gestations by using individual growth curves suggested by Rossavik for singleton gestations.

It should be noted that in twin pregnancies, especially in the third trimester, fetal crowding increases the likelihood that satisfactory measurements of both fetal heads cannot be obtained consistently. Yarkoni et al.[152] found that EFWs for both twins could be obtained from AC and BPD in only 54% of cases. Rodis et al.[123] could obtain EFW values from AC and BPD in only 63% of twins, versus 98% if AC and FL were used, because of such difficulties. Other authors have found that FL measurements are assessed with greater accuracy and reliability than BPD in twin pregnancies.[59,92,93] If accurate head measurements can be obtained, their use for EFW is appropriate, but an EFW based on AC and FL is more often and accurately obtained in twins.

The literature is divided on whether IUGR affects cerebellar growth in singleton gestations. Reece et al.[114] concluded that the transverse cerebellar diameter was unaffected by growth retardation. However, Hill et al.[69] found that the transverse cerebellar diameter was greater than 2 SD below the mean in 59% of fetuses with growth less than the fifth percentile. In twin gestations, Lettieri et al.[84] established a nomogram for the transverse cerebellar diameter and noted it to increase linearly with gestational age. Sixty-three percent of the fetuses with growth retardation had a transverse cerebellar diameter of less than or equal to the fifth percentile for gestational age. It would appear that IUGR may affect cerebellar growth in twins, particularly when the protective effect of head sparing asymmetry is lost.

Although a detailed discussion of twin delivery management is beyond this chapter's intent, Lodeiro et al.[88] noted the utility of the biophysical profile in the surveillance of twin gestations. It should be noted that normal values and ranges for the amniotic fluid index (AFI) have not been established for twin gestations. It is probable that both the upper and lower limit of the AFI should be somewhat higher than for singleton gestations. A subjective assessment of the relative amniotic fluid volume surrounding each twin should be performed routinely, with particular attention given when either TTS (oligohydramnios in the donor) or IUGR is suspected.

Although the next section of this chapter focuses on discordant fetal growth, the recent literature suggests that discordance is less important than is IUGR. Henriksen et al.[67] evaluated the following ultrasound values that are widely used as predictors for SGA infants in twin pregnancies: (1) the difference in biparietal diameter; (2) the difference in abdominal diameter; (3) the percentage difference in EFW; and (4) estimation of the weight deviation from the expected weight during pregnancy. Using relative operating characteristic (ROC) curves, EFW deviation was the most sensitive and specific of the methods. The authors stressed that fetal discordance is not the appropriate predictor of infants in twin pregnancies who are SGA at birth. Bronsteen, Goyert, and Bottoms[19] compared the prognostic value of IUGR, discordancy, and other classifications in 131 sets of surviving twins. A four-factor model for neonatal morbidity was developed from 161 potential outcome measures. Individual evaluation of each twin for IUGR using singleton growth curves was more effective than discordancy and other classifications in predicting neonatal morbidity. In fact, in the absence of IUGR, discordancy was not associated with neonatal morbidity increase. The authors suggest that evaluation of twin growth should concentrate on individual twin growth rather than discordancy. Patterson and Wood[107] noted that neither morbidity, neonatal death, nor anomalies were significantly related to level of discordance. They conclude that prematurity and birth weight below the tenth percentile may present a greater threat to twins than birth weight discordance.

Discordant Twin Growth

Multiple gestations offer the unique opportunity to simultaneously compare the growth of two genetically similar (if not identical) fetuses. A degree of reassurance is taken if the fetuses are growing at the same rate: that is, if their growth is concordant. Similarly, numerous authors have identified an increased need for concern if the estimated growth of twin fetuses is dissimilar: that is, if their growth is discordant. As mentioned in the previous section, the importance of accurate and timely identification of discordant growth lies primarily in its relationship to TTS (particularly when early in pregnancy), and to IUGR of the smaller twin. A risk for aneuploidy, anomaly, or viral syndrome affecting only one fetus must also be considered when discordant growth is identified. In the absence of these conditions, it would appear that even discordant fetal weights that exceed 20% to 25% are not of themselves associated with an increased risk. However, when this degree of discordance is present, it is likely that the smaller twin's weight will approach the tenth percentile, potentially show mild asymmetry, and be at increased risk to develop a significant growth disturbance.[28] Careful follow-up procedures are warranted to assess interval growth in these cases. At term, discordancy itself may not be a risk factor when the lighter twin weighs at least 2500 gm.[16]

Although there is no standard definition of what constitutes discordant growth, a number of ultrasonically derived measurements may be used for comparison of twin fetuses, with the larger twin as the standard (100%). The diagnosis of discordance has been based on numerous parameters. Crane, Tomich, and Kopta[35] first suggested that a BPD of greater than 2 SD below the mean or a BPD difference of 5 mm or greater is suggestive of discordant growth. However, Erkkola et al.[46] noted that this technique lacked sufficient sensitivity to be recommended, and most authors have abandoned this parameter. An AC difference of 20 mm or greater also suggests discordant growth in twins[5] and has been demonstrated to be more sensitive (72% to 80%) and specific (74% to 85%) than measuring the BPD difference in detecting twins with dissimilar birth weights.[20,137] EFWs based on BPD and AC[130] or AC and FL[63] nomograms have been reported to allow the most accurate identification of discordant fetal growth in twins.[137] The reported sensitivity of EFW to identify discordant birth weight is only fair and ranges from 25% to 55%.[91,24]

Blickstein[15] sent a questionnaire to 96 authors of twin-related obstetric articles. The views of the 61 respondents (33 from the United States) comprise this international census survey. The data suggest that a clear cut-off value for discordancy was still needed. Whereas most authors suggested that a birth weight (EFW) in the smaller twin that was 20% to 25% less than the larger twin's weight was an appropriate cut-off, Blickstein suggested that the data indirectly supported a two-grade definition, namely, mild (greater than 15% and less than 25% birth-weight disparity) and severe (greater than 25%) growth discordance. The sonographic diagnosis was done by comparing the EFWs of both twins (n = 35, 57.4% of respondents); three respondents (4.9%) compared the abdominal circumferences, one (1.6%) compared the biparietal diameters, and 16 (26.2%) based their sonographic diagnosis on more than one biometric criterion.

Rodis et al.[123] assessed 25 discordant twin pairs longitudinally, compared them with a group of 60 concordant twin pairs,

and noted that the smaller of each discordant pair exhibited a slower rate of intrauterine growth as early as 23 to 24 weeks' gestation, which was accentuated between 33 and 37 weeks. Their data suggest that if borderline discordance is noted before 33 weeks' gestation, it is apt to become significant when the disparity in growth rate widens. With this concern for late worsening of discordance, they have suggested that a significant growth disturbance in twin gestations exists in the following cases: (1) when either one or both of the twins fall below the tenth percentile in EFW (plotted on nomograms established for twins), (2) when the twins become greater than 20% discordant for EFW (regardless of weight percentile for either fetus), or (3) when a twin fetus fails to exhibit any growth over a 2-week interval (regardless of the percentage of discordancy between them).

Whereas many investigators consider a 20% to 25% difference of fetal weight to be the optimal parameter on which to base a diagnosis of discordance, it is this author's opinion that true discordance, which is significant and an indicator for an increased risk of IUGR, morbidity, and mortality for the smaller twin, is usually the consequence of relative UPI. This is particularly true for dichorionic twins. Eberle et al.[41] noted that among 18 discordant dichorionic twin pairs, 77.8% (14/18) of the lighter twins had more placental lesions than the heavier twins. Among 48 monochorionic twin pairs, regardless of birth weight discordance, no differences in placental abnormalities were observed. In dichorionic twins, significant birth weight discordance was attributable not to differences in placental weight but to a greater number of placental lesions in the lighter twin than in the heavier twin. With the current understanding of UPI and its pathogenesis, it is difficult to imagine truly discordant twins whose abdominal circumferences are not also discordant. Therefore if the EFWs are discordant but the abdominal circumferences are not, and if most of the weight estimate differences are the result of differences in the length of the femur or size of the fetal heads (HC or BPD), the difference in weight may be spurious and related to measurement error, dolichocephaly, or another factor that is less likely to be related to discordant placental perfusion. Although the clinical practice of assessing discordance based on percent deviation of EFW is generally sound, if there is not parallel discordance of the AC, a diagnosis of pathologically discordant twins may be incorrect and other factors influencing weight estimates should be considered.

Although concordant growth certainly should be expected if the twins are monozygotic, most twins are dizygotic (70%) and a range of growth dissimilarity can be anticipated in these cases purely because of the genetic differences between siblings. This phenomenon has been particularly demonstrated for unlike-sex twins. Blickstein and Weissman[17] studied 153 liveborn twin pairs of unlike sex. Male twins were heavier than their female cotwins, but the difference reached statistical significance in the male-first combination only. Two thirds of both combinations had male-female birth-weight differences of less than 15%. However, when compared with male discordant twins, significantly more female discordant twins were found in both the male-female and female-male combinations. Guttmacher and Kohl[61] studied 446 pairs of unlike-sex

twins and showed that dizygosity has a favorable positive influence on the birth weight of twins and that maleness increases the birth weight of twins. Corney et al.[31] studied 356 pairs and found that the combined birth weight of unlike-sex twins (n = 112) was significantly higher compared with pairs of like sex. They also found that males of unlike-sexed pairs were significantly heavier than their female cotwins and heavier than males of like-sex twins. Corey et al.[30] measured birth weights of 94 pairs of unlike-sex twins and compared them with the birth weights of 102 like-sex twins pairs. Overall, males were found to be significantly heavier than females, but these differences were not significant when compared within zygosity categories. Clearly a degree of tolerance is appropriate when dizygotic twins (particularly when they are discordant for sex) have discordant weights, especially when the smaller twin's EFW is above the tenth percentile for gestational age.

Once discordant growth is identified or suspected, antenatal follow-up evaluating subsequent growth and fetal well-being is necessary. In the previously mentioned international survey, 56 authors (91.8%) used sonographic biometry: biweekly evaluations were advocated by 30 (53.6%), and weekly evaluations were preferred by 23 authors (41%).[15] A biophysical profile was advocated by 44 participants (72.1%): 18 (41%) preferred twice weekly, and 22 (50%) advocated once weekly. Doppler velocimetry studies were suggested by 31 participants (50.8%). Nonstress testing (NST) was done twice weekly by 32 respondents (61.5%) and weekly by 11 (21.1%). Blickstein concluded that sonography (weekly to biweekly biometry plus weekly to twice weekly biophysical profile) and the twice weekly NST were most often recommended and that a consensus frequency of Doppler velocimetry assessments could not be defined. These recommendations largely parallel those found for singletons with IUGR.

A potential role for Doppler velocimetry and waveform analysis in the management of twin gestations complicated by either TTS or suspected IUGR has been suggested by several authors.* However, in light of the previous discussion, it would seem reasonable to conclude that for the approximate 80% of twins that are either dizygotic or dichorionic and not at risk for TTS, the role of Doppler in twin gestations is not different from its role in singleton gestations. Specifically, since IUGR is the specific risk for the smaller of discordant dichorionic twins, the role of Doppler in the identification and management of IUGR for twins is the same as in singleton gestations and well-described on p. 155. Several of these studies have suggested that discordant twins are often discordant for Doppler indices such as the S/D ratio or PI of the umbilical arteries and that such divergent values aid in the identification of the fetus at risk. However, it is likely that most of the smaller twins with discordant or frankly abnormal Doppler indices are also less than the tenth percentile of weight for gestational age and have abnormal indices, similar to singleton fetuses, because of the influence of UPI. A specific role for Doppler in the evaluation of the small twin fetus beyond its role in small singleton fetuses is not clearly proved. Whether a clinician can be reassured as to the health of the smaller of twin fetuses if its Doppler indices are normal is uncertain. The potential role of Doppler in the identification and management of TTS is discussed in that section of this chapter.

Prematurity and Twin Gestation: The Role of Cervical Cerclage

Prematurity is the most important cause of perinatal morbidity and mortality in twin gestation. In a recent analysis of data obtained from the National Center for Health Statistics for 1990 in the United States, 1/43 births (2.3%) (a marked rise from previous years) were twin births, and 47.9% were delivered before 37 weeks' gestation, versus 9.7% for singletons.[89] The observed rate of very low birth weight (VLBW) (less than 1500 gm) was 10% among twins versus 1% for singletons. The rate of low birth weight (LBW) (less than 2500 gm) among twins was 50.7% versus 5.9% for singletons. This fivefold increased risk of prematurity and ninefold increased risk of LBW warrants concern and has prompted attempts to reduce these risks.

Whereas a detailed discussion of prematurity prevention is beyond the scope of this chapter and addressed in Chapter 7, clinical and ultrasonographic assessment of the uterine cervix during singleton and twin pregnancy has been promoted as a means to identify an increased risk of preterm delivery both from preterm labor and incompetent cervix.† This section discusses this literature and the controversy it generates.

*References 37, 39, 53, 57, 78, 118, 128

†References 4, 58, 62, 71, 73, 80, 98, 99, 105, 111, 125, 133

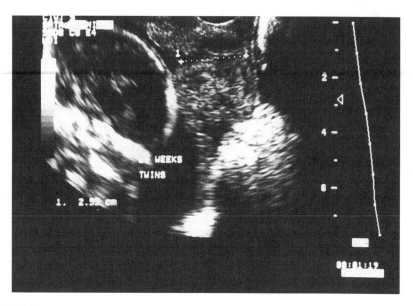

FIGURE 6-13 Cervical length measurement (2.55 cm) in a twin gestation (lower-limit normal).

Several investigators have measured the length of the cervix in pregnancy with transvaginal ultrasound during singleton pregnancies.[4,80,133] Similar normal measurements in twin gestations were not available at the time of this writing (Figure 6-13). Kushnir et al.[80] noted no differences between the measured cervical lengths of parous versus nonparous women in 166 obstetric patients. Before 32 weeks' gestation, in 5-week grouping intervals, the mean cervical lengths ranged from 43 to 48 mm ($\pm$10 to 18 mm) without specific trend. In this study they were somewhat longer than that reported by Smith et al.,[133] whose median cervical length in 132 low-risk patients was 37 mm and somewhat shorter than the mean before 34 weeks of 52 $\pm$ 12 mm reported by Ayers et al.[4] Other investigators caution that digital examination is inaccurate to measure cervical length and tends to underestimate it.[70,71] The assessment of cervical length by digital examination should not be compared with vaginal ultrasound determined normals, since this practice is expected to overestimate the rate of shortened cervical length. Other authors have noted the importance of funneling of the endocervical os, particularly when transfundal pressure is applied by the examiner[62] (Figure 6-14).

During ultrasound evaluation of the cervix, special care is warranted to avoid missing cervical shortening by inadequate duration of evaluation, overdistension of the bladder, or excess transducer pressure transabdominally that can falsely elongate the cervix.[80,105] Alternatively, a bladder that is emptied too well can falsely shorten the appearance of the cervix by allowing exaggerated anteflexion of the cervix.[80] Iams et al.[70] caution that the first measurement should be used when transvaginal measurement is made, stating that transducer pressure results in a 3 to 5 mm decrease in length with repeated measurements.

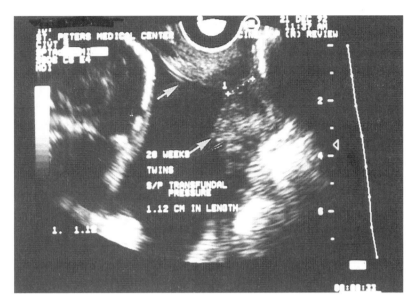

FIGURE 6-14   Cervical measurement in the same patient as Figure 6-13 after transfundal pressure was applied. Note the abnormal shortening and funnelling.

Several studies have evaluated the role of cerclage in twin gestation with and without the guidance of ultrasonographic cervical evaluation. Prophylactic cerclage in multiple gestation was evaluated in two studies dealing primarily with twins where patients were selected without ultrasound evaluation of cervical length. No beneficial effect was noted in one,[146] whereas in the other a significant prolongation of pregnancy was established.[153]

Michaels et al.[98] diagnosed 7/51 twin gestation patients (13.7%) to have cervical incompetency before 30 weeks' gestation (range 18 to 28 weeks with a mean of 24 weeks). The diagnosis of cervical incompetency was not based on cervical length alone but on a combination of cervical shortening, dilation, and membrane protrusion through the ultrasound internal os. For diagnosed patients these mean values were 1.9, 2.2, and 3.6 cm, respectively. There was a significant difference

in perinatal mortality when compared with controls. All twins in the study survived, but 9/153 twin control subjects were delivered at a mean gestational age of 22.7 weeks, with a loss of 17 infants. The authors conclude that although routine cerclage placement is not recommended for twin gestations, multiple gestations may benefit from ultrasound surveillance for cervical incompetency.

Although the results of this study are attractive and a 13.7% incidence of cervical incompetence among these twins does not seem unreasonable, the results are not conclusive. The mean values for this "incompetent" group do not provide a specific cut-off point for normal cervical length. Although each of the cerclage patients had a cervical length of less than 25 mm, the sensitivity and specificity of this possible cut-off point is unknown. Whereas funnelling is likely to be an abnormal finding in early pregnancy, a cut-off level for cervical dilation (range 1.2 to 3.5 cm in the cerclage patients) is likewise not identified. More importantly, as pointed out by Joffe et al.,[73] no prospective trials with and without cerclage have been performed when endocervical shortening has been demonstrated by ultrasonography. Most reports of successful pregnancy outcome after replacement of cerclage use the patients' earlier pregnancy outcomes for comparison. These comparisons are not valid, because several series' report that as many as 70% of patients who have a midtrimester loss are delivered of their infants at term with no treatment in their subsequent pregnancies. The question of whether to place a cerclage in the late second or early third trimester after the demonstration of significant shortening in cervical length remains difficult. A prospective, randomized study is needed in both twin and singleton gestations to evaluate the risks and benefits of cerclage in the prevention of preterm delivery when cervical shortening has been demonstrated by vaginal ultrasonographic assessment.

Ultrasound Evaluation of Fetal Presentation

Although it is beyond the scope of this chapter to discuss the route of delivery for twin gestations, the ultrasound surveillance of twins has allowed the accumulation of data regarding the rates of various combinations of twin presentations. Despite inconclusive data regarding the relative safety of carefully selected vaginal delivery attempts when the first twin is nonvertex, most nonvertex twins usually are delivered abdominally in the United States. The ACOG Technical Bulletin[2] supports this position. Although the literature regarding the appropriate route of delivery for term twin gestations when the first twin is vertex and the second twin is nonvertex largely supports vaginal delivery attempts, abdominal delivery is often selected not only for delivery of the second twin but, particularly in gestations complicated by prematurity, for both twins. Regardless of a practitioner's usual management of various combinations of presentation, it is important to know the probability that the observed presentation will change both antenatally and intrapartally after the birth of the first twin. This information is important to the proper counseling of couples with twin gestations.

Santolaya et al.[127] noted ultrasonographically the changes in fetal presentation throughout pregnancy in 332 sets of twins. At 26-30 weeks' gestational age, 78% of the leading twins were vertex, 75% were vertex at 31 to 34 weeks, and 81% were vertex at 35 to 38 weeks. The incidence of nonvertex presentation for either twin was 73.0%, 64.5%, and 59.5% at the same gestational ages. The total number of pregnancies in which either twin was nonvertex also decreased from 90.3% to 59.5% at term. The authors note that if vertex-vertex is a criterion for vaginal delivery before the 30th week of gestation, only 27% of twin pregnancies would be candidates for vaginal delivery. That number increases to between 41% and 49% at term.

Divon et al.[39] evaluated the rate of spontaneous version in twin gestations throughout the third trimester in 119 twin gestations. A spontaneous change from any presentation to any other presentation was considered a spontaneous version.

Birth weight discordancy was detected in 22 pregnancies (18.5%), but there was no significant association between the incidence of spontaneous version and birth weight discordancy. Neither placental location nor the amniotic fluid volume was significantly associated with the incidence of spontaneous version. The number of spontaneous versions observed with the first twin was significantly smaller than that observed for the second twin (21/119 [18%] versus 73/119 [61%]). Overall, the rate of spontaneous version decreased from 60% at 28 to 30 weeks' gestation to 25% to 30% at term. The lowest incidence of spontaneous version was observed in patients with a cephalic-cephalic presentation (7%). All other presentations were relatively unstable and demonstrated a 32% to 100% spontaneous version rate. The authors note that this rate is much higher than the 5% cephalic version reported in singleton breech presentations at term and suggest that the high rate of spontaneous version observed throughout the third trimester supports awaiting the onset of labor before a final decision regarding mode of delivery is made.[149] This author certainly supports this recommendation in most cases. For the discussion of intrapartum management and the presentation of the second twin following the delivery of the first, please consult Chapter 9.

Acknowledgments

Artwork was provided by Ms. Julie Anne Spinnato. Special thanks to Ms. Robin L. Newlon for secretarial and editorial assistance.

Bibliography

1. Allen SR et al: Ultrasonographic diagnosis of congenital anomalies in twins, *Am J Obstet Gynecol* 165:1056-1060, 1991.

2. American College of Obstetricians and Gynecologists: *ACOG technical bulletin no. 131*, August 1989, author.

3. Ash K, Harman CR, Gritter H: TRAP sequence: successful outcome with indomethacin treatment, *Obstet Gynecol* 76:960-962, 1990.

4. Ayers JWT et al: Sonographic evaluation of cervical length in pregnancy: diagnosis and management of preterm cervical effacement in patients at risk for premature delivery, *Obstet Gynecol* 71:939-944, 1988.

5. Barnea E et al: The value of biparietal diameter and abdominal perimeter in the diagnosis of growth retardation in twin gestations, *Am J Perinatol* 2:221-222, 1985.

6. Barss VA, Benacerraf BR, Frigoletto FD: Ultrasonographic determination of chorion type in twin gestation, *Obstet Gynecol* 66:779-783, 1985.

7. Belfort MA et al: The use of color flow Doppler ultrasonography to diagnose umbilical cord entanglement in monoamniotic twin gestations, *Am J Obstet Gynecol* 168:601-604, 1993.

8. Bendon RW, Siddiqi T: Clinical pathology conference: acute twin-to-twin in utero transfusion, *Pediatr Pathol* 9:591-598, 1989.

9. Benirschke K: The placenta in twin gestation, *Clin Obstet Gynecol* 33:1, 1990.

10. Benson CB, Doubilet PM, Laks MP: Outcome of twin gestations following sonographic demonstration of two heart beats in the first trimester, *Ultrasound Obstet Gynecol* 3:343-345, 1993.

11. Bessis R, Papiernik E: *Echographic imagery of amniotic membranes in twin pregnancies.* In Gedda L, Parisi P, editors: *Twin research,* vol 3, twin biology and multiple pregnancy, New York, 1981, Alan R. Liss.

12. Birnholz JC: Determination of fetal sex, *N Engl J Med* 309:942-944, 1983.

13. Blane CE et al: Sonographic detection of monoamniotic twins, *J Clin Ultrasound* 15:394, 1987.

14. Bleker OP, Breur W, Huidekoper BL: A study of birth weight, placental weight and mortality of twins as compared to singletons, *Br J Obstet Gynaecol* 86:111, 1979.

15. Blickstein I: The definition, diagnosis, and management of growth-discordant twins: an international census survey, *Acta Genet Med Gemellol (Roma)* 40:345-351, 1991.

16. Blickstein I, Shoham-Schwartz Z, Lancet M: Growth discordancy in appropriate for gestational age, term twins, *Obstet Gynecol* 72:582-584, 1988.

17. Blickstein I, Weissman A: Birth weight discordancy in male-first and female-first pairs of unlike-sexed twins, *Am J Obstet Gynecol* 162:661-663, 1990.

18. Bromley B et al: The natural history of oligohydramnios/polyhydramnios sequence in monochorionic diamniotic twins, *Ultrasound Obstet Gynecol* 2:317-320, 1992.

19. Bronsteen R, Goyert G, Bottoms S: Classification of twins and neonatal morbidity, *Obstet Gynecol* 74:98, 1989.

20. Brown CEL et al: Prediction of discordant twins using ultrasound measurement of biparietal diameter and abdominal perimeter, *Obstet Gynecol* 70:677-681, 1987.

21. Brown D et al: Twin-twin transfusion syndrome: sonographic findings, *Radiology* 170:61-63, 1989.

22. Bruner JP, Rosemond RL: Twin twin transfusion syndrome: a subset of the twin oligohydramnios-polyhydramnios sequence, *Am J Obstet Gynecol* 169:925-930, 1993.

23. Carlson N, Nageotte M: *Monoamniotic twin pregnancy: diagnosis by bubble dispersion,* SPO Ninth Annual Meeting, Abstract #248, New Orleans, La., February, 1989.

24. Chamberlain P, Murphy M, Comerford FR: How accurate is antenatal sonographic identification of discordant birthweight in twins? *Eur J Obstet Gynecol Reprod Biol* 40:91-6, 1991.

25. Chervenak FA et al: Twin gestation: antenatal diagnosis and perinatal outcome in 385 consecutive pregnancies, *J Reprod Med* 29:727-730, 1984.

26. Chervenak FA et al: Intrapartum management of twin gestation, *Obstet Gynecol* 65:119-124, 1985.

27. Chescheir NC, Seeds JW: Polyhydramnios and oligohydramnios in twin gestations, *Obstet Gynecol* 71:882-884, 1988.

28. Chitkara U et al: Twin pregnancy: routine use of ultrasound examinations in the prenatal diagnosis of intrauterine growth retardation and discordant growth, *Am J Perinatol* 2:49-54, 1985.

29. Chitkara U et al: Selective second-trimester termination of the anomalous fetus in twin pregnancies, *Obstet Gynecol* 73:690-694, 1989.

30. Corey LA et al: Effects of type of placentation on birthweight and its variability in monozygotic and dizygotic twins, *Acta Genet Med Gemellol (Roma)* 28:41-50, 1979.

31. Corney G et al: The effect of zygosity on birth weight of twins in Aberdeen and Northeast Scotland, *Acta Genet Med Gemellol (Roma)* 28:353-560, 1979.

32. Cox M et al: Spontaneous cessation of umbilical blood flow in the acardiac fetus of a twin pregnancy, *Prenat Diagn* 12:689-693, 1992.

33. Crade M, Nageotte MP, MacKenzie ML: The acardiac twin: a case report using color Doppler ultrasonography, *Ultrasound Obstet Gynecol* 2:364-365, 1992.

34. Crane JP: Sonographic evaluation of multiple pregnancy, *Semin Ultrasound CT MR* 5:114-156, 1984.

35. Crane JP, Tomich PG, Kopta M: Ultrasonic growth patterns in normal and discordant twins, *Obstet Gynecol* 55:678-683, 1980.

36. D'Alton ME, Dudley DK: The ultrasonographic prediction of chorionicity in twin gestation, *Am J Obstet Gynecol* 160:557-561, 1989.

37. Degani S et al: Doppler flow velocity waveforms in fetal surveillance of twins: a prospective longitudinal study, *J Ultrasound Med* 11:537-541, 1992.

38. DeLia JE, Cruikshank DP: Feticide versus laser surgery for twin-twin transfusion syndrome, *Am J Obstet Gynecol* 170:1480-1481, 1994.

39. Divon MY et al: Discordant twins: a prospective study of the diagnostic value of real-time ultrasonography combined with umbilical artery velocimetry, *Am J Obstet Gynecol* 161:757-760, 1989.

40. Divon MY et al: Twin gestation: fetal presentation as a function of gestational age, *Am J Obstet Gynecol* 168:1500-1502, 1993.

41. Eberle AM et al: Placental pathology in discordant twins, *Am J Obstet Gynecol* 169:931-935, 1993.

42. Eddleman KA et al: Clinical significance and sonographic diagnosis of velamentous umbilical cord insertion, *Am J Perinatol* 9:123, 1992.

43. Egan JFX et al: Correlation of uterine fundal height with ultrasonic measurements in twin gestations, *J Maternal Fetal Med* 3:18-22, 1994.

44. Elliot JP: Amniocentesis for twin-twin transfusion syndrome, *Contemp Ob/Gyn* Aug:30-47, 1992.

45. Englert Y et al: Morphologic anomalies in the placenta of IVF pregnancies, *Hum Reprod* 2:155, 1987.

46. Erkkola R et al: Growth discordancy in twin pregnancies: a risk factor not detected by

measurement of the biparietal diameter, *Obstet Gynecol* 66:203-206, 1985.

47. Ewigman B, LeFevre M, Hesser J: A randomized trial of routine prenatal ultrasound, *Obstet Gynecol* 76:189-194, 1990.

48. Finberg HJ: The "twin peak" sign: reliable evidence of dichorionic twinning, *J Ultrasound Med* 11:571-577, 1992.

49. Finberg HJ, Clewell WH: Definitive prenatal diagnosis of monoamniotic twins: swallowed amniotic contrast agent detected in both twins on sonographically selected CT images, *J Ultrasound Med* 10:513-516, 1991.

50. Foley MR et al: Use of the foley cordostat grasping device for selective ligation of the umbilical cord of an acardiac twin: a case report, *Am J Obstet Gynecol* 172:212-214, 1995.

51. Fox H: *Pathology of the placenta*, London, 1978, Saunders.

52. Fries MH et al: The role of velamentous cord insertion in the etiology of twin-twin transfusion syndrome, *Obstet Gynecol* 81:569-574, 1993.

53. Gerson A et al: Umbilical arterial systolic/diastolic values in normal twin gestation, *Obstet Gynecol* 72:205-208, 1988.

54. Gianopoulos J et al: Diagnosis of vasa previa with ultrasonography, *Obstet Gynecol* 69:488-491, 1987.

55. Gilbert WM et al: Morbidity associated with prenatal disruption of the dividing membrane in twin gestations, *Obstet Gynecol* 78:623-630.

56. Giles WB et al: Doppler umbilical artery studies in the twin-twin transfusion syndrome, *Obstet Gynecol* 76:1097-1099, 1990.

57. Giles WB et al: Placental microvascular changes in twin pregnancies with abnormal umbilical artery waveforms, *Obstet Gynecol* 81:556-559, 1993.

58. Goldman GA et al: Is elective cerclage justified in the management of triplet and quadruplet pregnancy? *Aust N Z J Obstet Gynaecol* 29:9, 1989.

59. Grumbach K et al: Twin and singleton growth patterns compared using US, *Radiology* 158:237-241, 1986.

60. Guaschino S et al: Growth retardation, size at birth, and perinatal mortality in twin pregnancy, *Int J Gynaecol Obstet* 25:399-403, 1987.

61. Guttmacher AF, Kohl SG: The fetus of multiple gestations, *Obstet Gynecol* 12:528-541, 1958.

62. Guzman ER et al: A new method using vaginal ultrasound and transfundal pressure to evaluate the asymptomatic incompetent cervix, *Obstet Gynecol* 83:248-252, 1994.

63. Hadlock FP et al: Sonographic estimation of fetal weight: the value of femur length in addition to head and abdomen measurements, *Radiology* 150:535-540, 1984.

64. Hamada H et al: Fetal therapy in utero by blockage of the umbilical blood flow of acardiac monster in twin pregnancy, *Nippon Sanka Fujinka Gakkai Zasshi* 41:1803-1809, 1989.

65. Hashimoto B et al: Ultrasound evaluation of polyhydramnios and twin pregnancy, *Am J Obstet Gynecol* 154:1069-1072, 1986.

66. Hellman LM, Kobayashi M, Cromb E: Ultrasonic diagnosis of embryonic malformations, *Am J Obstet Gynecol* 115:615-623, 1973.

67. Henriksen TB et al: Prediction of light-for-gestational age at delivery in twin pregnancies: an evaluation of fetal weight deviation and growth discordance measured by ultrasound, *Eur J Obstet Gynecol Reprod Biol* 47:195-200, 1992.

68. Hertzberg BS et al: Significance of membrane thickness in the sonographic evaluation of twin gestations, *Am J Roentgenol* 148:151-153, 1987.

69. Hill LM et al: The transverse cerebellar diameter cannot be used to assess gestational age in the small for gestational age fetus, *Obstet Gynecol* 75:329-332, 1990.

70. Iams JD et al: Cervical sonography in preterm labor, *Obstet Gynecol* 84:40-46, 1994.

71. Jackson GM, Ludmir J, Bader TJ: The accuracy of digital examination and ultrasound in the evaluation of cervical length, *Obstet Gynecol* 79:214-218, 1992.

72. Jauniaux E et al: Clinical and morphologic aspects of the vanishing twin phenomenon, *Obstet Gynecol* 72:577, 1988.

73. Joffe GM et al: Diagnosis of cervical change in pregnancy by means of transvaginal ultrasonography, *Am J Obstet Gynecol* 166:896-900, 1992.

74. Johnson JM et al: Maternal serum alpha-fetoprotein in twin pregnancy, *Am J Obstet Gynecol* 162:1020-1025, 1990.

75. Jou HJ et al: Doppler sonographic detection of reverse twin-twin transfusion after intrauterine death of the donor, *J Ultrasound Med* 5:307-309, 1993.

76. Kelly MP et al: Human chorionic gonadotropin rise in normal and vanishing twin pregnancies, *Fertil Steril* 56:221-224, 1991.

77. Kofinas AD, Penry M, Hatjis CG: Umbilical

vessel flow velocity waveforms in cord entanglement in a monoamnionic multiple gestation: a case report, *J Reprod Med* 36:314, 1991.

78. Kurmanavicius J et al: Umbilical artery blood flow velocity waveforms in twin pregnancies, *J Perinat Med* 20:307-312, 1992.

79. Kurtz AD et al: Twin pregnancies: accuracy of first trimester abdominal US in predicting chorionicity and amnionicity, *Radiology* 185:759-762, 1992.

80. Kushnir O et al: Vaginal ultrasonographic assessment of cervical length changes during normal pregnancy, *Am J Obstet Gynecol* 162:991-993, 1990.

81. Landy HJ et al: The 'vanishing twin': ultrasonographic assessment of fetal disappearance in the first trimester, *Am J Obstet Gynecol* 155:14-19, 1986.

82. Lavery JP, Gadwood KA: Amniography for confirming the diagnosis of monoamniotic twinning: a case report, *J Reprod Med* 35:911, 1990.

83. LeFevre ML et al: A randomized trial of prenatal ultrasonographic screening: impact on maternal management and outcome, *Am J Obstet Gynecol* 169:483-489, 1993.

84. Lettieri L et al: Transverse cerebellar diameter measurements in twin pregnancies and the effect of intrauterine growth retardation, *Am J Obstet Gynecol* 167:982-985, 1992.

85. Leveno KJ et al: Sonar cephalometry in twins: a table of biparietal diameters for normal twin fetuses and a comparison with singletons, *Am J Obstet Gynecol* 135:727-731, 1979.

86. Levi S: Ultrasonic assessment of the high rate of human multiple pregnancy in the first trimester, *J Clin Ultrasound* 4:3-5, 1976.

87. Lockwood C, Ghidini A, Romero R: Amniotic band syndrome in monozygotic twins: prenatal diagnosis and pathogenesis, *Obstet Gynecol* 71:1012, 1988.

88. Lodeiro JG et al: Fetal biophysical profile in twin gestations, *Obstet Gynecol* 67:824-827, 1986.

89. Luke B: The changing pattern of multiple births in the United States: maternal and infant characteristics, 1993 and 1990, *Obstet Gynecol* 84:101-106, 1994.

90. Luke B, Minogue J, Witter FR: The role of fetal growth restriction and gestational age on length of hospital stay in twin infants, *Obstet Gynecol* 81:949-953, 1993.

91. MacLean M et al: The ultrasonic assessment of discordant growth in twin pregnancies, *Ultrasound Obstet Gynecol* 2:30-34, 1992.

92. Maggio M et al: The first-trimester ultrasonographic diagnosis of conjoined twins, *Am J Obstet Gynecol* 152:833-835, 1985.

93. Mahony BS, Filly RA, Callen PW: Amnionicity and chorionicity in twin pregnancies: prediction using ultrasound, *Radiology* 155:205-209, 1985.

94. Mahony BS et al: The "stuck twin" phenomenon: ultrasonographic findings, pregnancy outcome, and management with serial amniocenteses, *Am J Obstet Gynecol* 163:1513-1522, 1990.

95. Mantoni M, Pedersen JF: Case report: monoamniotic twins diagnosed by ultrasound in the first trimester, *Acta Obstet Gynecol Scand* 59:551-553, 1980.

96. McLeod FN, McCoy DR: Monoamniotic twins with an unusual cord complication: case report, *Br J Obstet Gynaecol* 88:774, 1981.

97. Megory E et al: Pseudomonoamniotic twins with cord entanglement following genetic funipuncture, *Obstet Gynecol* 73:915-917, 1991.

98. Michaels WH et al: Ultrasound surveillance of the cervix in twin gestations: management of cervical incompetency, *Obstet Gynecol* 78:739-744, 1991.

99. Michaels WH et al: Ultrasound surveillance of the cervix during pregnancy in diethylstilbestrol-exposed offspring, *Obstet Gynecol* 73:230-239, 1989.

100. Monteagudo A, Timor-Tritsch IE, Sharma S: Early and simple determination of chorionic and amniotic type in multifetal gestations in the first fourteen weeks by high-frequency transvaginal ultrasonography, *Am J Obstet Gynecol* 170:824-829, 1994.

101. Moore TR, Gale S, Benirschke K: Perinatal outcome of forty-nine pregnancies complicated by acardiac twinning, *Am J Obstet Gynecol* 163:907-912, 1990.

102. Natsuyama E: Sonographic determination of fetal sex from twelve weeks of gestation, *Am J Obstet Gynecol* 149:748-757, 1984.

103. Nyberg DA et al: Entangled umbilical cords: a sign of monoamniotic twins, *J Ultrasound Med* 3:29, 1984.

104. Ohel G et al: Advanced ultrasonic placental maturation in twin pregnancies, *Am J Obstet Gynecol* 156:76-78, 1987.

105. Parulekar SG, Kiwi R: Dynamic incompetent cervix uteri, *J Ultrasound Med* 7:481-485, 1988.

106. Patten RM et al: Disparity of amniotic fluid volume and fetal size: problem of the stuck twin—ultrasound studies, *Radiology* 172:153-157, 1989.

107. Patterson RM, Wood RC: What is twin birthweight discordance? *Am J Perinatol* 7:217-219, 1990.

108. Persson PH, Kullander S: Long-term experience of general ultrasound screening in pregnancy, *Am J Obstet Gynecol* 146:942-947, 1983.

109. Plattner G et al: Fetal sex determination by ultrasound scan in the second and third trimesters, *Obstet Gynecol* 61:454-458, 1983.

110. Porreco RP, Barton SM, Haverkamp AD: Occlusion of umbilical artery in acardiac acephalic twin, *Lancet* 337:326-327, 1991.

111. Quinn MJ: Vaginal ultrasound and cervical cerclage: a prospective study, *Ultrasound Obstet Gynecol* 2:410-416, 1992.

112. Radestad A, Thomassen PA: Acute polyhydramnios in twin pregnancy: a retrospective study with special reference to therapeutic amniocentesis, *Acta Obstet Gynecol Scand* 69:297-300, 1990.

113. Reece EA et al: Can ultrasonography replace amniocentesis in fetal gender determination during the early second trimester? *Am J Obstet Gynecol* 156:579-581, 1987.

114. Reece EA et al: Fetal cerebellar growth unaffected by intrauterine growth retardation: a new parameter for prenatal diagnosis, *Am J Obstet Gynecol* 157:632-638, 1987.

115. Reece EA et al: A prospective longitudinal study of growth in twin gestations compared with growth in singleton pregnancies. I. The fetal head, *J Ultrasound Med* 10:439-443, 1991.

116. Reece EA et al: A prospective longitudinal study of growth in twin gestations compared with growth in singleton pregnancies. II. The fetal limbs, *J Ultrasound Med* 445-450, 1991.

117. Reisner DP et al: Stuck twin syndrome: outcome in thirty-seven consecutive cases, *Am J Obstet Gynecol* 169:991-995, 1993.

118. Rizzo G, Arduini D, Romanini C: Cardiac and extracadiac flows in discordant twins, *Am J Obstet Gynecol* 170:1321-1327, 1994.

119. Robinson HP, Caines JS: Sonar evidence of early pregnancy failure in patients with twin conceptions, *Br J Obstet Gynaecol* 84:22-25, 1979.

120. Robinson LK, Jones KL, Benirschke K: The nature of structural defects associated with velamentous and marginal insertion of the umbilical cord, *Am J Obstet Gynecol* 146:191, 1983.

121. Rodis JF et al: Antenatal diagnosis and management of monoamniotic twins, *Am J Obstet Gynecol* 157:1255-1257, 1987.

122. Rodis JF et al: Intrauterine fetal growth in concordant twin gestations, *Am J Obstet Gynecol* 162:1025-1029, 1990.

123. Rodis JF et al: Intrauterine fetal growth in discordant twin gestations, *J Ultrasound Med* 9:443-448, 1990.

124. Rudnicki M, Vejerslev LO, Junge J: The vanishing twin: morphologic and cytogenetic evaluation of an ultrasonographic phenomenon, *Gynecol Obstet Invest* 31:141-145, 1991.

125. Rush RW et al: A randomized controlled trial of cervical cerclage in women at high risk of spontaneous preterm delivery, *Br J Obstet Gynaecol* 91:724-730, 1984.

126. Sanders SP et al: Prenatal diagnosis of congenital heart defects in thoracoabdominally conjoined twins, *N Engl J Med* 313:370-374, 1985.

127. Santolaya J et al: Twin pregnancy: ultrasonographically observed changes in fetal presentation, *J Reprod Med* 37:328-330, 1992.

128. Shah YG et al: Doppler velocimetry in concordant and discordant twin gestations, *Obstet Gynecol* 80:272-276, 1992.

129. Shalev E et al: Short communication: first-trimester ultrasonic diagnosis of twin reversed arterial perfusion sequence, *Prenat Diagn* 12:219-222, 1992.

130. Shepard MJ, Richards VA, Berkowitz RL: An evaluation of two equations for predicting fetal weight by ultrasound, *Am J Obstet Gynecol* 147:47-54, 1982.

131. Sherer DM et al: Marked growth discordancy in three sets of twins associated with velamentous insertion of the umbilical cord of the smaller twin, *J Maternal Fetal Med* 2:165-169, 1993.

132. Shimizu T, Gaudette S, Nimrod C: Transverse cerebellar diameter in twin gestations, *Am J Obstet Gynecol* 167:1004-1008, 1992.

133. Smith CV et al: Transvaginal sonography of cervical width and length during pregnancy, *J Ultrasound Med* 11:465-467, 1992.

134. Stefos T et al: Individual growth curve standards in twins: prediction of third-trimester growth and birth characteristics, *Am J Obstet Gynecol* 161:179-183, 1989.

135. Stiller RJ et al: Amniotic fluid alpha-fetoprotein concentrations in twin gestations: dependence on placental membrane anatomy, *Am J Obstet Gynecol* 158:1088-1092, 1988.

136. Stiller RJ et al: Prenatal identification of twin reversed arterial perfusion syndrome in the first trimester, *Am J Obstet Gynecol* 160:1194-1196, 1989.

137. Storlazzi E et al: Ultrasonic diagnosis of discordant fetal growth in twin gestations, *Obstet Gynecol* 69:363-367, 1987.

138. Suttor J, Arab H, Manning FA: Monoamniotic twins: antenatal diagnosis and management, *Am J Obstet Gynecol* 155:836-837, 1986.

139. Townsend RR, Filly RA: Sonography of nonconjoined monoamniotic twin pregnancies, *J Ultrasound Med* 7:655, 1988.

140. Townsend RR, Simpson GF, Filly RA: Membrane thickness in ultrasound prediction of chorionicity of twin gestations, *J Ultrasound Med* 7:327-332, 1988.

141. Turner RJ et al: Magnetic resonance imaging and ultrasonography in the antenatal evaluation of conjoined twins, *Am J Obstet Gynecol* 155:645-649, 1986.

142. Urig MA, Clewell WH, Elliott JP: Twin-twin transfusion syndrome, *Am J Obstet Gynecol* 163:1522-1526, 1990.

143. Varma TR: Ultrasound evidence of early pregnancy failure in patients with multiple conceptions, *Br J Obstet Gynaecol* 86:290-292, 1979.

144. Ville Y et al: Endoscopic laser coagulation of umbilical cord vessels in twin reversed arterial perfusion sequence, *Ultrasound Obstet Gynecol* 4:396-398, 1994.

145. Watson WJ: Early-second-trimester fetal sex determination with ultrasound, *J Reprod Med* 35:247-249, 1990.

146. Weekes ARL, Menzies DN, DeBoer CH: Relative efficacy of bed rest, cervical suture and no treatment in the management of twin pregnancy, *Br J Obstet Gynaecol* 84:161-164, 1977.

147. Weir PE, Ratten GJ: Acute polyhydramnios—a complication of monozygous twin pregnancy, *Br J Obstet Gynaecol* 86:849-853, 1979.

148. Weissman A et al: The first-trimester growth-discordant twin: an ominous prenatal finding, *Obstet Gynecol* 84:110-114, 1994.

149. Westgren M et al: Spontaneous cephalic version of breech presentation in the last trimester, *Br J Obstet Gynaecol* 92:19-22, 1985.

150. Winn HN et al: Ultrasonographic criteria for the prenatal diagnosis of placental chorionicity in twin gestations, *Am J Obstet Gynecol* 161:1540-1542, 1989.

151. Yamada A et al: Antenatal diagnosis of twin-twin transfusion syndrome by Doppler ultrasound, *Obstet Gynecol* 78:1058-1061, 1991.

152. Yarkoni S et al: Estimated fetal weight in the evaluation of growth in twin gestations: a prospective longitudinal study, *Obstet Gynecol* 69:636-639, 1987.

153. Zakut H, Insler V, Serr DM: Elective cervical suture in preventing premature delivery in multiple pregnancy, *Isr J Med Sci* 13:488-492, 1977.

154. Zucchini S et al: Transvaginal ultrasound diagnosis of twin reversed arterial perfusion syndrome at 9 weeks' gestation, *Ultrasound Obstet Gynecol* 3:209-311, 1993.

Assessment of Fetal Well-Being

Kirk D. Ramin, Susan M. Ramin, and Larry C. Gilstrap III

Although the news of a twin or higher-order multiple pregnancy is often exciting for the woman and her family, such news often causes anxiety and concern for the clinician. Concern on the clinician's part surrounds both the marked increase in perinatal and maternal morbidity and mortality. Although significant progress has been made in both perinatal and neonatal medicine with improvement in overall neonatal outcome, there has been little improvement in the outcome in multiple pregnancies. For example, it has been well documented that the rate of spontaneous abortion is significantly increased in twin pregnancies. Moreover, Spellacy, Handler, and Fene,[24] in a comparison of twin pregnancies with singleton pregnancies reported perinatal mortality rates of 54/1000 versus 10.4/1000 livebirths, respectively. The perinatal mortality rate for the second twin is higher than for the first twin. Additionally, perinatal death is significantly increased for monozygotic twins when compared with dizygotic twins. Kovacks, Kirschbaum, and Paul[12] reported that the perinatal death rate for monozygotic twins was 2.5 times that for dizygotic twins. Probably the most important factor affecting outcomes of multiple pregnancies is the length of gestation. As the number of fetuses increases, the average duration of the gestation decreases dramatically. Caspi et al:[4] reviewed multiple gestations and concluded that the average gestational length for singleton pregnancies was approximately 39 weeks, compared with 35 weeks for twins, 33 weeks for triplets, and only 29 weeks for quadruplets. Other causes of adverse outcomes in these pregnancies include congenital anomalies, hypertension, dysfunctional growth, and abnormal vascular supply or vascular anastomosis. These complications are discussed in detail in Chapter 7.

With the above factors in mind, the need and the indication for antepartum surveillance of multiple gestations can easily be appreciated. Although the American College of Obstetricians and Gynecologists[1] includes multiple gestations with significant discordant growth as an indication for antepartum fetal testing, many cli-

nicians consider multiple gestation in and of itself a significant complication of pregnancy worthy of antepartum fetal surveillance, even in the absence of discordant growth.

The primary focus of this section is on the various modalities (excluding ultrasound, Doppler, and prenatal diagnosis, which are discussed on p. 135) of fetal well-being in multiple gestations. Since there is a paucity of scientific data regarding the efficacy of such testing in multiple pregnancies, much of the available information is "extrapolated" from databases on singleton pregnancies. Specifically, the following tests are discussed: fetal movement assessment, the contraction stress test (CST), the nonstress test (NST), vibratory acoustic stimulation, and the biophysical profile (BPP).

Fetal Movement

The literature is replete with studies regarding the efficacy of maternal-fetal movement assessment in surveying fetal well-being.[17,18] However, these studies primarily address the singleton pregnancy and to the authors' knowledge, there are no randomized, prospective trials of fetal movement assessment in multiple gestation as the primary means of antepartum assessment of fetal well-being. In a randomized study of fetal movement by Neldam[18] involving over 2000 pregnant women, there were 8 fetal demises in the control group and no deaths in the monitored group. All fetuses weighed more than 1500 gm and had no congenital anomalies. In contrast, a study by Grant et al.,[10] involving 68,000 women with uncomplicated pregnancies allocated to either routine fetal movement assessment or to standard

TABLE 6-1

Rates of Antepartum Late Fetal Death per 1000 Normally Formed Singleton Births

RATE	CLUSTERS		DIFFERENCES IN MEANS (95% CI)
	COUNTING (N = 33)	CONTROL (N = 33)	
All	2.90 (0.33)	2.67 (0.27)	0.24 (−0.50-0.98)
Potentially avoidable	2.17 (0.30)	2.23 (0.25)	−0.06 (−0.76-0.64)
Unexplained	1.77 (0.28)	1.85 (0.24)	−0.08 (−0.80-0.64)

From Grant A et al: Lancet 2:345, 1989.

prenatal care between 28 and 32 weeks' gestation, the death rates for infants from the two groups did not differ significantly. Interestingly, the authors noted that despite routine counting of fetal movements, most of the fetuses were dead by the time the mothers received medical attention. They calculated that 1250 women would have to undergo routine counting to prevent one explained antepartum fetal demise. This should not be surprising, considering the low incidence of fetal demise in this population. It is also important to note that these women did not have a significantly increased number of ultrasound scans, antepartum admissions, inductions, or elective cesarean sections. Considering these facts, along with the fact that fetal movement assessment by the patient does not engender additional medical costs, it is the authors' opinion that such effort is justifiable (if indeed one fetal death could be prevented for every 1250 women so monitored). Data concerning antepartum late fetal death per 1000 singleton births from this latter study are illustrated in Table 6-1.

Moore and Piacquadio[17] also evaluated fetal movement screening to reduce the incidence of unexplained antepartum fetal deaths. As controls they used 2519 pregnancies in which no formal fetal movement assessment had been performed before delivery. The fetal mortality rate among this group was 8.7 deaths per 1000 births. They then prospectively enrolled 1864 women who recorded the length of time required to appreciate 10 fetal movements. The mean (±standard deviation [SD]) interval for this time was 20.9 ± 18.1 minutes. They instructed women in whom 2 hours had elapsed without 10 fetal movements to report to the delivery unit for further evaluation. The fetal mortality rate among this group was 2.1/1000 births ($p < 0.01$ compared with controls). However, they did note that introduction of such a screening method resulted in a 13% increase in utilization of other antepartum fetal tests. Moreover, interventions for fetal compromise prompted by inadequate fetal activity tripled during the study period. They concluded that a "count-to-10" fetal movements screening program was simple to implement and effective in reducing fetal mortality. Again, it should be noted that this study involved singleton pregnancies.

Importantly, the establishment of a time limit at which a fetus must have 10 movements is somewhat arbitrary. In the study by Moore and Piacquadio,[17] the authors used 2 hours as the outer limit for which a fetus should move 10 times, since this encompassed five SDs from the "norm." One can interpret this 2-hour limit as being the extreme position from the mean for most fetuses and thereby exclude the need for further intervention or additional antepartum fetal surveillance. Although no prospective, randomized studies exist concerning fetal movement evaluation and multiple pregnancy, many physicians use antepartum movement assessment as an adjunct to other antepartum testing modalities.

Several concerns arise when considering fetal movement in a multiple gestation. The first is the ability of the mother to distinguish which fetus is actively moving, which is difficult at best in twin gestations and probably not possible with three or more fetuses. Secondly, it is commonly reported that women with multiple gestations and overdistention of the uterus have decreased ability to detect not only contractions but also fetal movement. Additionally, sensitivity to fetal movement may be significantly decreased when the pregnancy is complicated by hydramnios or oligohydramnios. Regardless of these shortcomings of fetal movement assessment in multiple pregnancies, the most common method of assessment of movement is to have a woman lie on her left side and count distinct movements until a perception of the desired number of movements has occurred over a given time. One protocol is summarized in Box 6-1 and generally consists of detecting five movements in 30 to 60 minutes. For twins this is performed for each fetus, if possible. For three or more fetuses, keeping track

BOX 6-1

Protocol for Assessment of Fetal Movement in Twins

- The patient should be in the left lateral recumbent position.
- Distinct fetal movements should be noted for each fetus.
- Each fetus should move at least five times within 30 minutes.
- Counts should be continued for up to 60 minutes if each fetus has not moved at least five times.*
- The patient should notify health care personnel if there are less than five fetal movements within 60 minutes.
- Assessment should be at least twice daily (for example, in the morning and at night).
- In the presence of three or more fetuses, it is helpful to establish a mean number of fetal movements over 1 to 2 hours and to have the patient report a discernible decrease in fetal movement. This varies among patients.

*Counting for each fetus when there are three or more is difficult if not impossible for most patients.

of the number of movements for each fetus is extremely difficult if not impossible for the majority of women. In general, it is best to use other antepartum tests along with fetal movement assessment when evaluating the well-being of fetuses in high-order multiple pregnancies. In this latter circumstance, one alternative is to have the mother begin counting fetal movements over 1 to 2 hours and arrive at a mean number of movements for that amount of time in her particular gestation. The mother is then instructed to report a discernible change in these fetal movements. This varies from patient to patient.

In light of the above findings and the shortcomings of all antepartum fetal testing, evaluation of fetal movement may be thought of as a significant adjunct to the assessment of overall fetal well-being because it is simple, of little or no cost, relatively easy to teach, and involves the mother and possibly her spouse to a greater degree in the pregnancy. In short, it allows the mother to participate in the monitoring of the well-being of her fetuses and in so doing, it may help alleviate some of her anxiety associated with her multiple pregnancy.

Contraction Stress Test

One of the earliest tests developed to monitor fetal well-being was the CST. Ray et al.[20] described the use of oxytocin-induced uterine contractions as a method of assessing uteroplacental insufficiency (UPI). This test became known as the oxytocin challenge test (OCT) and was widely used throughout the United States in the 1970s.[6] This test is based on the premise that fetuses in an environment of UPI manifest persistent late decelerations with contractions.[8,13,20] Although the literature is replete with articles regarding the use of the CST as an antepartum monitoring tool, there is less than unanimity of opinion regarding the clinical utility or efficacy of this modality in singleton pregnancies, let alone multiple pregnancies.[8,19,20,25]

The CST can be performed in several ways. For example, contractions can be induced either with oxytocin or through nipple stimulation. This latter test is also known as the nipple stimulation test. Huddleston, Sutliff, and Robinson[11] reported a 100% success rate for producing adequate contractions in 193 high-risk pregnancies by using intermittent nipple stimulation. There were no unexplained stillbirths in this series. A successful CST may also be obtained with spontaneous contractions.[8] The criteria used for interpretation of the CST is summarized in Box 6-2.

In a prospective (but not randomized) multicenter study of antepartum fetal testing in high-risk women, Freeman, Anderson, and Dorchester[9] reported the pregnancy outcomes of 4626 women who underwent the CST and 1542 women who underwent the NST for primary surveillance. These authors reported a significant decrease in fetal deaths in the CST group (0.4/1000 versus 3.2/1000; p < 0.05). Multiple gestations were not included in either arm of this study. In fact, there are no randomized prospective studies of the CST in multiple gestations.

One reason for the lack of data for multiple pregnancies is that this complication of pregnancy is a relative contraindication for either oxytocin– or nipple-stimulation–induced contractions. The reasons for this are twofold. First and foremost is the fact

BOX 6-2

Interpretation of the CST

- Negative: no late decelerations
- Positive: late decelerations after 50% or more of the contractions, even if the contraction frequency is less than three per 10 minutes
- Suspicious (equivocal): intermittent late or significant variable decelerations
- Unsatisfactory: fewer than three contractions per 10 minutes or poor quality tracing

From American College of Obstetricians and Gynecologists: Technical Bulletin No. 188, January 1994.

that women with multiple pregnancies are at significant risk for preterm labor, and induction of contractions may increase this risk. Moreover, many of these women also have dilated and partially effaced cervices. Secondly, the uterus is relatively overdistended and thus more susceptible to uterine rupture or placental abruption (especially with three or more fetuses). However, since most women with multiple gestations have recurrent episodes of contractions, a CST can often be accomplished without these concerns. The CST appears to be a useful adjunct to fetal evaluation in this latter scenario.

Nonstress Test

The NST evolved from the widespread use of the CST. Several advantages to using antepartum fetal heart rate tracings have been noted. First was the simplicity of the test in that is was noninvasive, low cost, did not require admission to labor and delivery, and could be performed in women in whom a CST might be contraindicated. Certainly women with multiple pregnancies are at increased risk for preterm labor and subsequent delivery and as such meet one of the relative contraindications to labor-induced CST. Moreover, the CST was associated with a high rate of false positive results.[7] By the start of the 1980s, the NST had largely replaced the CST as the primary means of antepartum surveillance and is widely used today. The rationale (at least from a scientific standpoint) for this widespread switch from the CST to the NST is unclear (that is, considering that the CST supposedly detects UPI). The rationale for the NST is that the fetal heart rate accelerates with fetal movement, provided that the fetus is not acidotic or neurologically depressed. This fetal heart rate reactivity implies normal fetal autonomic function and includes both sympathetic and parasympathetic pathways. Besides acidosis and neurologic depression, loss of reactivity or acceleration may also be associated with fetal sleep cycles.

There are several definitions of fetal heart rate reactivity in the interpretation of the NST. The NST is interpreted as reactive (normal) if there are two or more fetal heart rate accelerations peaking at least 15 bpm above the baseline and lasting 15 seconds from baseline to baseline within 20 minutes,[7] with or without fetal movement perceived by the mother. The NST is considered nonreactive when there is insufficient fetal heart rate acceleration over a 40 minutes.

Unlike the CST, there are several reports that have evaluated the efficacy of the NST in multiple gestations.[2,3,5,14,22] In an early report of 50 women with multiple gestations by Bailey et al.,[2] there were five women in whom one of the twin fetuses had a nonreactive NST, and four of these fetuses died. Devoe and Azor[5] reported on simultaneous NST monitoring in 24 sets of twins (Figures 6-15 and 6-16). These authors concluded that a reactive test was predictive of a good outcome and a nonreactive test was less specific.

Blake et al.[3] used the NST in 94 women with multiple gestations and reported an overall perinatal mortality rate similar to that of singleton pregnancies. Moreover, the perinatal mortality rate was 6 times greater with a nonreactive NST compared with a reactive test. Eighteen of the 25 women with a nonreactive NST also were evaluated by CST. Of these, 11 (61%) were found to have a positive CST and were de-

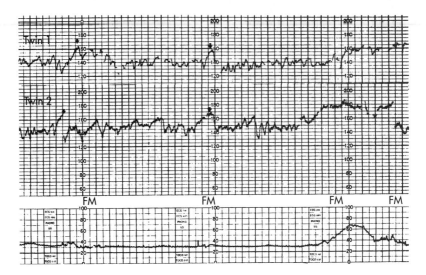

FIGURE 6-15 Nonstress tests in twin gestation at 37 weeks, showing concordant fetal heart rate patterns. Note the synchrony of accelerations *(arrows)* and similarity of baseline variability patterns. Fetal movements *(FM)* are indicated by remote-event marker. *(From Devoe LD, Azor H: Obstet Gynecol 58:450, 1981.)*

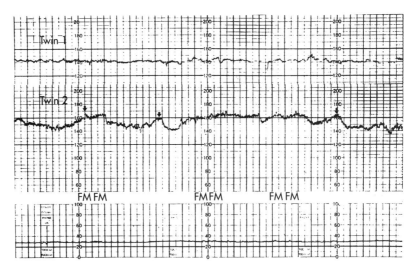

FIGURE 6-16 Nonstress tests in twin gestation at 36.5 weeks, showing nonconcordant fetal heart rate patterns. Accelerations *(arrows)* are present in lower tracing only. Fetal movements *(FM)* are indicated by remote-event marker. *(From Devoe LD, Azor H: Obstet Gynecol 58:450, 1981.)*

TABLE 6-2

Measures of Efficacy for Perinatal Outcome Predicted by NST in Multiple Gestations				
PREDICTED PARAMETER	SENSITIVITY (%)	SPECIFICITY (%)	PREDICTIVE VALUE OF REACTIVE TEST (%)	PREDICTIVE VALUE OF NONREACTIVE TEST (%)
Any perinatal complication	50.0	96.1	88.7	76.0
Fetal distress in labor	70.0	97.4	96.2	77.7
Growth retardation	26.0	89.0	88.0	28.0
Perinatal mortality	50.0	87.8	98.8	8.0

From Blake GD et al: Obstet Gynecol 63:528, 1984.

livered of their infants immediately. The remaining seven women were followed-up conservatively. The sensitivity, specificity, and predictive value of reactive and non-reactive tests in this study are summarized in Table 6-2.

In a randomized, prospective study by Sherman et al.,[22] the efficacy of the NST in predicting pregnancy outcome in twin gestations in 665 women was evaluated. The women received either prenatal care and NSTs or prenatal care alone. The groups were similar demographically. Fetal demise of one or both twins occurred in 10 pregnancies receiving prenatal care alone, compared with one in the group who received NSTs. Although a trend was evident with decreased fetal deaths in the NST group, this difference was not statistically significant (p = 0.062). A confounding variable detected in their data evaluation was that birth weight was statistically higher in the NST group. Other authors have shown a similar trend in decreasing perinatal mortality in women with twin gestations who were undergoing antepartum NST. Obviously a large prospective randomized trial is necessary to

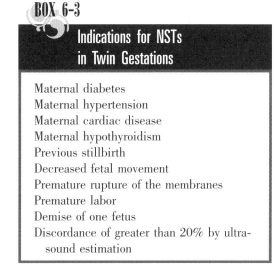

BOX 6-3

Indications for NSTs in Twin Gestations

Maternal diabetes
Maternal hypertension
Maternal cardiac disease
Maternal hypothyroidism
Previous stillbirth
Decreased fetal movement
Premature rupture of the membranes
Premature labor
Demise of one fetus
Discordance of greater than 20% by ultrasound estimation

From Sherman SJ et al: J Reprod Med 37:804, 1992.

establish the efficacy of NST in reducing the fetal death rate in twin gestations.

Sherman et al.[22] also summarized the indications for NSTs in twin gestations (Box 6-3). When NST is performed in pregnancy, a therapeutic dilemma arises when the results are nonreactive. Although a CST may logically follow a nonreactive NST in a singleton pregnancy, there is concern about the induction of

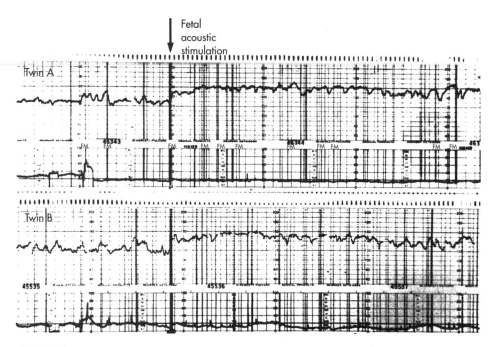

FIGURE 6-17   Fetal vibratory acoustic stimulation of a twin gestation at 33 weeks with simultaneous electronic FHR monitoring with two separate cardiotocometers. Note the synchronous FHR accelerations of both twins in response to stimulus *(arrow)*.

contractions in the setting of a multiple gestation because of the risk of preterm labor. Others have used fetal acoustic stimulation as an alternative to CST in these patients. This test would seem to especially lend itself to multiple pregnancies when the CST is contraindicated. This test is discussed in the following section.

Fetal Vibratory Acoustic Stimulation

Smith et al.[23] prospectively randomized women with a standard NST to those who had both the NST and fetal acoustic stimulation. They used a model 5C artificial larynx to stimulate the fetus. In these singleton gestations the incidence of a nonreac-

tive test was statistically significant at 14% in the control group and 9% in the study group. Additionally, a significant reduction in testing time was also observed by reducing the number of prolonged tests in those fetuses that had initially nonreactive tests. Sherer et al.[21] evaluated fetal vibratory acoustic stimulation in seven normal twin gestations with simultaneous fetal heart rate monitoring. In these gestations, sixteen stimulations were performed and all resulted in immediate synchronous fetal heart rate acceleration in both fetuses (Figures 6-17 and 6-18). Interestingly, these synchronous fetal heart rate accelerations occur in contrast to naturally occurring fetal heart rate accelerations that are nonsynchronous in nature among twins. The authors of the study concluded

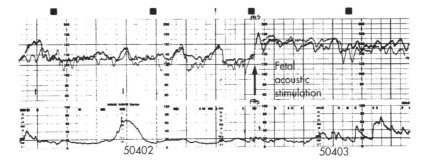

FIGURE 6-18 Twin gestations at 37 weeks. Simultaneous FHR monitoring with a single cardiotocograph. Note two distinctly separate FHR recordings with synchronous FHR accelerations in response to stimulus *(arrow)*, as opposed to the four coinciding, yet nonsynchronous, FHR accelerations that occur spontaneously before the vibratory acoustic stimulation. *(From Sherer DM et al: Am J Obstet Gynecol 164:1104, 1991.)*

that this synchronous fetal heart rate acceleration suggested that different mechanisms are responsible for spontaneous and evoked movements in twin gestations.

Fetal Biophysical Profile

The fetal BPP usually consists of five measurements: the NST, fetal breathing movements, fetal limb movements, fetal tone, and amniotic fluid assessment. A sixth measurement, placental grading, is used by some clinicians. A score of 2 is given for each normal variable, and a 0 is given for each abnormal variable. Thus a maximum score is 10 or 12.

Manning et al.[16] reported their results from almost 30,000 pregnancies evaluated by the BPP (more than 70,000 tests). Of the 29 fetuses with a score of 0, 14 died (11 were stillbirths).

Lodeiro et al.[15] reported on the use of the BPP in 49 women with twin gestations. These authors included placental grading and thus had 6 measurements. These authors used a score of 0, 1, or 2 for

each measurement, for a maximum score of 12. The sensitivity and specificity of this test were 83% and 100%, respectively. The positive and negative predictive values were 100% and 98%, respectively. Moreover, the false positive rate was 0% and the false negative rate was only 2%. These authors concluded that the BPP was a useful modality for the evaluation of twin gestations when used with an NST.

Sonography is no doubt one of the most useful tools for the antepartum evaluation of multiple gestations. The use of sonography and Doppler assessment in multiple gestations is summarized in Chapter 6.

Summary

There is no unanimity of opinion regarding which antenatal test is most effective in the evaluation of fetal assessment in pregnancies complicated by multiple fetuses (the same may be said for singleton pregnancies). Moreover, there is little scientific data on which to base firm recommendations.

Clinicians should generally use the specific test that best fits their patient population and ability (that is, equipment and personnel).

Some form of fetal movement assessment is recommended in all pregnancies complicated by multiple gestation. Generally, this testing can be routinely started at approximately 32 weeks' gestation. In pregnancies with other additional risk factors, testing may be indicated as early as 27 to 28 weeks' gestation. Some clinicians prefer to use the NST when further assessment is indicated, although a CST may prove useful in the presence of spontaneous contractions. A BPP may also prove useful in the evaluation of multiple gestations in which one or more of the fetuses has a nonreactive NST.

It should be obvious from this review that further studies are urgently needed to determine the ideal test for antepartum assessment of fetal well-being in multiple gestations. It is of paramount importance that these studies are prospective, randomized, and of sufficient power to address the questions.

References

1. American College of Obstetricians and Gynecologists: *Antepartum surveillance, Technical Bulletin No. 188*, January 1994.
2. Bailey D et al: Antepartum fetal heart rate monitoring in multiple pregnancy, *Br J Obstet Gynaecol* 87:561, 1980.
3. Blake GD et al: Evaluation of nonstress fetal heart rate testing in multiple gestations, *Obstet Gynecol* 63:528, 1984.
4. Caspi E et al: The outcome of pregnancy after gonadotropin therapy, *Br J Obstet Gynaecol* 83:967, 1976.
5. Devoe LD, Azor H: Simultaneous nonstress fetal heart rate testing in twin pregnancy, *Obstet Gynecol* 58:450, 1981.
6. Dilts PV: Current practices in antepartum and intrapartum fetal monitoring, *Am J Obstet Gynecol* 126:491, 1976.
7. Evertson LR et al: Antepartum fetal heart rate testing. I. Evolution of the nonstress test. *Am J Obstet Gynecol* 133:29, 1979.
8. Freeman RK: The use of the oxytocin challenge test for antepartum clinical evaluation of uteroplacental respiratory function, *Am J Obstet Gynecol* 121:481, 1975.
9. Freeman RK, Anderson G, Dorchester W: A prospective multiinstitutional study of antepartum fetal heart rate monitoring. I. Risk of perinatal mortality and morbidity according to antepartum fetal heart rate test results, *Am J Obstet Gynecol* 143:771, 1982.
10. Grant A et al: Routine formal fetal movement counting and risk of antepartum late death in normally formed singletons, *Lancet* 2:345, 1989.
11. Huddleston JF, Sutliff JG, Robinson D: Contraction stress test by intermittent nipple stimulation, *Obstet Gynecol* 63:669, 1984.
12. Kovacs BW, Kirschbaum TH, Paul RH: Twin gestations. I. Antenatal care and complications, *Obstet Gynecol* 74:313, 1989.
13. Kubli FW, Kaeser O, Hinselmann M: *Diagnostic management of chronic placental insufficiency*. In Pecile A, Finzi C, editors: *The Foeto-Placental Unit*, Amsterdam, 1969, Excerpta Medica.
14. Lenstrup C: Predictive value of antepartum nonstress testing in multiple pregnancies, *Acta Obstet Gynecol Scand* 63:597, 1984.
15. Lodeiro JG et al: Fetal biophysical profile in twin gestation, *Obstet Gynecol* 67:824, 1986.
16. Manning FA et al: Fetal assessment based on biophysical profile scoring. III. Positive predictive accuracy of the very abnormal test, *Am J Obstet Gynecol* 162:398, 1990.
17. Moore TR, Piacquadio K: A prospective evaluation of fetal movement screening to reduce the incidence of antepartum fetal death, *Am J Obstet Gynecol* 160:1075, 1989.
18. Neldam S: Fetal movements as an indicator of fetal well-being, *Lancet* 1:1222, 1980.
19. Peck TM: Physician's subjectivity in evaluating oxytocin challenge tests, *Obstet Gynecol* 56:13, 1980.
20. Ray M et al: Clinical experience with the oxytocin challenge test, *Am J Obstet Gynecol* 114:1, 1972.
21. Sherer DM et al: Fetal vibratory acoustic stimulation in twin gestation with simultaneous fetal heart rate monitoring, *Am J Obstet Gynecol* 164:1104, 1991.

22. Sherman SJ et al: Nonstress test assessment of twins, *J Reprod Med* 37:804, 1992.
23. Smith CV et al: Fetal acoustic stimulation testing. II. A randomized clinical comparison with the nonstress test, *Am J Obstet Gynecol* 155:131, 1986.
24. Spellacy WN, Handler A, Fene CD: A case-control study of 1253 twin pregnancies from a 1982-1987 perinatal data base, *Obstet Gynecol* 75:168, 1990.
25. Staisch KJ, Westlake JR, Bashore RA: Blind oxytocin challenge test and prenatal outcome, *Am J Obstet Gynecol* 138:399, 1980.

Multiple Pregnancy Reduction and Selective Termination

Joanne Stone and Richard L. Berkowitz

Natural History of Multiple Gestations

The incidence of multiple pregnancies has increased dramatically since the introduction of ovulation induction (OI) therapy and assisted reproductive techniques (ART). From 1978 to 1988, twin births have increased by 33%, and triplet and higher-order multiple births have increased by 101%.[36] The incidence of multiple gestation after OI ranges from 6% to 8% with clomiphene citrate and 15% to 53% with the use of gonadotropins.[54] Although twins account for the majority of infants from multiple pregnancies that occur after infertility treatment, the occurrence of pregnancies with three or more fetuses can no longer be considered rare events. In these patients the incidence of high-order multiple births containing three or more fetuses ranges from 1% to 20%, depending on the particular medications used and the techniques employed.[54,55]

The advancements made in the treatment of infertility are paralleled by the increased risks associated with multiple gestation. Although accurate information on the natural outcome of multiple pregnancies is incomplete, perinatal and maternal morbidity and mortality are known to increase with increasing numbers of fetuses.[29,45] Published studies generally contain relatively small numbers of patients, and most do not provide long-term follow-up information on the outcomes of survivors. Information available on early fetal losses in multiple gestation is limited because the majority of published series only report on pregnancies that continue beyond 20 weeks. However, two recent studies do provide insight into early fetal losses among patients carrying two or more fetuses. Seoud et al.[56] reported the outcome of twin, triplet, and quadruplet gestations that occurred after in vitro fertilization at the Jones Institute for Reproductive Medicine between 1982 and 1990. Among patients with previously documented fetal heart activity, 17/165 patients with twins (10.3%), 2/26 with triplets (7.7%), and 1/5 with quadruplets (20%) lost their entire pregnancies before 20 weeks' gestation. Similarly, Lipitz et al.[35] reported that 13.2% of 106 women carrying viable triplets lost all of their fetuses before 20 weeks' gestation.

Undoubtedly the most common and most significant complication of multiple pregnancy is preterm delivery. Gestational age at delivery and birth weight are the two most important factors affecting perinatal mortality and neonatal and infant morbidity.[36] Low birth weight (LBW) infants (less than 2500 gm) are 40 times as likely to die in the neonatal period and 3 times as likely to exhibit neurodevelopmental handicaps as infants of normal weight.[36]

The length of gestation and infants' birth weights of multiple pregnancies are inversely proportional to the number of fetuses carried in the uterus. The average gestational ages at delivery of twins, triplets, and quadruplets are 35, 33, and 30 weeks,[9] and the average birth weights are 2473, 1666, and 1414 gm, respectively.[56]

In 1988 Pons et al.[46] reported on 21 triplet pregnancies that were studied from 1975-1986. Twelve of these 21 sets of triplets were conceived spontaneously, and the rest resulted from OI therapy. Seven (33.3%) sets were delivered between 29 and 32 weeks, 13 sets (62%) were delivered between 33 and 36 weeks, and 1 set was delivered at term. Three infants in this series died because of complications of prematurity.

In 1989 Lipitz et al.[35] published data on the outcome of 78 sets of triplets that were delivered at a single center between 1975 and 1988. Preterm delivery occurred in 86% of all of these pregnancies; 26% were delivered before 32 weeks, and 9% were delivered before 27 weeks. The mean length of gestation was 33.2 weeks, and the perinatal and neonatal mortality rates were 93/1000 and 51/1000, respectively. Follow-up data for a minimum of 1 year were available for 38 of the 48 infants with birth weights below 1500 gm. Eleven percent of these infants had severe neurologic disabilities and included one infant with spastic diplegia and normal intelligence and three with spastic quadriplegia and marked developmental delay. An additional 21% of infants had mild developmental problems, including abnormalities of muscle tone or attention deficit disorders.

A study by Newman, Hamer, and Clinton Miller[43] published in 1989 reviewed the outcome of 198 women who were delivered of triplets between 1985 and 1988 at 24 centers in the United States. All patients were followed-up with home uterine activity monitoring, and 58% of them received prophylactic tocolytic medications. Despite a goal of outpatient management, 88 women (44%) required antepartum hospitalization on 110 occasions for reasons other than preterm labor. Preterm labor occurred in 88% of the patients in spite of this aggressive management. Seven percent of patients were delivered of their infants before 29 weeks, 14% between 29 and 31 weeks, and 75% between 32 and

37 weeks. The corrected perinatal mortality rate was 50/1000. Interestingly, there was no increase in gestational age at delivery or birth weight for the infants of the 115 women who received prophylactic tocolysis over the infants of the 83 women who did not receive these medications. A compilation of data from studies on the natural history of triplet gestations is provided in Table 6-3.

A paucity of reports exists on the natural history of pregnancies containing four or more fetuses. In 1990 Lipitz et al.[34] reported their experience with 11 high-order multiple pregnancies between 1975 and 1989 that reached at least 13 weeks' gestation. The series contains eight sets of quadruplets, two sets of quintuplets, and one set of sextuplets. All of the infants were delivered before 37 weeks, 73% before 34 weeks, and 27% before 29 weeks. The fetal loss rate was 23%, and the perinatal mortality rate was 12%. Thirty of 37 neonatal survivors were followed-up for at least 2 years. Seventy percent appeared to have normal development, whereas 30% had evidence of neurodevelopmental abnormalities.

Gonen et al.[23] reported on 1 quintuplet, 5 quadruplet, and 24 triplet gestations delivered between 1978 and 1988. The mean gestational ages at delivery were 29, 30, and 32.4 weeks, respectively. Follow-up data for a period from 1 to 10 years were available for 85/88 infants. Ten infants (12%) had mild hypotonia as well as a mild delay in gross motor development. Seven infants (8%) had a mild language delay, and two (2%) had a mild delay in cognitive development. The authors considered these findings functional and transient in nature. One infant had a mild spasic diple-

gia, and another had a moderate spastic diplegia as well as delays in social-adaptive and language development.

In 1990 Collins and Bleyl[11] reviewed the outcome of 71 quadruplet pregnancies. Data were collected by sending out a questionnaire to mothers who participated in a support group for women with high-order multiple gestations. The study has been criticized for its methodology, poor response rate, and potential ascertainment bias. The mean gestational age at delivery was 31.4 weeks. In 75% of cases, delivery occurred before 34 weeks, in 47% it was before 32 weeks, and in 13% it was before 28 weeks. The perinatal and neonatal mortality rates were 15% and 12%, respectively. Not surprisingly, the majority of neonatal losses occurred in the patients whose infants were delivered before 28 weeks.

A recent study of quadruplet pregnancies published in 1992 by Elliot and Radin[15] compared 10 sets of quadruplets reaching at least 20 weeks of gestation and managed by one perinatal team with 57 sets of quadruplets managed at various institutions across the United States. Data on the latter group were obtained from the records of a perinatal service, which supplied home uterine activity monitoring to these 57 patients. The mean gestational age at delivery of the 10 sets of quadruplets was 32.5 weeks, as opposed to 30.2 weeks in the other group. Accurate neonatal and follow-up data on the latter group were not available, but among the 10 sets of quadruplets, 38% had respiratory distress syndrome (RDS) and no neonatal deaths were reported. Table 6-4 reviews recent publications on the outcome of quadruplet pregnancies.

TABLE 6-3

Natural History of Triplet Gestations

AUTHOR	YEARS	NUMBER	MEAN GA[a] AT DELIVERY (WK)	GA AT DELIVERY (%)		
				<37 WK	<32 WK	<28 WK
Itzkowic[30]	1946-1976	59	33	83	25	10
Syrop and Varner[57]	1946-1983	20	33	75	—	15
Holcberg et al.[27]	1960-1979	31	32	87	36	16
Pons et al.[46]	1975-1986	4	36	95	33	0
Lipitz et al. (1989)[33]	1975-1988	78	33	86	26	10
Keith et al.[32]	1981-1986	13	33	85	46	0
Creinin, Katz, and Laros[12]	1981-1988	13	34	92	15	0
Jonas and Lumley[31]	1982-1990	133	33	92[b]	32[b]	14[b]
Lipitz et al. (1994)[35]	1984-1992	106	34	92	24	—
Newman, Hamer, and Clinton Miller[43]	1985-1988	198	34	96	20	7[c]
Boulot et al.[7]	1985-1991	48	34	53	16	2
Peacemen et al.[44]	1988-1991	15	35	60	13	0
Totals		735	33.5	88	25	9

[a]GA, gestational age; [b]Reported as <2500 gm, <1500 gm, and <1000 gm; [c]<29 weeks.

Whereas prematurity is the most common complication associated with multiple pregnancies, the maternal risks associated with multiple gestation are also significantly increased over those observed in singleton gestations.[15] Up to 32% of women carrying multiple fetuses are reported to develop pregnancy-induced hypertension; 25% develop anemia, 21% suffer a postpartum hemorrhage, and 13% require blood transfusion.[11]

Although advances in perinatal and neonatal care have reduced the morbidity and mortality associated with multiple gestation, the outcome of high-order multiple births is still worse than that for either singletons or twins. In 1990 Sassoon et al.[53] published a study in which 15 triplet pregnancies were compared with 15 twin pregnancies matched for age, race, socio-economic status, mode of delivery, number of previous term deliveries, and a history of previous preterm birth. Preterm labor occurred significantly more often in triplet than in twin gestations (80% versus 40%), as did preterm delivery (87% versus 27%). The mean length of neonatal hospitalization was significantly longer in triplets than in twins (29 days versus 9 days), and triplets had a fivefold increased risk of requiring neonatal intensive care compared with twins. No significant differences were detected in major neonatal complications such as RDS or intraventricular hemorrhage.

Seoud et al.[56] reported on the outcomes of 103 twin, 15 triplet, and 4 quadruplet pregnancies conceived through in vitro fertilization (IVF) between 1982 and 1990. The mean gestational ages at delivery were

TABLE 6-3

Natural History of Triplet Gestations—cont'd

AUTHOR	MEAN BW[d] (GM)	MEAN MATERNAL HOSPITAL STAY (DAYS)	CORRECTED PNM[e] PER 1000 BIRTHS >500 gm
Itzkowic[30]	—	—	93
Syrop and Varner[57]	1539	—	216
Holcberg et al.[27]	1711	34	312
Pons et al.[46]	1710	35	78
Lipitz et al. (1989)[33]	—	—	232
Keith et al.[32]	1779	10	—
Creinin, Katz, and Laros[12]	1875	25	0[f]
Jonas and Lumley[31]	1720	32	108[g]
Lipitz et al. (1994)[35]	1780	—	50
Newman, Hamer, and Clinton Miller[43]	1871	15[h]	50
Boulot et al.[7]	1870	—	59
Peacemen et al.[44]	1957	27	22
Totals	1796	23	123

[d]*BW*, birth weight; [e]*PNM*, perinatal mortality; [f]Excluding 3 sets of triplets delivered between 23 and 24 weeks; [g]Includes stillborns >400 grams or >20 weeks; [h]Mean per each hospitalization.

36 weeks for twins versus 32 and 31 weeks for triplets and quadruplets. The mean birth weights were 2473, 1666, and 1414 gm, respectively. The mothers of 42% of the twins, 92% of the triplets, and 75% of the quadruplets experienced preterm labor. The average length of the neonatal hospital stay was 12 days for the twins, 17 days for the triplets, and 58 days for the quadruplets. The corrected perinatal mortality rates (excluding losses occurring before 28 weeks) for twins, triplets, and quadruplets were 38.5/1000, 0/1000, and 0/1000, respectively.

Thus the data on the natural history of twins, triplets, and higher-order multiple births indicate that the risk of adverse outcome increases with increasing fetal numbers. Patients who have finally become pregnant after a long history of infertility may find that they have conceived more fetuses than can be successfully carried to viability or to a gestational age at which the risk of preterm delivery and its associated morbidity is acceptable. These patients must choose one of three difficult options. One possibility is to terminate the entire pregnancy, a choice that is usually unacceptable for couples with a history of infertility and who have tried desperately to achieve pregnancy. A second option is to continue the pregnancy and take the risk of delivering severely preterm infants at high risk for long-term morbidity. The third option is to undergo a procedure called multifetal pregnancy reduction (MPR), in which the number of fetuses is reduced to decrease the risk of preterm delivery and optimize the chances of a successful outcome. If a woman is car-

TABLE 6-4

Natural History of Quadruplet Gestations

AUTHOR	YEARS	NUMBER	MEAN GA[a] AT DELIVERY (WK)	GA AT DELIVERY (%)		
				<37 WK	<32 WK	<28 WK
Lipitz et al.[34]	1975-1989	8	31	100	50	25
Gonen et al.[23]	1978-1988	5	30	100	—	—
Collins and Bleyl[11]	1980-1998	71	31[b]	94	59	20
Jonas and Lumley[31]	1982-1990	6	31	100	50	33
Vervliet et al.[61]	1985-1988	5	32	100	67	33
Elliott and Radin[15]	1986-1991	10	33	100	30	0
Totals		105	31	96	55	20

[a]GA, Gestational age; [b]29.7 after excluding patients with a spontaneous demise of one fetus.

rying five or more fetuses, the decision to undergo MPR is usually not difficult because the chances of a favorable outcome under these circumstances is extremely small. However, for patients carrying triplets or quadruplets the decision is more complex.

Multifetal Pregnancy Reduction

In an attempt to decrease the perinatal morbidity and mortality associated with multiple pregnancies, several techniques have been used to reduce the number of living fetuses within the uterus. Three approaches to MPR are described.

TRANSVAGINAL ASPIRATION

In 1986 Dumez and Oury[14] first described 15 cases of MPR performed between 9 and 10 weeks of gestation. The patients had 3 to 6 fetuses and had their pregnancies reduced to 4 singletons, 10 sets of twins, and 1 set of triplets. The procedures were performed by dilating the cervix and aspirat-

ing the gestational sacs transvaginally under ultrasound guidance. At the time of publication, 11 pregnancies were completed and 4 were still in progress. Of the 10 completed pregnancies, 4 patients had their infants delivered at term, 3 had them delivered between 33 and 36 weeks, 1 had them delivered at 30 weeks, and 2 lost their pregnancies in the second trimester.

In 1989 Itskovitz et al.[28] described two patients in whom transvaginal ultrasound-guided aspiration of gestational sacs was performed at 7 weeks. One patient required placement of a cerclage at 18 weeks and treatment for multiple episodes of preterm labor, but eventually was delivered of her infant at 36 weeks. The second patient's infant was delivered at term after an uneventful prenatal course.

Boulot et al.[7] published a series of 61 women who underwent MPR—35 by the transabdominal approach and 26 by transcervical sac perforation. The loss rate before 24 weeks was 13.1% and did not vary significantly with the approach used.

TABLE 6-4

Natural History of Quadruplet Gestations—cont'd

AUTHOR	MEAN BW[c] (gm)	MEAN MATERNAL HOSPITAL STAY (DAYS)	CORRECTED PNM[d] PER 1000 BIRTHS <500 gm
Lipitz et al.[34]	—	—	290[e]
Gonen et al.[23]	1172	49	0
Collins and Bleyl[11]	1482	—	67
Jonas and Lumley[31]	1357	47[f]	—
Vervliet et al.[61]	1422	—	—
Elliott and Radin[15]	1536	45	0
Totals	1416	47	75

[c]BW, birth weight; [d]PNM, perinatal mortality; [e]Includes >400 gm and excludes one fetus with trisomy 18 syndrome; [f]Includes only hospitalization in which delivery occurred.

TRANSVAGINAL INTRATHORACIC POTASSIUM CHLORIDE INJECTION

In 1990 Gonen, Blankier, and Casper[22] reported six cases of transvaginal MPR. The reductions were performed between 8 and 13 weeks' gestation and were guided by transvaginal ultrasound. The procedures were performed by inserting a needle into the gestational sac via a needle-guide fixed to the vaginal transducer. The needle was then directed into the fetal thorax, and KCl was injected until asystole was observed. Two of the six pregnancies in this small series were ongoing at the time of publication. One patient developed fever and chorioamnionitis 2 days after the procedure, which led to a septic abortion, and three patients were delivered of healthy infants.

In 1993 Timor-Tritsch et al.[60] reported the outcomes of 134 patients undergoing MPR by transvaginal puncture and KCl injection. Of the 134 cases, 100 women had been delivered of their infants at the time of publication and 15 had ongoing

pregnancies beyond 24 weeks. The uncorrected loss rate was 12.6%. There was no difference in the loss rate in those patients whose fetus in the sac over the internal os was targeted for reduction (as opposed to patients with other targeted fetuses). Three clinically apparent infections were detected, two of which responded to antibiotics and enabled the patients to have otherwise uncomplicated prenatal courses. Evacuation of the uterine contents was required in the third woman because of uncontrolled infection.

TRANSABDOMINAL INTRATHORACIC POTASSIUM CHLORIDE INJECTION

In 1988 Berkowitz et al.[4] reported the first series of ultrasound-guided transabdominal MPR by intrathoracic KCl injection. In this series of 12 pregnancies, the first three procedures were performed by transcervical aspiration. However, after the third patient experienced placental separation and excessive vaginal bleeding during the procedure, the subsequent nine procedures were performed by transabdominal intrathoracic injection of KCl. In this series, eight patients were delivered of at least one healthy fetus, and four lost their entire pregnancies. In an extended series published in 1993, Berkowitz et al.[5] reported their experience with 200 cases of transabdominal MPR. This series consisted of 88 sets of triplets, 89 sets of quadruplets, 16 sets of quintuplets, and 7 pregnancies containing between six and nine fetuses. In five cases the pregnancies were reduced to triplets at the patients' requests, and in six cases the pregnancies were reduced to singleton pregnancies for medical reasons. All patients underwent an extensive counseling session in which the risks and benefits of the procedure were discussed in detail. Under ultrasound guidance, a 22-gauge spinal needle was inserted into the fetal thorax and 2 to 3 mEq of KCl were injected. Asystole was observed for 3 minutes before the removal of the needle. This procedure was repeated for each fetus that was terminated. Unless significant discrepancies in the size of the fetuses existed or gross anomalies were detected, the selection of the fetuses to be terminated was based on the technical ease with which the procedure could be performed. The fetus in the sac over the internal os was left alone. In this series of 200 patients, 181 were delivered of one or more viable infants after 24 weeks' gestation and 19 lost their entire pregnancies. Three of these 19 losses occurred within 4 weeks of the procedure, six losses occurred from 4 to 8 weeks later, and 10 happened more than 8 weeks after the procedure had been performed. The loss rates were 7.9% for women with three or four fetuses at the time of the procedure,

12.5% for those with five fetuses, and 42.9% for those with six or more fetuses.

Other authors have presented their experience with transabdominal MPR, and the results are similar.[6,13,59,62] Recently Evans et al.[17] published the collaborative experience of transabdominal reductions at six worldwide centers. This study reported the outcomes of 463 completed pregnancies. The procedures were performed with a 100% technical success rate. Of the 463 pregnancies, 388 (83.8%) ended with infants delivered after 24 weeks. The risks of fetal loss were 3.9% and 4.6% at 2 and 4 weeks postprocedure, and the overall loss rate was 16.2% at 24 weeks. Interestingly, the authors reported that the incidence of obstetric complications such as premature rupture of membranes, preeclampsia, fetal growth retardation, and other maternal and obstetric problems was similar to that reported for spontaneously conceived twins.

Table 6-5 summarizes the data on the outcome of MPR performed at several centers and with different techniques. In another collaborative multicenter study, Evans et al.[18] compared the outcome of transabdominal versus transcervical and transvaginal MPR. The study included 846 transabdominal procedures and 238 done by either the transcervical or the transvaginal route. The starting and finishing numbers were higher in the transabdominal group, as was the gestational age at the time of procedure. There was no significant difference in loss rates before 24 weeks between the two groups. Not surprisingly, when the transabdominal group was divided into procedures performed in the early and late years of each group's experience, a steep learning curve

TABLE 6-5

Summary of Publications of Multifetal Pregnancy Reduction

AUTHOR	NUMBER	METHOD	COMPLETE LOSS RATE <24 WK (%)	LOSS RATE WITHIN 4 WEEKS OF PROCEDURE	INFECTIONS (%)	MEAN GA* AT DELIVERY
Wapner et al.[62]	32	TA KCl	3	0	0	—
Tabsch[59]	28	TA KCl	0	0	0	35
Boulot et al.[7]	61	35 TA KCl 26 TC sac perforation	13	3	0	36
Donner et al.[13]	26	23 TA KCl	14	0	0	36
Berkowitz et al.[5]	200	TA KCl	10	2	0	36
Timor-Tritsch et al.[60]	134	TV KCl	13†	6	2	—

*GA, gestational age; TA, transabdominal; TC, transcervical; TV, transvaginal; †81% delivered at 36 weeks or more.

for loss rates was demonstrated. The loss rate in the early years was 16.2% versus 8.8% in the later years. There were not enough cases to assess a learning curve in the transcervical and transvaginal group.

LONG-TERM FOLLOW-UP

Since MPR is a fairly new procedure, little long-term follow-up data are available. However, a study by Brandes et al.[8] in 1990 reported on the psychomotor and physical development of seven children born to three women who had undergone MPR. Follow-up examinations were performed between 12 and 38 months. The children were matched to controls for birth weight, gestational age, sex, mode of delivery, parity, age at examination, and maternal age and education. No differences were detected in the physical and psychomotor development between the two groups.

TIMING

Transabdominal MPRs are generally performed between 10 and 13 weeks' gesta-

tion, whereas the transvaginal technique is usually carried out earlier. Transabdominal MPR procedures performed before 10 weeks are technically more difficult because of the small fetal size, the greater distance between the fetus and the maternal abdominal wall, and the limitations in the resolution of transabdominal ultrasound. Additionally, there are several other reasons that the time between 10 and 13 weeks' gestation is believed to be the optimal time to perform these procedures. Before this time, the spontaneous loss of an embryo may occur, possibly alleviating the need to perform the reduction procedure. In fact, Seoud et al.[56] reported that of 26 patients with triplet gestations and documented fetal cardiac activity in all three sacs, 11 patients (30%) spontaneously lost one or more (but not all) fetuses. Unfortunately the authors do not provide the gestational ages at which the fetal demises occurred. Additionally, waiting until the eleventh or twelfth week of pregnancy increases the chances that an underlying growth delay in one of the fetuses may be revealed. Since fetuses with a significant lag in crown-rump length (CRL) are at increased risk of spontaneous death and chromosomal anomalies, those fetuses would be targeted for reduction.[37,42] Moreover, the chances that morphologic abnormalities may be detected by ultrasound are better at a slightly greater gestational age. However, waiting longer than 12 weeks has few advantages because the chances for the spontaneous loss of one fetus are probably small, and the risk of developing disseminated intravascular coagulopathy from a larger mass of retained dead fetal tissue may be increased.

MATERNAL SERUM ALPHA FETOPROTEIN

Maternal serum alpha fetoprotein (MSAFP) levels have been studied in 57 patients who underwent first-trimester MPR at the Mount Sinai Medical Center.[38] The mean interval between reduction and MSAFP determination was 4.4 weeks. All patients demonstrated higher MSAFP values than patients with twins of the same gestational age at the time of testing. The mean MSAFP in these 57 patients was 11.6 multiples of the median (MOM) (ranging from 3.9 to 47 MOM). A positive correlation between the MSAFP MOM and the number of dead fetuses was demonstrated. The elevations in MSAFP levels are not necessarily indicative of a morphologic abnormality in the surviving fetuses and most likely result from the release of material from the dead embryos. It is currently recommended that patients undergoing MPR have a detailed ultrasound examination of the surviving fetuses performed in the mid-second trimester and that MSAFP values be ignored.

TRIPLETS: THE DECISION TO REDUCE

At this time it is unclear whether MPR from triplets to twins results in an improvement in long-term neonatal outcome. Although pregnancy reduction to twins decreases the incidence of premature delivery, the beneficial effects on the long-term outcome of these infants is less certain. Four recent studies compare the perinatal morbidity and mortality in patients undergoing MPR from triplet to twin gestations with patients who kept triplets and did not undergo the procedure. The results are summarized in Table 6-6.

Three of the four studies showed an increase in gestational age at the time of delivery among patients undergoing MPR, and all four studies demonstrated an increase in birth weight in these patients compared with the patients carrying triplets. Two studies reported a decline in the complete loss rate at less than 24 weeks' gestation, but the other two reported opposite findings. All four studies documented a decrease in the proportion of patients with infants delivered before 32 weeks when patients underwent MPR. All four studies also demonstrated a decrease in neonatal respiratory complications, and two of three studies demonstrated a decrease in the incidence of intraventricular hemorrhage among patients who underwent MPR. Additionally, three studies reported a decrease in perinatal mortality among those patients who underwent MPR compared with patients who retained their triplet gestations. Although MPR from triplets to twins appears to decrease the short-term morbidity associated with multiple pregnancies, it is still unclear whether the long-term outcome of survivors is improved. Further studies containing much larger numbers of patients with

TABLE 6-6

Perinatal Outcome of Triplets Versus MPR Twins

AUTHOR	STUDY GROUP	NUMBER	MEAN GA* DELIVERY AT (WK)	LOSS RATE <24 WK (%)	BW (gm)	% REQUIRING MECHANICAL VENTILATION	PNM PER 1000
Porreco, Shannon Burke, and Hendrix[48]	Triplets	11	36	0	2239	9	0
	Reduced twins	13	36	8	2727	8	0
Macones et al.[40]	Triplets	14	31	7	1593	5†	210
	Reduced twins	47	36	0	2279	14	30
	Nonreduced twins	63	35	1	2292	23	40
Boulot et al.[6]	Triplets	48	34	6	1870	45	59
	Reduced twins	32	37	18	2340	15‡	38
Lipitz et al.[35]	Triplets	106	34	21	1780	29	109
	Reduced twins	34	37	9	2350	7	48

*GA, gestational age; BW, birth weight; PNM, perinatal mortality; †RDS; ‡Respiratory disorders.

long-term follow-up data are necessary to adequately resolve this issue. The compelling social and financial issues, as well as concerns for maternal morbidity, appear to make it justifiable to continue to offer MPR to women carrying three fetuses until all the necessary data are available for analysis.

Selective Termination

Women undergoing infertility treatment receive frequent ultrasound examinations, and as a consequence, multiple gestations are often diagnosed in the first trimester. Furthermore, improvements in screening with both ultrasound and prenatal genetic diagnostic modalities have resulted in an increase in the detection of fetal abnormalities in multiple gestations. Until fairly recently, when a chromosomal abnormality, congenital malformation, or genetic disorder was discovered in one fetus of a multiple gestation, the parents were faced with a decision to either terminate the entire pregnancy or do nothing and allow the delivery of one or more healthy fetuses as well as an abnormal child. The development and refinement of a procedure known as selective termination enables couples to choose a third option: the termination of the abnormal fetus and the continuation of the pregnancy.

In 1978 Aberg et al.[1] reported the first successful selective termination of a twin pregnancy that was discordant for Hurler's syndrome. Since that time, a variety of methods for performing this procedure have been described, including cardiac tamponade,[65] intracardiac air embolization,[52] fetoscopic umbilical cord ligation,[49] and intracardiac KCl injection.

In 1989 Chitkara et al.[10] reported on 17 patients who underwent second-trimester selective termination. In the first seven cases, termination was achieved by cardiac puncture with either exsanguination (one patient), air embolization (five patients), or cardiac tamponade (one patient). Four of these pregnancies were lost completely, and three had successful outcomes. The remaining 10 procedures were performed by intracardiac KCl injection, and all of these pregnancies resulted in the births of healthy singletons. Between 1986 and 1993, 54 transabdominal selective terminations with KCl injection have been performed at the Mount Sinai Medical Center (unpublished data). In 48 of these 54 cases, twin gestations were reduced to singletons; in five cases triplets were reduced to either twins or singletons; and in one case quadruplets were reduced to triplets. Three of the 54 pregnancies were lost entirely 3 to 3.5 weeks after the procedure, for a loss rate of 5.6%. The remaining 51 pregnancies were all successfully completed, with a mean gestational age at delivery of 36.3 weeks.

Evans et al.[19] compiled data on 183 completed cases of selective termination from 9 centers in four countries and utilizing a variety of techniques. These cases included 169 twins, 11 triplets, and 3 quadruplets. Indications for the procedures included 96 chromosome abnormalities, 76 structural abnormalities, and 11 mendelian disorders detected in the anomalous fetuses. The procedures were technically successful in 100% of cases. Twenty-three of the 183 pregnancies (12.6%) were lost completely before 24 weeks' gestation. If the procedures were performed before or at 16 weeks, the loss rate was 5.4%, but this figure rose to 14.4% if the procedures were performed at 17 weeks or later. Of all the viable pregnancies, 83.8% had infants delivered after 33 weeks, and 4.3% had infants delivered between 25 and 28 weeks.

Not all patients with a multiple gestation discordant for a fetal abnormality are candidates for a selective termination. Several issues must be considered when a patient's appropriateness and feasibility for undergoing the procedure are being evaluated. These include proper identification of the abnormal fetus, sac chorionicity, and severity or lethality of the diagnosed condition.

IDENTIFICATION OF THE ABNORMAL FETUS

Cases in which the abnormal fetus manifests morphologic abnormalities pose few problems, because the targeted fetus can be readily identified with ultrasound. However, cases in which a chromosomal abnormality has been detected by prenatal genetic analysis of amniotic fluid, chorionic villi, or fetal blood and the fetus demonstrates no sonographic signs of an abnormality may be more difficult. Under these circumstances, if the gender of the fetuses is discordant, visualization of the fetal genitalia will establish which fetus should be targeted for termination. If the fetuses are of the same sex and information on the placental locations and relative position of the amniotic sacs was carefully recorded at the time of initial genetic testing, these data may be used to correctly identify the abnormal fetus. If, on the other hand, this information is not available, it is essential to perform amniocentesis, a placental biopsy, or fetal blood sampling to identify the karyotypically abnormal fetus with certainty. Complete confidence in knowing which fetus is abnormal is mandatory before the performance of the termination procedure. Furthermore, at the Mount Sinai Medical Center a confirmatory specimen of either amniotic fluid or fetal blood is always sent for genetic analysis on the completion of a selective termination to verify that the correct fetus was terminated.

DETERMINING CHORIONICITY

The need to establish chorionicity is an essential component in counseling patients for both MPR and selective termination. The incidence of monochorionicity in the general population is 1/240 or 0.4%.[39] Interestingly, Wenstrom et al.[63] studied the incidence of monochorionic gestations in 218 pregnancies conceived with the help of ART and found the incidence to be 3.2%, which is 8 times higher than the background rate.

The death of one fetus of a monochorionic pair may have severe repercussions for the surviving twin. The high incidence of subsequent fetal death and the potential for morbidity in the surviving fetus are the major causes of concern when one fetus dies in this setting. Enbom[16] reviewed 14 reports of deaths in monochorionic pregnancies and found that 46% of the surviving twins either died or suffered major morbidity. Szymonowicz, Preston, and Yu[58] reviewed the literature on the morbidity in the surviving twins from monozygotic gestations complicated by fetal death of one twin and found that 72% of survivors had central nervous system (CNS) abnormalities, 19% had gastrointestinal compromise, and 15% had renal impairment, whereas only 17% of the infants were completely normal. Although some literature suggests that fetal death in the first or early second trimester may not result in damage to the survivor, Anderson et al.[2] reported neurologic damage to the surviving fetus in four twin pregnancies complicated by fetal demise occurring at 13 to 21 weeks.

Several factors are believed to contribute to the morbidity and mortality encountered by the survivors. The insult that initially led to the demise of one fetus may cause hypoxia and hypotension in the other fetus. Additionally, the existence of vascular connections between the fetuses' circulatory systems may lead to thromboembolism secondary to disseminated intravascular coagulopathy (DIC). Patients undergoing KCl injection to terminate one fetus of a monochorionic pair are subject not only to the aforementioned risks, but also to the risk of immediate fetal death of the nonreduced twin secondary to exsanguination into the low pressure system formed by the dead twin. In fact, Timor-Tritsch et al.[60] reported that of three patients undergoing transvaginal MPR with known monochorionic-diamniotic twins, all 3 procedures resulted in the death of the second twin within 4 days.

Thus establishing chorionicity before performing either MPR or selective termination is an integral part of determining a patient's candidacy for the procedure. Ultrasound has been demonstrated to be fairly accurate in determining chorionicity in the second and third trimesters.[3,64] Sonographic findings consistent with dichorionicity are a thick, four-layered dividing membrane, two discrete placental locations, and the twin peak sign.[20] Recently Monteagudo, Timor-Tritsch, and Sharma[41] reported on the accuracy of first-trimester transvaginal ultrasound in determining chorionicity in multiple gestations. The amnion was described as being a thin membrane bordered on one side by the sonolucent amniotic fluid and on the other by the extraembryonic space containing the yolk sac. The chorion was described as being a thicker, echogenic structure surrounding the extraembryonic space and the amniotic sac. The presence of both a chorion and an amnion was further delineated by the shape of the junction between the membranes and the uterine wall. A wedge-shaped junction (the twin peak sign) was considered to represent a fusion of two chorionic membranes, and a T-shaped junction was thought to reflect the fusion of two amniotic membranes. In this publication, transvaginal ultrasound correctly identified chorionicity in all 43 pregnancies studied, as confirmed by pathologic evaluation of the placentas after delivery. If despite thorough sonographic evaluation the chorionicity cannot be definitely determined, zygosity studies on amniotic fluid cells utilizing analysis of chromosomal banding patterns may be performed to calculate the probability that the pregnancy contains a monochorionic or dichorionic gestation.

For patients undergoing first-trimester MPR, determination of chorionicity by ultrasound evaluation is performed before the procedure. If the diagnosis of a monochorionic pair is made in a triplet or higher-order multiple gestation, either both fetuses of the monochorionic pair should be targeted for reduction or both should be left alone. Because of the increased risks for intrauterine growth retardation (IUGR), twin-twin transfusion syndrome (TTS), congenital anomalies, and perinatal morbidity and mortality associated with monochorionic gestations, reduction of both monochorionic fetuses may be preferable. In patients diagnosed with monochorionic twins who are discordant for a fetal anomaly, selective termination with KCl injection would not be an appropriate option because of the risk of subsequent fetal death or damage to the surviving twin. One technique developed to eliminate the risk of damage to the surviving fetus in this setting is the delivery of the abnormal fetus through a hysterotomy.[50] However, this procedure requires the use of general anesthesia, a large uterine incision, and disruption of the fetal membranes, and it carries an extremely high risk of premature labor. Intraarterial injection of either thrombogenic coils or fibrin in the umbilical cord of the abnormal fetus has also been attempted, but this carries the risk of recanalization of the umbilical cord.[25,26,51,47] Recently, successful fetoscopic ligation of the umbilical cord in a patient diagnosed with twin reversed-arterial perfusion (TRAP) sequence has been reported.[49]

Any patient who has been diagnosed as having a multiple gestation should have the membrane's chorionicity determined at the time of the initial ultrasound examination. The type of placentation has important implications in the counseling of patients and the management of their pregnancies. Careful mapping of the amniotic cavities and placental locations before any prenatal diagnostic procedure should always be performed.

FETUSES WITH LETHAL ANOMALIES

In the situation where one fetus has been diagnosed as having a lethal anomaly such as anencephaly or renal agenesis, performing a selective termination and subjecting the normal fetus to the risks of an invasive procedure is unwarranted. The one exception to this philosophy is if the condition of the abnormal fetus poses an increased risk of preterm delivery to the normal twin. For example, if a fetus with anencephaly has associated hydramnios, it poses a significant risk of premature labor and delivery to the healthy twin. Under these circumstances, selective termination might be an appropriate course of action to consider.

THE RISK OF DISSEMINATED INTRAVASCULAR COAGULOPATHY

The demise of one fetus in a multiple gestation poses the theoretic risk to the mother of developing DIC. This phenomenon is presumed to be caused by the release of thromboplastic material from the dead fetus into the maternal circulation.

In the Mount Sinai experience, two patients developed laboratory evidence of hypofibrinogenemia between 11 and 14 weeks after the procedure was performed. One of these cases resolved spontaneously, and the other case occurred so close to term that delivery was undertaken and no further treatment was necessary.

Chitkara et al.[10] followed-up all of their 17 patients undergoing selective termination with bimonthly coagulation studies (fibrinogen level, platelet count, and circulating fibrinogen degradation products) throughout the pregnancy. None of the patients developed clinical or laboratory evidence of DIC. This finding was confirmed in the collaborative series by Evans et al.[19]

Conclusion

In summary, both MPR and selective termination are procedures developed to minimize the risk of serious perinatal morbidity associated with either preterm delivery or the care of a severely handicapped child.

MPR offers an acceptable option to patients faced with the significant risks as-sociated with carrying three or more fetuses. Clearly the outcome of patients carrying quadruplets and other higher-order multiple gestations is improved by reducing the number of fetuses contained in the uterus. The impact of MPR on the long-term morbidity of triplet gestations is less clear, although an improvement on short-term morbidity is apparent. Additionally, new data on the background loss rate of women carrying triplets suggests that the procedure-related risk of MPR is less than what was previously thought. Until advancements in reproductive technology eliminate the iatrogenic occurrence of multiple gestations and progress in perinatal care eliminates the threat of preterm delivery, MPR offers hope for an improved outcome in a situation fraught with potential difficulties.

For patients confronted with the unfortunate circumstance of carrying a multiple gestation in which the fetuses are discordant for genetic diseases, chromosomal abnormalities, or morphologic anomalies, selective termination offers a reasonable alternative to either doing nothing, or terminating the pregnancy completely. Although data collected at the Mount Sinai Medical Center and from centers around the world confirm the success and relative safety of selective termination in dichorionic gestations, more work needs to be done in the area of selective feticide of monochorionic gestations.

References

1. Aberg A et al: Cardiac puncture of fetus with Hurler's disease avoiding abortion of unaffected co-twin, *Lancet* 2:990, 1978.
2. Anderson RL et al: Central nervous system damage and other anomalies in surviving fetus following second trimester antenatal death of co-twin, *Prenat Diagn* 10:513-518, 1990.

3. Barss VA, Benacerraf BR, Frigoletto FD: Ultrasonographic determination of chorion type in twin gestation, *Obstet Gynecol* 66:779-783, 1985.

4. Berkowtiz RL et al: Selective reduction of multifetal pregnancies in the first trimester, *Lancet* 318:1043-1047, 1988.

5. Berkowitz RL et al: First-trimester transabdominal multifetal pregnancy reduction: a report of two hundred completed cases, *Am J Obstet Gynecol* 169:17-21, 1993.

6. Boulot P et al: Effects of selective reduction in triplet gestation: a comparative study of 80 cases managed with or without this procedure, *Fertil Steril* 60:497-503, 1993.

7. Boulot P et al: Multifetal pregnancy reduction: a consecutive series of 61 cases, *Br J Obstet Gynaecol* 100:63-68, 1993.

8. Brandes JM et al: The physical and mental development of co-sibs surviving selective reduction of multifetal pregnancies, *Hum Reprod* 5:1014-1017, 1990.

9. Caspi E et al: The outcome of pregnancy after gonadotrophin therapy, *Br J Obstet Gynaecol* 83:967-973, 1976.

10. Chitkara U et al: Selective second-trimester termination of the anomalous fetus in twin pregnancies, *Obstet Gynecol* 73:690, 1989.

11. Collins MS, Bleyl J: Seventy-one quadruplet pregnancies: management and outcome, *Am J Obstet Gynecol* 162:1384-1392, 1990.

12. Creinin M, Katz M, Laros R: Triplet pregnancy: changes in morbidity and mortality, *J Perinatol* XI:207-212, 1991.

13. Donner C et al: Multifetal pregnancy reduction: a Belgian experience, *Eur J Obstet Gynecol Reprod Biol* 38:183-187, 1990.

14. Dumez Y, Oury JF: Method for first trimester selective abortion in multiple pregnancy, *Contrib Gynecol Obstet* 15:50-53, 1986.

15. Elliott JP, Radin TG: Quadruplet pregnancy: contemporary management and outcome, *Obstet Gynecol* 80:421-424, 1992.

16. Enbom JA: Twin pregnancy with intrauterine death of one twin, *Am J Obstet Gynecol* 152:424-429, 1985.

17. Evans MI et al: Efficacy of transabdominal multifetal pregnancy reduction: collaborative experience among the world's largest centers, *Obstet Gynecol* 82:61-66, 1993.

18. Evans MI et al: Transabdominal versus transcervical and transvaginal multifetal pregnancy reduction: international collaborative experience of more than one thousand cases, *Am J Obstet Gynecol* 170:902-909, 1994.

19. Evans MI et al: Efficacy of second trimester selective termination for fetal abnormalities: international collaborative experience among the world's largest centers, *Am J Obstet Gynecol* (In press).

20. Finberg HJ: The "twin peak" sign: reliable evidence of dichorionic twinning, *J Ultrasound Med* 11:571-577, 1992.

21. Golbus MS et al: Selective termination of multiple gestations, *Am J Med Genet* 31:339-348, 1988.

22. Gonen Y, Blankier J, Casper RF: Transvaginal ultrasound in selective embryo reduction for multiple pregnancy, *Obstet Gynecol* 75:720-722, 1990.

23. Gonen R et al: The outcome of triplet, quadruplet, and quintuplet pregnancies managed in a perinatal unit: obstetric, neonatal, and follow-up data, *Am J Obstet Gynecol* 162:454-459, 1990.

24. Gonen R et al: The outcome of triplet gestations complicated by fetal death, *Obstet Gynecol* 75:175-178, 1990.

25. Grab D et al: Twin, acardiac, outcome, *Fetus* 2(1):11-13, 1992.

26. Hamada H et al: Fetal therapy in utero by blockage of the umbilical blood flow of acardiac monster in twin pregnancy, *Nippon Sanka Fujinka Gakkai Zasshi* 41:1803-1809, 1989.

27. Holcberg G et al: Outcome of pregnancy in 31 triplet gestations, *Obstet Gynecol* 59:472-476, 1982.

28. Itskovitz J et al: Transvaginal ultrasonography-guided aspiration of gestational sacs for selective abortion in multiple pregnancy, *Am J Obstet Gynecol* 160:215-217, 1989.

29. Itzkowic D: A survey of 59 triplet pregnancies, *Br J Obstet Gynaecol* 86:23-28, 1979.

30. Itzkowic D: A survey of 59 triplet pregnancies, *Br J Obstet Gynaecol* 86:2302-2308, 1986.

31. Jonas HA, Lumley J: Triplets and quadruplets born in Victoria between 1982 and 1990: the impact of IVF and GIFT on rising birthrates, *Med J Austr* 158:659-663, 1993.

32. Keith LG et al: The Northwestern University triplet study II: fourteen pregnancies delivered between 1981 and 1986, *Acta Genet Med Gemellol (Roma)* 37:65-75, 1988.

33. Lipitz S et al: The improving outcome of triplet pregnancies, *Am J Obstet Gynecol* 161:1279-1284, 1989.

34. Lipitz S et al: High-order multifetal gestation: management and outcome, *Obstet Gynecol* 76:215-218, 1990.

35. Lipitz S et al: A prospective comparison of the

outcome of triplet pregnancies managed expectantly or by multifetal reduction to twins, *Am J Obstet Gynecol* 170:874-879, 1994.

36. Luke B, Keith LG: The contribution of singletons, twins, and triplets to low birth weight, infant mortality and handicap in the United States, *J Reprod Med* 37:661-666, 1992.

37. Lynch L, Berkowitz RL: First trimester growth delay in trisomy 18, *Am J Perinatol* 6:234, 1989.

38. Lynch L, Berkowitz RL: Maternal serum alphafetoprotein and coagulation profiles after multifetal pregnancy reduction, *Am J Obstet Gynecol* 169:987-990, 1993.

39. Mac Gillvray I: Epidermiology of twin pregnancy, *Semin Perinatol* 10:4-8, 1986.

40. Macones GA et al: Multifetal reduction of triplets to twins improves perinatal outcome, *Am J Obstet Gynecol* 169:982-986, 1993.

41. Monteagudo A, Timor-Tritsch IE, Sharma S: Early and simple determination of chorionic and amniotic type in multifetal gestations in the first fourteen weeks by high-frequency transvaginal ultrasonography, *Am J Obstet Gynecol* 170:824-829, 1994.

42. Nazari A et al: Relationship of small-for-dates sac size to crown-rump length and spontaneous abortion in patients with a known date of ovulation, *Obstet Gynecol* 78:369-373, 1991.

43. Newman RB, Hamer C, Clinton Miller M: Outpatient triplet management: a contemporary review, *Am J Obstet Gynecol* 161:547-555, 1989.

44. Peacemen AM et al: Antepartum management of triplet gestations, *Am J Obstet Gynecol* 167:1117-1120, 1992.

45. Petrikowsky B, Vintzileos A: Management and outcome of multiple pregnancies of higher fetal order: literature review, *Obstet Gynecol Surv* 44:578, 1989.

46. Pons JC et al: Management of triplet pregnancy, *Acta Genet Med Gemellol (Roma)* 37:99-103, 1988.

47. Porreco RP, Barton SM, Haverkamp AD: Occlusion of umbilical artery in acardiac, acephalic twin, *Lancet* 337:326-327, 1991.

48. Porreco RP, Shannon Burke M, Hendrix ML: Multifetal reduction of triplets and pregnancy outcome, *Obstet Gynecol* 78:335-339, 1991.

49. Quintero RA et al: Brief Report: umbilical-cord ligation of an acardiac twin by fetoscopy at 19 weeks gestation, *N Engl J Med* 330:469-471, 1994.

50. Robie GF, Payne GG Jr, Morgan MA: Selective delivery of an acardiac acephalic twin, *N Engl J Med* 320:512-513, 1989.

51. Roberts RM et al: Twin, acardiac, ultrasound guided embolization, *Fetus* 1:5-10, 1991.

52. Rodeck CH et al: Selective feticide of the affected twin by fetoscopic air embolism, *Prenat Diagn* 2:189, 1982.

53. Sassoon DA et al: Perinatal outcome in triplet versus twin gestations, *Obstet Gynecol* 75:817-820, 1990.

54. Schenker JG, Yarkoni S, Granat M: Multiple pregnancies following induction of ovulation, *Fertil Steril* 35:105-123, 1981.

55. Seibel MM: In vitro fertilization, gamate intrafallopian transfer, and donated gametes and embryos, *N Engl J Med* 318:828-34, 1988.

56. Seoud MAF et al: Outcome of twin, triplet, and quadruplet in vitro fertilization pregnancies: the Norfolk experience, *Fertil Steril* 57:825-834, 1992.

57. Syrop CH, Varner MW: Triplet gestation: maternal and neonatal implications, *Acta Genet Med Gemellol (Roma)* 34:81-88, 1985.

58. Szymonowicz Q, Preston M, Yu VVM: The surviving monozygotic twin, *Arch Dis Child* 61:454-458, 1986.

59. Tabsh KMA: Transabdominal multifetal pregnancy reduction: report of 40 cases, *Obstet Gynecol* 75:739-741, 1990.

60. Timor-Tritsch IE et al: Multifetal pregnancy reduction by transvaginal puncture: evaluation of the technique used in 134 cases, *Am J Obstet Gynecol* 168:799-804, 1993.

61. Vervliet J et al: Management and outcome of 21 triplet and quadruplet pregnancies, *Eur J Obstet Gynecol Reprod Biol* 33:61-69, 1989.

62. Wapner RJ et al: Selective reduction of multifetal pregnancies, *Lancet* i:90-93, 1990.

63. Wenstrom KD et al: Increased risk of monochorionic twinning associated with assisted reproduction, *Fertil Steril* 60:510-514, 1993.

64. Winn HN et al: Ultrasonographic criteria for the prenatal diagnosis of placental chorionicity in twin gestations, *Am J Obstet Gynecol* 161:1540-1542, 1989.

65. Wittman BK et al: The role of feticide in the management of severe twin transfusion syndrome, *Am J Obstet Gynecol* 155:1023, 1986.

7 Maternal Complications

Daniel W. Skupski and Frank A. Chervenak

Clinicians' knowledge of the possible dangers to maternal health that result from multiple gestation has advanced rapidly during the last 10 to 15 years. This is a direct result of the increased use of assisted reproductive techniques (ART), which has led to an increased incidence of multiple pregnancies. The numerous maternal complications that are known to carry an increased incidence in multiple gestations are listed in Box 7-1. As further studies progress, more may be added to this list. Multiple gestation is certainly not a benign event to maternal health. All mothers who are discovered to have more than one fetus should be counseled regarding the detrimental effects on personal health that may ensue as a result of multiple gestation. Furthermore, it is essential that patients submitting to impregnation by ART are counseled beforehand about the likelihood of multiple gestation and its possible ill effects on maternal health.

Of course, all complications of pregnancy may occur during multiple gestation. This chapter is limited to those maternal complications that are known or are suspected to be increased in incidence when more than one fetus is present. Specifically, this chapter reviews: (1) those maternal problems that are either known or suspected to have an increased inci-

dence during a multiple gestation; (2) fetal conditions unique to multiple pregnancies that may affect maternal status; (3) management strategies for multiple pregnancies, whether of proven or unproven value, that may result in maternal morbidity; and (4) the current knowledge of maternal complications in high-order multiple gestations (quadruplets or higher).

Maternal Complications of Multiple Gestation

CARDIOPULMONARY

Given that there is an increased rate of preterm labor in patients with multiple gestations, it should not be surprising that the use of intravenous tocolysis is also increased in these patients. Intravenous tocolysis, particularly with beta-mimetic agents, is associated with a host of serious cardiovascular and metabolic side effects, which are listed in Box 7-2. All of the cardiovascular complications that are discussed in the following section are principally seen with the use of intravenous tocolysis. Multiple gestation adds an additional strain on the maternal cardiovascular system that produces a propensity toward the development of these cardiovascular complications.

BOX 7-1

Maternal Complications of Multiple Gestation

Increased Incidence Compared with Singleton Pregnancies

CARDIOPULMONARY

Pulmonary edema
Complications of tocolysis
Pregnancy-induced hypertension
Preeclampsia

OBSTETRIC

Preterm labor
Preterm delivery
Cervical effacement and dilation
Increased incidence of cesarean delivery
    and subsequent complications
Increased use of tocolysis
Antepartum hemorrhage
Abruptio placenta
Uterine rupture
Postpartum hemorrhage
Puerperal infection
Increased hospitalization

GASTROINTESTINAL

Acute fatty liver of pregnancy
Cholestasis of pregnancy

HEMATOLOGIC

Anemia

BOX 7-2

Cardiovascular and Metabolic Complications of Intravenous Tocolysis

Hyperglycemia
Hypokalemia
Sodium retention
Water retention
Decreased urine output
Tachycardia
Hypotension
Volume overload
Arrhythmias
Mycardial ischemia
Pulmonary edema
Respiratory arrest*

*associated with extremely high levels of magnesium (>13mg/dl).

Pulmonary edema

Pulmonary edema is the most common life-threatening complication of intravenous tocolysis, occurring in as many as 3% to 9% of women undergoing beta mimetic therapy.[14,82,125] Of the reported cases of pulmonary edema, multiple gestation appears to have been a predisposing factor in over 19% of cases.[63] Patients with multiple gestations undergo intravenous toco-lysis more often than patients with singleton pregnancies and thus are at increased risk for pulmonary edema. The most common symptoms are shortness of breath and tachypnea, although pulmonary edema may be present in the absence of symptoms.

Pulmonary edema occurs when there is high cardiac output with either of the following conditions: (1) cardiac failure and increased intravascular capillary hydrostatic pressure that drive fluid out of the pulmonary vasculature or (2) increased permeability or damage to the pulmonary capillary endothelium that allows fluid to leak out. The combination of pregnancy, multiple gestation, labor, and the administration of tocolytic agents can more than triple cardiac output over nonpregnant levels (Figure 7-1). It is therefore not surprising that cardiac failure and pulmonary edema may occur in this setting. Risk

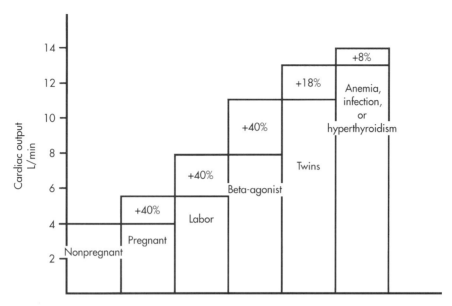

FIGURE 7-1 Cumulative effects of pregnancy and various pregnancy complications on cardiac output. *(From Clark SL et al, editors: Critical care obstetrics, ed 2, Cambridge, Mass., 1991, Blackwell Scientific Publications.)*

factors for the development of pulmonary edema in pregnancy are shown in Box 7-3.

Intravascular volume overload can occur in the setting of intravenous tocolysis particularly when large volumes of intravenous fluids have been administered. Volume overload has been reported to be a precipitating factor in the development of pulmonary edema in at least 24% of the reported cases.[63] The determining factors are related to the type of tocolytic medication used, the preexisting status of the vascular volume, and the ability of both cardiac and renal dynamics to withstand and adjust to the insult of the intravascular volume load. Beta mimetic agents allow volume overload to occur in two ways. First, as a direct result of the stimulation of arginine vasopressin, urine volume is decreased. Second, beta mimetic agents stimulate the renin-angiotensin system, leading to a selective vasospasm of the re-

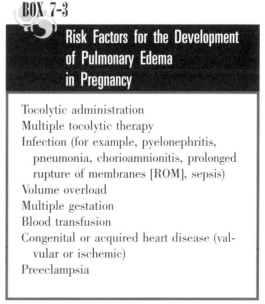

BOX 7-3

Risk Factors for the Development of Pulmonary Edema in Pregnancy

Tocolytic administration
Multiple tocolytic therapy
Infection (for example, pyelonephritis, pneumonia, chorioamnionitis, prolonged rupture of membranes [ROM], sepsis)
Volume overload
Multiple gestation
Blood transfusion
Congenital or acquired heart disease (valvular or ischemic)
Preeclampsia

From Clark SL et al, editors: Critical care obstetrics, ed 2, Cambridge, Mass., 1991, Blackwell Scientific Publications.

nal arteries, a decrease in renal perfusion, and thus a further decrease in urine output. Salt and water retention occurs, predisposing the patient to volume overload. Additionally, the beta-1 chronotropic and inotropic effects of beta sympathomimetic medications lead to an increase in cardiac output.[63] This may predispose the patient to cardiac failure, which, alone or in combination with volume overload, may precipitate pulmonary edema.

Incipient or overt infection has been suggested to be a cause of transient injury to the pulmonary capillary endothelium, allowing increased permeability and predisposing the patient to pulmonary edema. Infection has been reported to be a precipitating factor in about 29% of reported cases of pulmonary edema associated with tocolytic therapy.[63] Additionally, studies of the association of pulmonary disease with pyelonephritis in pregnancy support the role of infection as a cause for pulmonary injury.[31]

The administration of steroid medications to the mother in an effort to enhance fetal lung maturation has been associated with the development of pulmonary edema. These cases seem to have been limited to patients receiving beta mimetic agents. The mineralocorticoid (salt-and-water-retaining) effects of the steroid medications used for enhancement of fetal lung maturation are much weaker than the same effects of beta mimetic agents. Thus authorities are divided as to whether steroid medications in this setting are a predisposing or additive factor in the development of pulmonary edema.

The appearance of pulmonary edema in patients with preeclampsia is presumed to be either from excessive afterload, from volume overload (as previously described), or both. Aggressive intravenous fluid administration in the setting of preeclampsia is therefore contraindicated, because the combination of increased afterload (caused by the vasospasm seen in preeclampsia) and increased preload (caused by volume overload) may be particularly dangerous.

Management. Treatment of any of the complications of tocolytic therapy begins with discontinuation of therapy. Additionally, standard therapy for pulmonary edema should be instituted. This includes oxygen administration, intravenous furosemide, and intravenous morphine sulfate. Response to therapy can initially be based on the patient's symptoms, but subsequent serial monitoring of other diagnostic tests should be performed to monitor the patient's response. These tests include arterial blood gas measurements, a chest x-ray, serum electrolyte measurements, and an electrocardiogram (ECG). The patient should be monitored in an intensive care setting. Consultation with specialists in internal medicine, pulmonary medicine, cardiology, and respiratory therapy is appropriate. Careful recording of fluid intake and output is also essential. Invasive hemodynamic monitoring is indicated if there is not a rapid response to the initial therapeutic steps.

For the prevention of pulmonary edema, prudent—and not aggressive—intravenous fluid administration in the setting of intravenous tocolysis is warranted. Additionally, beta mimetics should be administered by a controlled infusion with 5% dextrose in water to avoid the exacerbation of salt and water retention that occurs when balanced salt solutions are used.[63] This in combination with careful fluid intake and output monitoring, as well as frequent auscultation of the lungs, helps prevent volume overload and thus decreases the risk of the development of pulmonary edema. Finally, it is prudent to avoid intravenous tocolysis in most cases where there is either maternal infection or maternal hypertension.

Pulmonary edema is a life-threatening situation. Steps for prevention, early recognition, and a prompt response by the obstetric team are required to prevent pulmonary edema from progressing to maternal death.

Myocardial ischemia

The advent of ART has led to an increasing number of women of advanced reproductive age who are able to become pregnant. These women are at increased risk for underlying myocardial ischemia, which can be recognized by the "stress tests" of pregnancy, multiple gestation, and (particularly) intravenous tocolysis.

In the apparently healthy woman of somewhat more advanced years, multiple gestation poses an increased risk for cardiovascular complications. This is because the appearance of preterm labor and the necessity for intravenous tocolysis are increased in multiple gestation, and it is the combination of multiple gestation and tocolysis that places a marked increased demand on cardiac reserve.

It is principally with intravenous tocolysis, and more particularly with beta mimetic agents, that myocardial ischemia and infarction are seen. Patients with a history of cardiovascular disease or a history of cardiovascular risk factors are at risk for myocardial ischemia and infarction at any time during pregnancy. However, women with undiscovered (underlying) myocardia ischemia, women of more

advanced age, and even apparently healthy and younger women can suffer from myocardia ischemia or infarction during pregnancy. This is particularly true for patients with multiple pregnancies who are undergoing intravenous tocolysis. In a patient with documented ischemic cardiac disease, tocolysis is strongly contraindicated if preterm labor ensues.

Chest pain is a symptom in one out of five women undergoing intravenous beta mimetic tocolysis.[63] A significant proportion of these patients are shown to have ischemic ECG changes, including ST segment depression and elevation, T-wave changes, peaked P waves, left axis deviation, and arrhythmias. Additionally, the majority of patients (78%) who undergo beta mimetic tocolysis have nonspecific ST- and T-wave ECG changes consistent with ischemia.[63]

Management. We perform a baseline ECG in all patients undergoing beta mimetic tocolysis. Any symptom of chest pain, pressure, or shortness of breath is an indication to discontinue tocolytic therapy. In this setting, routine treatment of myocardial ischemia including oxygen administration and serial ECG monitoring, should be undertaken. If chest pain or pressure persists, sublingual nitroglycerin is appropriate and consideration should be given to obtaining serum cardiac enzymes in an effort to document myocardial damage. However, it should be understood that 10% of patients in preterm labor have elevated levels of the serum creatine kinase muscle-brain (MB) fraction (CK_2) that is thought to be fetal in origin.[5,100,124] This makes the measurement of CK isoenzymes much less specific for myocardial necrosis during pregnancy. In the setting of continued symptoms, consultation with a cardiologist should also be obtained. In most cases, symptoms resolve after discontinuation of the tocolytic agent.

Myocardial ischemia also places the patient at increased risk for the development of life-threatening arrhythmias.

Cardiac arrhythmias

The increased use of tocolysis in women with multiple gestations means that these patients may also be at increased risk for the development of cardiac arrhythmias. Cardiac arrhythmias that have been reported to occur during beta mimetic therapy include supraventricular tachycardia, atrial fibrillation, and premature ventricular contractions.[63] Prompt discontinuation of tocolysis is often all that is needed to treat the arrhythmia. Other precipitating causes, such as hypokalemia, hypoxemia, and myocardial infarction, should be identified and treated. Standard therapies for cardiac arrhythmias should be instituted if no response is seen after discontinuation of the tocolytic agent. Of course, immediate consultation with a cardiologist is encouraged.

Maternal death

In addition to the cardiovascular risk factors (see the section on pulmonary edema), multiple gestation may also be a risk factor for maternal death. Maternal death associated with beta mimetic tocolysis has been reported to occur in at least 3 patients with multiple gestation.[38,73,91] However, reviews of maternal mortality have not included multiple gestation either as a risk factor for or as a cause of maternal death.*

*References 4, 9, 36, 47, 60, 91, 94, 96, 97, 131, 139, 148, 149, 151

OBSTETRIC

Antenatal complications have been shown to be increased in incidence in twin gestations compared with singleton gestations.[84] Many of these complications have been reported to have not only an increased rate in twin pregnancies, but an even further increase in incidence in triplet pregnancies. A discussion of these obstetric complications follows.

Preterm labor

Preterm labor is markedly increased in multiple gestations, with an incidence ranging from 20% to 75%.[18,81,119] The incidence of preterm labor in multiple gestations increases in direct proportion to the number of fetuses present, and the average number of completed weeks of gestation at delivery is inversely related to the number of fetuses.[21] Many theories for the cause of preterm labor in multiple gestation have been put forward, including uterine overdistension, increased intraamniotic pressure, increased readiness of the myometrium, and uteroplacental insufficiency.[104]

Prevention of preterm labor has been evaluated in many ways. Knowledgeable risk assessment combined with serial cervical examinations that are performed either manually or with transvaginal ultrasound may help identify infants at highest risk for premature birth.[2,28,113] Additionally, patient education, antepartum care in a special clinic, and early referral to a specialist are measures that are commonly employed to identify preterm labor as early as possible. Home uterine activity monitoring (HUAM) is a noninvasive modality that combines frequent contact with the health care provider and early identification of premature uterine activity.[80] Although some controversy exists, these authors believe that outpatient uterine monitoring may be of value.[61,74,79,103] HUAM procedures may identify the fetuses in multiple gestations that need the initiation of the more invasive methods of combatting prematurity.

Bed rest: The value of bed rest in the prevention of prematurity is controversial because of confusion in the literature that stems from a lack of unanimity among protocols and a predominance of retrospective data. Since up to 81% of perinatal mortality in twins occurs before the 29th week of gestation, bed rest is needed before this point.[26] Bed rest in a hospital is disruptive and costly, and given a lack of clear benefit in the scientific literature, not indicated. However, certain complications, such as premature cervical dilation, recurrent uterine contractions, and suspected discordant growth, may warrant prolonged hospitalization for rest or closer observation.

Tocolysis: The classic approach to preterm labor in the patient with a multiple pregnancy is tocolysis. Numerous medications and routes of administration are available and detailed elsewhere.[19,39,106,120] There is also research on newer medications for the control of preterm labor, including oxytocin antagonists, calcium channel blockers, antiprostaglandin agents, and nitric oxide.

The efficacy of the classic approach of tocolysis as a treatment for preterm labor has recently been challenged.[18,102] Despite this, long experience has shown the efficacy of tocolytic agents in decreasing uterine activity. Thus tocolysis is appropriate for the multiple pregnancies before 34 weeks' gestation in the following circumstances: (1) preterm labor as defined by regular uterine contractions with evidence of cervical change on serial examinations; (2) regular uterine contractions with a cervix dilated to 1 to 3 cm and more than 80% effaced; (3) an increase in baseline uterine activity as determined by electronic uterine activity monitoring, either at home or in hospital, that is not responsive to rest and hydration; and (4) in an effort to obtain 24 to 48 hours of delay in delivery for the fetal benefit of maternally administered steroids to be realized. Of course, because of the higher blood volume and increased cardiac output in patients with multiple pregnancies, careful monitoring of fluid status is paramount, as detailed in Chapter 5.

Prophylactic oral tocolytic agents have not been shown to be of benefit in most studies to date, and the present consensus does not support their use.[22,111,140]

Steroids: Although it is not a treatment for preterm labor, the use of maternally administered steroids for fetal benefit is becoming more widespread. Recently, the National Institutes of Health sponsored a multidisciplinary conference that discussed the use of steroids and attempted to encourage their use.[105] Although the use of steroids in multiple pregnancies has not been documented to be efficacious for the decrease of respiratory distress syndrome (RDS), the numbers of patients have been small.[27] There are major theoretical benefits of the use of steroids to several fetal organ systems, including a decrease in RDS, intracranial hemorrhage (ICH), and necrotizing enterocolitis (NEC). Thus the use of steroids in the multiple pregnancy complicated by preterm labor is indicated.

Cesarean delivery

Perhaps the most common maternal complication of multiple gestation is the increase in incidence of cesarean sections, primarily as a result of malpresentation. There are numerous maternal complications with an increased incidence in patients undergoing cesarean sections as compared with patients who deliver vaginally. These include but are not limited to the following complications: puerperal infection (such as endometritis, pelvic abscess, wound infection, and septic pelvic thrombophlebitis), wound dehiscence and evisceration, deep venous thrombosis, ileus, bowel obstruction, bladder catheter drainage, intraperitoneal or retroperitoneal hemorrhage, and an increased need for transfusion of blood products. Documentation of an increased rate of these complications in patients with multiple gestations is lacking for many of these problems.

We have previously recommended an intrapartum management plan for twin gestations that may allow a decrease in the rate of cesarean deliveries performed because of malpresentation.[24] This plan anticipates vaginal delivery for vertex/vertex twin presentations, vaginal delivery of Twin A with intrapartum external cephalic version of Twin B for vertex/nonvertex twin presentations, and cesarean delivery for nonvertex presentations of Twin A. Decreasing the cesarean delivery rate for twin pregnancies is appropriate to prevent maternal morbidity.

Although not universally accepted, most authorities agree that elective cesarean delivery is the appropriate delivery route for higher-order multiple gestations (triplets or more).

Preeclampsia and eclampsia

The incidence of preeclampsia in twin pregnancies has been reported in various studies to be between 6% and 37% (Table 7-1). Most authorities agree that the incidence of preeclampsia is increased in multiple gestation. However, it should be noted that most of the early studies on hypertension in twin gestation suffered from several flaws. Most were retrospective reviews that were not looking specifically at preeclampsia; each study defined hypertension (or preeclampsia) in different ways; and several factors known to have a significant influence on the rate of preeclampsia (age, race, and parity) were uncontrolled. More recent controlled reviews have documented an increase in preeclampsia in twin pregnancies.[84,141] The reported rates of preeclampsia in triplet pregnancies range from 5% to 46%.* It is not known whether increasing numbers of fetuses within the uterus may lead to an increase in the rate of preeclampsia.

Eclampsia has not been shown to be increased in multiple gestation. The only reports of eclampsia in multiple pregnancy are from 1941 to 1955.[15,85,104,116,129] The incidence of eclampsia in twin pregnancies in the studies ranged from 0% to 2.9%. No comparison with any singleton gestation population was undertaken in any of the reports. The relative rarity of eclampsia means that large numbers of patients would be required to adequately study this problem. At the present time this has not been carried out. A recent review of eclampsia at one institution showed that 9/254 cases of eclampsia (3.5%) occurred in twin pregnancies.[139]

*References 34, 69, 76, 107, 128, 133, 145

TABLE 7-1

Incidence of Preeclampsia in Multiple Gestation: Literature Review

STUDY	YEAR	POPULATION	RESULT	RATE OF INCREASE
Guttmacher[62]‡	1939	Twins		3-fold
Russel[130]‡	1952	Twins	20%	
Bender[8]‡	1952	Twins		3-fold
Aaron and Halperin[1]	1955	Twins	5%	
Kurtz, Keating, and Loftus[85]	1955	Twins	<20%	
Anderson[3]	1956	Twins	<20%	
Bulfin and Lawler[15]‡	1957	Twins	31.2%	
MacGillivray	1958	Twins		5-fold
Graves, Adams, and Schreier[58]‡	1962	Twins	37%	
Farrell[46]	1964	Twins	8.3%	
Kohl and Casey[83]‡	1975	Twins		2-fold
McFarlane and Scott[98]‡	1976	Twins	18%	3-fold
Daw[34]	1978	Triplets	21%	
Itzkowic[76]	1979	Triplets	19%	
Houlton, Marivate, and Philpott[71]	1981	Twins	10%	
Ron-El et al.[128]	1981	Triplets	8%	
Holcberg et al.[69]	1982	Triplets	46%	
McMullen, Norman, and Marivale[99]‡	1984	Twins	37%	2-fold
Syrop and Varner[145]	1985	Triplets	20%	
Thompson, Lyons, and Makowski[146]‡	1987	Twins	17.9%	
Newman, Hamer, and Miller[107]	1989	Triplets	15%	
Kovacs, Kirschbaum, and Paul[84]*‡	1989	Twins	23%	4-fold
Spellacy, Handler, and Kerre[141]*	1990	Twins	13%	2.5-fold
Sassoon et al.[133]	1990	Both	13%	
Howarth, Pattinson, and De Jong[72]	1991	Twins	8%	

*denotes a controlled study—random singleton population chosen for comparison; ‡denotes studies with an increased rate of preeclampsia in twins.

Interested readers are referred to Roberts for an excellent review of the diagnosis and management of preeclampsia and eclampsia.[123]

Abruptio placentae and placenta previa

An increased rate of antepartum hemorrhage has been reported for twin gestations.[72,84] These studies were retrospective chart reviews that used discharge diagnoses or face sheet coding to determine the presence of complications in twin and singleton pregnancies. The cause of antepartum hemorrhage, if determined, was not reported. This increased rate of antepartum hemorrhage is probably primarily the result of abruptio placentae and *not* placenta previa, as evidenced by an increased rate of abruption found in a controlled study that compared a large number of singleton and twin pregnancies.[141] In this study it was also determined that placenta previa was not increased in incidence for the twin pregnancies.[141]

The diagnosis and management of abruptio placentae is elegantly reviewed by Green.[59]

Uterine rupture

The rate of uterine rupture is increased in patients with twin gestations who have had previous cesarean sections. The reported rate of uterine rupture for patients with a previous uterine incision during a subsequent twin gestation is 4%.[143] This is increased to approximately 2 times the rate for uterine rupture in singleton gestations with previous uterine incisions. The diagnosis rests on evaluation of maternal symptoms, the presence of fetal heart rate (FHR) abnormalities, and intrauterine pressure manometry. Catastrophic uterine rupture requires prompt action on the part of the clinician to prevent both maternal and fetal morbidity or mortality. Immediate laparotomy for a cesarean section should be undertaken as soon as the diagnosis is strongly suspected, such as when severe abdominal pain occurs during a pregnancy in a woman with a previous uterine incision, when severe variable FHR decelerations or bradycardia appear during continuous FHR monitoring, or when maternal hemodynamic instability (from intraperitoneal hemorrhage and hypovolemia) develops.

Postpartum hemorrhage

The incidence of postpartum hemorrhage has been reported to be increased in multiple gestations, occurring in as many as 27.8% of twin gestations[15] and 35% of triplet gestations.[145] Controlled studies have not addressed this issue.[84,141] It is generally accepted that overdistension of the uterus, such as seen in hydramnios, macrosomia, and multiple gestation, increases the incidence of uterine atony and thus increases the incidence of postpartum hemorrhage. Patients who have been delivered of multiple fetuses should therefore be watched closely not only for the development of uterine atony or postpartum hemorrhage, but also for its recurrence at any time during the first 24 to 48 hours after delivery. Uterine massage performed often by a knowledgeable attendant during the first few hours after delivery may help prevent uterine atony. Treatment includes manual uterine evacuation and massage, intravenous oxytocin, intramuscular methylergonovine, and intramuscular prostaglandin $F_{2\alpha}$. One or more of these measures should be instituted immediately for any marked increase in vaginal bleeding after the delivery of multiple fetuses.

The diagnosis and management of obstetric hemorrhage, including postpartum hemorrhage, is found in an excellent review by Hayashi.[66]

Preterm premature rupture of the amniotic membranes

Although preterm premature rupture of the amniotic membranes (PROM) has been reported to be increased in twin pregnancies,[146] controlled studies have not shown an increased risk of preterm PROM in multiple gestation.[84,141] However, when preterm PROM does occur, increased risks of chorioamnionitis and maternal sepsis ensue, just as they do in singleton pregnancies. The occurrence of preterm PROM in a multiple gestation and thus the presence of one or more intact amniotic sacs at risk for infection leads to a unique management dilemma. This is discussed in Chapter 7.

GASTROINTESTINAL

Acute fatty liver of pregnancy

A high incidence of twin gestations has been reported in patients afflicted with acute fatty liver of pregnancy (AFLP). This is a rare condition, reported in as many as 1/13,000 pregnancies.[114] AFLP is a cause of jaundice in the third trimester, and patients often experience nausea and vomiting. If AFLP is undiagnosed or untreated, severe abdominal pain and headache follow. Any or all of the following symptoms or conditions may ensue if AFLP is untreated: somnolence, coma, liver rupture, liver failure, hypoglycemia, disseminated intravascular coagulation (DIC), oliguria, renal failure, metabolic acidosis, multisystem organ failure, maternal death, fetal distress, and fetal demise.[101,118,137] Coagulopathy, hypoglycemia, and renal failure are causes of maternal death in this disease.

AFLP is a fulminant disease that has historically been associated with poor maternal and perinatal outcome. Maternal mortality has been reported to be as high as 75%, and the rate of fetal mortality is 71%.[33] It has been suggested that the high rate of fetal mortality is the result of uteroplacental insufficiency (UPI).[101] Mortality from this disease has decreased in recent years, probably because of earlier diagnosis and advances in intensive care medicine.[147] The key to early diagnosis and thus the improvement of the mother's chance for survival in AFLP is increased awareness of all physicians in-

volved in the care of a pregnant patient. Nausea and vomiting in the third trimester should not be overlooked or passed off as normal or as a result of the increased incidence of heartburn that is seen in pregnancy. All pregnant patients with nausea and vomiting in the third trimester should be examined, and consideration should be given to obtaining serum chemistry values to rule out the diagnosis of AFLP.

Features of preeclampsia are present in 40% of AFLP cases, indicating that there may be a link between these two diseases. Liver histology suggests that they are separate entities.[35] The differential diagnosis includes acute viral hepatitis, intrahepatic cholestasis of pregnancy, and severe preeclampsia. A pathognomic feature of the disease is a centrilobular pattern of microvesicular fat deposition in hepatocytes. Computed tomography (CT) and magnetic resonance imaging (MRI) are helpful in establishing the presence of fatty infiltration of the liver in cases where the diagnosis is uncertain.[45,56,92]

Four series of cases of AFLP at large institutions have shown a high incidence of AFLP in twin gestations, with 7/42 cases of AFLP (16.7%) occurring in twin pregnancies.[16,33,114,147]

Management. Management of AFLP involves support in an intensive care setting. Because of the high rates of fetal mortality if AFLP is left untreated, immediate delivery is paramount. This requires a cesarean section whenever advanced cervical dilation and rapid progress in labor are not evident. The association of fetal distress and fetal death with AFLP mandates careful fetal monitoring.[101]

The principles of resuscitation and intensive care support are fully applied in the case of the patient with AFLP. This begins with adequate airway and ventilation support for the patient in hepatic coma. Adequate nutrition should also be provided. Nasogastric tube administration of concentrated glucose solutions provides this, and it will correct the severe hypoglycemia seen in AFLP. Exclusion of protein from the diet and decreasing ammonia production by colonic bacteria by both neomycin and magnesium citrate administration are important. Coagulation abnormalities need to be anticipated and corrected with administration of vitamin K, platelets, and fresh frozen plasma. Consultations with specialists in internal medicine and gastroenterology are appropriate.

Intensive care treatment of patients with AFLP has resulted in markedly increased maternal and fetal survival rates, with recent series showing maternal mortality of 8% to 10%[11,37,70,126] compared with historical reports of 75% to 80%.[75,109,114,138]

The prognosis for women who recover from the acute phase of AFLP is usually excellent. The recurrence of AFLP is low and has been reported in only 2 cases.[6,135]

Cholestasis of pregnancy

Certain populations, particularly in Sweden and Chile, have a genetic predisposition to intrahepatic cholestasis of pregnancy.[10,122] Although it has not been shown that multiple gestation increases the risk or incidence of intrahepatic cholestasis of pregnancy in the general population, it has been shown to do so in one of the genetically susceptible populations in Chile.[55] The incidence increased in this study from less than 10% in singleton pregnancies to 20.9% in twin pregnancies.

Intrahepatic cholestasis of pregnancy is a disorder of the third trimester of pregnancy that is characterized by severe, generalized pruritus and mild jaundice. It has been shown to occur earlier than the third trimester, and has even been induced by the use of oral contraceptive medications.[10,50,121] The recurrence rate is high and has been reported to be 70.5% in Chile.[55]

Patients generally have insidious pruritus that is first noticed at night. Jaundice develops in approximately 50% of cases about 2 weeks later, persisting until 2 to 3 days after delivery. The pruritus is usually progressive and excoriations are common. Patients are almost always otherwise asymptomatic.

The differential diagnosis includes viral hepatitis, acute fatty liver of pregnancy, and cholelithiasis. The diagnosis rests on the demonstration of elevated levels of serum bile acids. Cholic acid, deoxycholic acid, and chenodeoxycholic acid are increased to 10 to 100 times their normal levels, and they should be at least 3 times their normal levels to confirm the diagnosis.[43,53,150] The extreme pruritus seen is thought to be from deposition of these bile acids in the skin.

There have been conflicting reports regarding the preterm birth rate in intrahepatic cholestasis of pregnancy, but it is generally thought to be increased.[50,77,78] Intrapartum fetal distress, stillbirth, and perinatal mortality are increased.[48] The reason for fetal demise is unknown.

Management. The management of intrahepatic cholestasis of pregnancy involves two goals. First, careful antepartum fetal monitoring is necessary to attempt to decrease the rate of stillbirths. Serious consideration should be given to inducing labor at term or when amniotic fluid studies show fetal lung maturity.

Second, attempts at achieving patient comfort (reducing pruritus) are important. The only proven effective therapy is cholestyramine resin, an anionic binding resin taken orally that reduces the intestinal reabsorption of bile acids, thus decreasing serum bile acid levels and hopefully also reducing pruritus. Bloating can be a limiting side effect. Dosage is usually started at 4 to 8 gm/day in three or four divided doses and increased gradually (to minimize bloating) to 16 gm/day. Up to 30 gm/day may need to be given to control pruritus. Vitamin K should also be administered parenterally, since the gastrointestinal absorption of Vitamin K is impaired with the use of cholestyramine resin. Antihistamines are completely ineffective for pruritus in this disorder. Often there are significant laboratory delays in obtaining serum bile acid results. If intrahepatic cholestasis is strongly suspected, cholestyramine resin may be instituted as soon as possible so the pruritus may thus be more effectively reduced. Phenobarbital has also been used for pruritus refractory to cholestyramine resin or for those patients who cannot tolerate cholestyramine resin.[12,44,86]

Recently, ursodeoxycholic acid (UDCA) has become available for the treatment of the pruritus of intrahepatic cholestasis of pregnancy.[29,49,112,115] UDCA has been available for the treatment of other cholestatic liver diseases and has been found to be without significant adverse effects in both adults and children.[89,110,115] UDCA is administered orally. Dosage of UDCA has ranged from 450 mg/day to 1 gm/day, in three divided doses.[49,112] Both the pathophysiologic nature of intrahepatic cholestasis of pregnancy and the mechanism of action of UDCA are unknown, but it is thought that that UDCA may act in one of two ways: (1) through the replacement of other endogenous bile acids that are less hydrophilic and more cytotoxic, mainly at the site of the liver cell membrane,[52,68] and (2) through inhibition of the intestinal absorption of less hydrophilic bile acids.[95,142] There has been a favorable initial experience, with success in eradicating pruritus in 10/12 patients and in one case at The New York Hospital.[29,49,112,115] UDCA still requires further study for determination of both its safety in pregnancy and its efficacy in decreasing pruritus.

HEMATOLOGIC

Anemia

Anemia, defined as a hemoglobin level of less than 10 gm/dl or a hematocrit value of less than 30%, happens more often in multiple gestation. Anemia has been reported to happen 2.4 times more often in mothers with twin pregnancies than in those with singleton pregnancies,[141] although this has not been a universal finding.[84] The increased incidence of both antepartum and postpartum hemorrhage (see below) also adds circumstantial evidence that women with multiple pregnancies are at increased risk for anemia. There is some evidence that an increasing order of multiple gestation may increase the risk of anemia; one study reported a 35% incidence of anemia in a population of 15 triplet pregnancies.

Severe anemia can be defined as a hematocrit value of less than 22%, an anemia that requires blood transfusion, or an anemia associated with cardiorespiratory

BOX 7-4

Complications of Blood Transfusion

TRANSFUSION REACTIONS

Fever
Chills
Pruritis
Urticaria
Anaphylaxis

ISOIMMUNIZATION

Usually atypical antibody formation)

BLOOD-BORNE INFECTION

Hepatitis B infection
Hepatitis C infection
Hepatitis D co-infection
Cytomegalovirus infection
Human immunodeficiency virus (HIV)
Other blood-borne infection

BOX 7-5

Complications of Severe Anemia

Dizziness
Fatigue/Malaise
Syncope
Tachycardia
Shortness of breath
Chest pain

In addition to severe anemia, predisposing risk factors or severe hypovolemia usually need to be present for the following problems to occur:
Myocardial infarction
Cardiac arrhythmias
Acute renal tubular necrosis (ATN)
Cerebrovascular accident (CVA)
Note: Severe anemia has been shown *not* to be associated with an increased risk of postsurgical infectious complications.

symptoms or decompensation. It is suspected, but has not been shown, that severe anemia is also increased in multiple pregnancy. Additionally, an increased need for blood transfusion has not been documented for mothers with multiple gestation. The risk of transmission of blood-borne infection associated with blood transfusion and complications of severe anemia have also not been documented to be increased in multiple gestation (Boxes 7-4 and 7-5).

In multiple gestations there is an additional increase in blood volume above that seen in singleton pregnancies. Thus the dilutional anemia associated with pregnancy, often aggravated by the iron deficiency that can accompany pregnancy, is accentuated in multiple gestations. However, if the hemoglobin level falls below 10 gm/dl or if the hematocrit value goes below 30%, many authorities believe that a workup for anemia is indicated. The most likely causes of such an anemia in pregnancy include iron deficiency, folate deficiency, vitamin B_{12} deficiency, α- or β-thalassemia trait, sickle-cell disease, and glucose-6-phosphatase deficiency (with exposure to a medication or environmental agent that may produce hemolysis). The initial workup may vary according to the measurement of the mean cell volume and the race and nutritional status of the patient, but it may include assessments of the following values: serum iron level, total iron-binding capacity, haptoglobin level, serum folate, and vitamin B_{12} levels, transferrin and ferritin levels, and hemoglobin electrophoresis. Consultation with a hematologist also may be indicated.

Follow-up during the pregnancy is crucial to assessing the adequacy of treatment and to counseling the patient on the risk of severe anemia requiring blood transfusion. Follow-up after the pregnancy is important to assess the adequacy of red blood cell and hemoglobin replacement, particularly if the patient is likely to become pregnant again soon.

INFECTIONS

Puerperal infection

Maternal febrile morbidity after cesarean section has been reported to be increased in incidence in multiple gestations, with a rate as high as 84.4%.[146] In a recent controlled study comparing women with twin and singleton pregnancies who underwent cesarean sections, endometritis was increased nearly threefold (13.1% versus 4.7%) and abdominal wound infections were increased nearly twofold (5.6% versus 3.0%).[144] The etiologic factors are unknown, but a large placental bed or possibly immunologic factors have been suggested.

Treatment of puerperal infection is based on the principles of initial broad spectrum antibiotic coverage, which is subsequently tailored to the culture and sensitivity results that are obtained from cultures of the infected area. Abscess formation is treated by incision and drainage when antibiotic therapy has not succeeded in eradicating the infection (see Chapter 10).

Pyelonephritis

Early studies of multiple gestations seemed to suggest that there was an increased rate of pyelonephritis in these pregnancies. Most recent controlled studies have documented that there is *not* an increased incidence of pyelonephritis in multiple pregnancies.[84,141]

ENDOCRINE COMPLICATIONS

Gestational diabetes

For a host of anecdotal and theoretical reasons, gestational diabetes was previously presumed to be increased in multiple pregnancies. Recent controlled studies have shown that gestational diabetes does *not* have an increased incidence in multiple gestations.[84,141]

Fetal Conditions that May Affect Maternal Status

Many pathologic conditions of the fetus or fetuses are unique to multiple gestations. These conditions, listed in Table 7-2, may predispose the gravida to maternal complications that are rare in singleton pregnancies or are only seen in the unique circumstances of a multiple pregnancy.

DISCORDANT GROWTH

Careful serial ultrasonographic monitoring of multiple gestations is recommended. Discrepancies in growth between fetuses may occur and may place the gravida at increased risk for preeclampsia.[133,146] Intensive antepartum fetal surveillance is necessary in the presence of growth discordance, and there is an increased reliance on bed rest as an intervention, which is discussed in a later section of this chapter.

HYDRAMNIOS

Preterm labor undoubtedly follows the appearance and rapid progression of hy-

TABLE 7-2

Fetal Conditions In Multiple Gestation That May Affect Maternal Status

CONDITION	MATERNAL MORBIDITY
Discordant growth	Increased risk of pre-eclampsia
	Complications of bed rest (see Table 7-3)
Hydramnios	Respiratory embarrassment
	Preterm labor
	Complications of tocolysis
Stuck twin syndrome	Preterm labor
	Chorioamnionitis (if serial amniocenteses are performed)
Fetal malformation	Complications of cesarean section
Conjoined twins	Increased classical cesarean
	Complications of cesarean section
	Soft tissue trauma to the birth canal if vaginal delivery ensues.
Single fetal death	Consumptive coagulopathy
	Complications of bedrest (see Table 7-3)

dramnios in a multiple gestation. Hydramnios in a multiple gestation also places a marked stress on the vital capacity of the lungs. Shortness of breath and respiratory embarrassment are rare maternal complications that may ensue. If respiratory decompensation occurs, options for therapy include amniocentesis for amniotic fluid volume reduction or early delivery. Large-volume therapeutic amniocentesis can be performed for the relief of respiratory embarrassment or for the treatment of preterm labor.[41] The risks of this procedure are minimal (1.5%), particularly if the fluid volumes are limited to less than 5 L removed during one procedure. It is recommended that the amniotic fluid volume be decreased to a normal level (that is, either a single fluid pocket level that is less than 8 cm or an amniotic fluid index that is less than 25 cm). This should be done by removing fluid at a rate in the range of 30 to 60 ml/min.[41] This procedure can be repeated as often as every 2 days, although it is not usually necessary. This procedure can also be performed in cases of hydramnios in twin gestations,[40] and for the rare case of twin-twin transfusion syndrome (TTS) (see the following section).

STUCK TWIN SYNDROME

Hydramnios in one amniotic sac is a finding that is often present when the "stuck" twin syndrome occurs (named for the severe oligohydramnios present in the other sac that causes the fetus to appear to be adherent to the uterine wall). Preterm labor is invariable as this syndrome progresses. The patient is thus at increased risk for tocolysis and all the complications that may occur with the use of tocolysis. The occurrence of shortness of breath or respiratory embarrassment is more unlikely because the stuck twin syndrome tends to become apparent during the late second or early third trimester when uterine size is smaller and less likely to impinge on respiratory capacity. Options for therapy are reviewed in Chapter 8.

FETAL MALFORMATION

There is an increased rate of fetal malformation in multiple gestations.[117] This leads to an increased incidence of cesarean sections, as discussed previously.

CONJOINED TWINS

The occurrence of conjoined twins necessitates a cesarean section. An increased risk for classical cesarean section is also present. The need for a classical cesarean section depends on the size of the fetuses and type of conjoining that is present. If vaginal delivery ensues, damage to soft tissues of the maternal birth canal is likely.[93]

SINGLE FETAL DEATH

Fetal death is increased in incidence in multiple gestations. One study reported a rate of fetal death in twin gestations of 3.7% compared with 0.98% in singleton pregnancies.[84] When this occurs, the surviving fetus is at increased risk for adverse outcomes, including encephalomalacia and death.[7,42]

A maternal complication that must not be overlooked is the development of coagulopathy. The development of coagulation derangements is a distinct rarity in the setting of multiple gestation. There have been only 3 reported cases of maternal consumptive coagulopathy in multiple gestation, despite numerous series investigating this problem.* In most cases, these are probably transient alterations in coagulation factors, with a progressive fall in fibrinogen and a rise in fibrin split products, that resolve over the course of several weeks. If the mother's circulatory system is intact (providing for a low risk of

*References 20, 25, 26, 32, 51, 87

hemorrhage), some authors have advocated heparin therapy to reverse the coagulopathy and prevent complications to either the mother or the surviving fetus.[127] Although heparin therapy is well known in the setting of a singleton fetal demise, the efficacy of this therapy for the gravida with a multiple gestation is unproven. In a patient with a multiple pregnancy and a single fetal death, it is appropriate to monitor coagulation factors for the development of consumptive coagulopathy for as long as 6 weeks after the event. Intensive antepartum surveillance is indicated, since the cause of the death of one fetus may also affect the surviving fetus. Heparin therapy should be considered in a patient being monitored for coagulopathy whose fibrinogen levels fall below 100 mg/dl. Again, it is paramount that the use of heparin only be considered in a patient with an intact circulatory system.

Other than premature iatrogenic delivery (with all the attendant fetal complications of prematurity), there is no therapy that can prevent these maternal or fetal complications. Delivery after documentation of pulmonary maturity is appropriate.

Management Strategies that May Result in Maternal Morbidity

There are several widely available management strategies for multiple gestation, all designed to decrease the incidence or severity of premature delivery. The efficacy of each of the following management strategies remains to be proven. Maternal complications that may ensue during the course of these management strategies are

TABLE 7-3

Management Strategies that May Result in Maternal Morbidity

MANAGEMENT	MATERNAL MORBIDITY
Bed rest or hospital- ization	Maternal exhaustion in labor
	Deep venous thrombosis
	Infection with resistant or hospital-acquired organ- isms
Oral tocolysis	Tachyphylaxis
	Pulmonary edema
	Cardiac arrhythmias
Uterine activity monitoring	Increased hospitalization
	Increased tocolysis with attendant complications (see Boxes 7-2 and 7-3)
Cervical cerclage	Maternal sepsis
	Preterm PROM
	Cervical trauma
	Cervical dystocia
	Cervical stenosis
	Vesicovaginal fistula
	Uterine rupture
	Anesthetic complications

not well documented to have an increased incidence, but they are listed in Table 7-3.

BED REST OR HOSPITALIZATION

Recommendations by the physician for bed rest, either at home or in the hospital, are not uncommon for the patient with multiple gestation. Numerous trials, as well as metaanalysis, have not shown bed rest to influence the length of gestation or the rate of preterm deliveries, although a modest decrease in nonproteinuric hypertension was observed.[30,64,134] In the only

report of maternal complications of bed rest for multiple gestations, Hartikainen-Sorri and Jouppila[64] reported that patients with twin pregnancies who were hospitalized for bed rest had no difference in complications of pregnancy (such as premature contractions, cervical opening, rupture of membranes, maternal hypertension, and fetal distress) when compared with a group who received routine outpatient care.[134]

TOCOLYSIS

Preterm labor occurs at an increased rate in multiple gestations, thus subjecting women with multiple fetuses to an increased use of tocolysis. A host of serious cardiopulmonary side effects or complications may accompany tocolysis, as reviewed in the first half of this chapter.

HOME UTERINE ACTIVITY MONITORING

The role of HUAM in the management or prevention of preterm labor and in association with multiple gestation is still evolving. Further refinements in the existing knowledge are needed to define the role of HUAM. It should be noted that increased hospitalization may accompany the use of HUAM. This topic is reviewed in detail in Chapter 5.

CERVICAL CERCLAGE

The value of cervical cerclage for the prevention of preterm delivery in multiple gestation remains unproven in numerous trials, including an extensive series of metaanalyses.[57] Complications of placement of a cervical cerclage are unusual (reported rates are low), but they are listed in Table 7-3.

High-Order Multiple Gestations

High-order multiple gestations comprise an ever-increasing proportion of births in the United States.[17] Any assessment of the relative rates of maternal complications in high-order multiple gestations is limited by their relative rarity. In published reports, maternal complications in these patients have been mostly limited to spontaneous abortion, preterm labor, preterm PROM, preeclampsia, and increased rates of cesarean sections necessitated by malpresentation.[17,90,136] Because of their rarity, it is not known whether some of the complications previously reviewed (such as preeclampsia, intrahepatic cholestasis of pregnancy, and AFLP) are increased in high-order multiple gestations.

Psychologic Impact of Multiple Gestation

The psychologic stress imposed on a new mother with the birth of twins, triplets, or an even greater number of infants should not be underestimated. Many new mothers of multiple infants feel completely overwhelmed after they are discharged from the hospital. The difficulties that a patient encounters should be anticipated and carefully reviewed with the patient during the course of her antepartum care. Additionally, there are several well-known organizations that provide information, education, and support to new mothers who have delivered multiple infants, and patients should be encouraged to use these services.

Conclusion

There are numerous maternal complications of multiple gestation that can involve virtually all maternal organ systems and produce a critically ill patient. Knowledge of these complications is essential for the care of the patient with a multiple gestation. When maternal complications of multiple gestation ensue, prompt action by the obstetric team is paramount to successful management.

References

1. Aaron JB, Halperin J: Fetal survival in 374 twin deliveries, *Am J Obstet Gynecol* 69:794-804, 1955.
2. Anderson HF et al: Prediction of risk for preterm delivery by ultrasonographic measurement of cervical length, *Am J Obstet Gynecol* 163:859-867, 1990.
3. Anderson WJR: Stillbirth and neonatal mortality in twin pregnancy, *J Obstet Gynaecol Br Emp* 59:510-517, 1956.
4. Atrash HK et al: Maternal mortality in the United States, 1979-1986, *Obstet Gynecol* 76:1055-1066, 1990.
5. Bardeguez A et al: Umbilical artery creatine kinase brain-band isozyme as a predictor of neonatal periventricular-intraventricular hemorrhage, *Am J Obstet Gynecol* 160:202-206, 1989.
6. Barton JR et al: Recurrent acute fatty liver of pregnancy, *Am J Obstet Gynecol* 163:534, 1990.
7. Bejar R et al: Antenatal origin of neurologic damage in newborn infants. Part I. Preterm Infants, *Am J Obstet Gynecol* 159:357, 1988.
8. Bender S: Twin pregnancy, *J Obstet Gynaecol Br Emp* 59:510-517, 1952.
9. Benedetti TJ, Starzyk P, Frost F: Maternal deaths in Washington state, *Obstet Gynecol* 66:99-101, 1985.
10. Berg B et al: Cholestasis of pregnancy: clinical and laboratory studies, *Acta Obstet Gynecol Scand* 65:107, 1986.
11. Bernuau J et al: Nonfatal acute fatty liver of pregnancy, *Gut* 24:340, 1983.
12. Bloomer JR, Bower JL: Phenobarbital effects in cholestasis liver disease, *Ann Intern Med* 82:310, 1975.

13. Bloss JD et al: Pulmonary edema as a delayed complication of ritodrine therapy: a case report, *J Reprod Med* 32:469-471, 1987.

14. Bowen RE et al: ARDS associated with the use of sympathomimetics and glucocorticoids for the treatment of premature labor, *Crit Care Med* 11:671-672, 1983.

15. Bulfin MJ, Lawler PE: Problems associated with toxemia in twin pregnancies, *Am J Obstet Gynecol* 73:37-42, 1957.

16. Burroughs AK et al: Idiopathic acute fatty liver of pregnancy in 12 patients, *Q J Med, New Series LI*, 20:481-497, 1982.

17. Callahan TL et al: The economic impact of multiple-gestation pregnancies and the contribution of assisted-reproduction techniques to their incidence, *N Engl J Med* 331:244-249, 1994.

18. The Canadian Preterm Labor Investigators Group: Treatment of preterm labor with the beta-adrenergic agonist ritodrine, *N Engl J Med* 327:308-312, 1992.

19. Caritis S: A pharmacologic approach to the infusion of ritodrine, *Am J Obstet Gynecol* 158:380-384, 1988.

20. Carlson NJ, Towers CV: Multiple gestation complicated by the death of one fetus, *Obstet Gynecol* 73:685, 1989.

21. Caspi E et al: The outcome of pregnancy after gonadotropin therapy, *Brit J Obstet Gynaecol* 83:967, 1976.

22. Cetrulo CL, Freeman RK: Ritodrine for the prevention of premature labor in twin pregnancies, *Acta Genet Med Gemellol (Roma)* 25:321, 1976.

23. Chervenak FA et al: Antenatal diagnosis and perinatal outcome in a series of 385 consecutive twin pregnancies, *J Reprod Med* 29:727, 1984.

24. Chervenak FA et al: Intrapartum management of twin gestation, *Obstet Gynecol* 65:119, 1985.

25. Chescheir NC, Seeds JW: Spontaneous resolution of hypofibrinogenemia associated with death of a twin in utero: a case report, *Obstet Gynecol* 159:1183, 1988.

26. Chitkara U et al: Selective second-trimester termination of the anomalous fetus in twin pregnancies, *Obstet Gynecol* 73:690, 1989.

27. Collaborative Group on Antenatal Steroid Therapy: Effects of antenatal dexamethasone administration on the prevention of respiratory distress syndrome, *Am J Obstet Gynecol* 141:276, 1981.

28. Creasy RK, Gummer BA, Liggins GC: System for predicting spontaneous preterm birth, *Obstet Gynecol* 55:692-695, 1980.

29. Crosignani A et al: Failure of ursodeoxycholic acid to prevent a cholestatic episode in a patient with benign recurrent intrahepatic cholestasis: a study of bile acid metabolism, *Hepatology* 13:1076-1083, 1991.

30. Crowther C, Chalmers I: *Bed rest and hospitalization during pregnancy*. In Chalmers I, Enkin M, Keirse MJNC, editors: *Effective care in pregnancy and childbirth*, vol 1, *Pregnancy*, Oxford, 1988, Oxford University Press.

31. Cunningham FG, Lucas MJ, Hankins GDV: Pulmonary injury complicating antepartum pyelonephritis, *Am J Obstet Gynecol* 156:797, 1987.

32. Cunningham FG et al: Williams *obstetrics*, ed 19, Norwalk, Conn., 1993, Appleton and Lange.

33. Davies MH et al: Acute liver disease with encephalopathy and renal failure in late pregnancy and early puerperium: a study of fourteen patients, *Br J Obstet Gynaecol* 87:1005, 1980.

34. Daw E: *Triplet pregnancy*, *Br J Obstet Gynaecol* 85:505-509, 1978.

35. Duff P: *Acute fatty liver of pregnancy*. In Clark SL et al, editors: *Critical care obstetrics*, ed 2, Cambridge, Mass., 1991, Blackwell Scientific Publications.

36. Dye TD et al: Retrospective maternal mortality case ascertainment in West Virginia, 1985 to 1989, *Am J Obstet Gynecol* 167:72-76, 1992.

37. Ebert EC et al. Does early diagnosis and delivery in acute fatty liver of pregnancy lead to improvement in maternal and infant survival? *Dig Dis Sci* 29:453, 1984.

38. Edoute Y et al: Peripartum congestive cardiomyopathy and endocardial fibroelastosis associated with ritodrine treatment: a case report, *J Reprod Med* 32:793-800, 1987.

39. Elliott JP: Magnesium sulfate as a tocolytic agent, *Am J Obstet Gynecol* 147:277-280, 1984.

40. Elliott JP, Urig MA, Clewell WH: Aggressive therapeutic amniocentesis in the treatment of acute twin-twin transfusion syndrome, *Obstet Gynecol* 77:537-540, 1991.

41. Elliott JP et al: Large volume therapeutic amniocentesis in the treatment of hydramnios, *Obstet Gynecol* 84:1025-1027, 1994.

42. Embom JA: Twin pregnancy with intrauterine death of one twin, *Am J Obstet Gynecol* 152:424, 1985.

43. Engstrom J et al: Recurrent cholestasis of pregnancy: treatment with cholestyramine of one case with an unusually early onset, *Acta Obstet Gynecol Scand* 49:29, 1970.

44. Espinoza J, Barnaf L, Schnaidt E: The effect of phenobarbital on intrahepatic cholestasis of pregnancy, *Am J Obstet Gynecol* 199:234, 1974.

45. Farine D et al: Magnetic resonance imaging and computed tomography scan for the diagnosis of acute fatty liver of pregnancy, *Am J Perinatol* 78:316, 1990.

46. Farrell AGW: Twin pregnancy: a study of 1000 cases, *S Afr J Obstet Gynaecol* 2:35-41, 1964.

47. Fianu S: Maternal mortality in Sweden, 1955-1974, *Acta Obstet Gynecol Scand* 57:129-131, 1978.

48. Fisk NM, Storey Gn: Fetal outcome in obstetric cholestasis, *Br J Obstet Gynaecol* 95:1137, 1988.

49. Floreani A et al: Ursodeoxycholic acid in intrahepatic cholestasis of pregnancy, *Br J Obstet Gynaecol* 101:64-65, 1993.

50. Furhoff Ak, Hellstrom K: Jaundice in pregnancy: a follow-up study of the series of women originally reported by L. Thorling. I. The pregnancies, *Acta Med Scand* 193:259, 1973.

51. Fusi L, Gordon H: Twin pregnancy complicated by single intrauterine death: problems and outcomes with conservative management, *Br J Obstet Gynaecol* 97:511, 1990.

52. Galle PR et al: Ursodeoxycholate reduces hepatotoxicity of bile salts in primary human hepatocytes, *Hepatology* 12:486-491, 1990.

53. Ghent CN, Bloomer JR, Koatska G: Elevations in skin tissue levels of bile acids in humans with cholestasis: relation to serum levels and to pruritus, *Gastroenterology* 73:125, 1977.

54. Gonik B: *Intensive care monitoring of the critically ill pregnant patient.* In Creasy RK, Resnik R, editors: *Maternal fetal medicine: principles and practice,* ed 3, Philadelphia Pa., 1994, W.B. Saunders.

55. Gonzalez MC et al: Intrahepatic cholestasis of pregnancy in twin pregnancies, *J Hepatol* 9:84-90, 1989.

56. Goodacre RL et al: The diagnosis of acute fatty liver of pregnancy by computed tomography, *J Clin Gastroenterol* 10:680, 1988.

57. Grant A: *Cervical cerclage to prolong pregnancy.* In Chalmers I, Enkin M, Kierse MJNC, editors: *Effective care in pregnancy and childbirth*, vol 1, *Pregnancy*, Oxford, 1988, Oxford University Press.

58. Graves LR, Adams JQ, Schreier PC: The fate of the second twin, *Obstet Gynecol* 19:246-250, 1962.

59. Green JR: *Placenta previa and abruptio placentae.* In Creasy RK, Resnik R, editors: *Maternal fetal medicine: principles and practice.* ed 3, Philadelphia, 1994 W.B. Saunders.

60. Grimes DA, The morbidity and mortality of pregnancy: still risky business, *Am J Obstet Gynecol* 170:1489-1494, 1994.

61. Grimes DA, Schulz KF: Randomized controlled trials of home uterine activity monitoring: a review and critique, *Obstet Gynecol* 79:137-142, 1992.

62. Guttmacher AF: An analysis of 573 cases of twin pregnancy. II. The hazards of pregnancy itself, *Am J Obstet Gynecol* 38:277-288, 1939.

63. Hankins GDV: *Complications of beta-sympathomimetic tocolytic agents.* In Clark SL et al, editors: *Critical care obstetrics,* ed 2, Cambridge, Mass., 1991, Blackwell Scientific Publications.

64. Hartikainen-Sorri AL, Jouppila P: Is routine hospitalization needed in antenatal care of twin pregnancy? *J Perinat Med* 12:31-34, 1984.

65. Hatjis CG, Swain M: Systemic tocolysis for premature labor is associated with an increased incidence of pulmonary edema in the presence of maternal infection, *Am J Obstet Gynecol*, 159:723-728, 1988.

66. Hayashi R: *Obstetric hemorrhage and hypovolemic shock.* In Clark SL et al, editors: *Critical care obstetrics,* ed 2, Cambridge, Mass., 1991, Blackwell Scientific Publications.

67. Hendricks SK, Keroes J, Katz M: Electrocardiographic changes associated with ritodrine-induced maternal tachycardia and hypokalemia, *Am J Obstet Gynecol* 154:921-923, 1986.

68. Heuman DM et al: Conjugates of ursodeoxycholate protect against cholestasis and hepatocellular necrosis caused by more hydrophobic bile salts: in vivo studies in the rat, *Gastroenterology* 100:203-211, 1991.

69. Holcberg G et al: Outcome of pregnancy in 31 triplet gestations, *Obstet Gynecol* 59:472-476, 1982.

70. Hou SH et al: Acute fatty liver of pregnancy: survival with early cesarean section, *Dig Dis Sci* 29:444, 1984.

71. Houlton MCC, Marivate M, Philpott RH: The prediction of fetal growth retardation in twin pregnancy, *Br J Obstet Gynaecol* 88:264-273, 1981.

72. Howarth GR, Pattinson RC, De Jong G: Total perinatal-related wastage in twin pregnancies, *S Afr Med J* 80:31-33, 1991.

73. Hudgens DR, Conradi SE: Sudden death associated with terbutaline sulfate administration, *Am J Obstet Gynecol* 169:120-121, 1993.

74. Iams JD et al: A prospective random trial of home uterine activity monitoring in pregnancies at increased risk of preterm labor, *Am J Obstet Gynecol* 157:638-643, 1987.

75. Iber FL: Jaundice in pregnancy: a review, *Am J Obstet Gynecol* 91:721, 1965.

76. Itzkowic D: A survey of 59 triplet pregnancies, *Br J Obstet Gynaecol* 86:23-28, 1979.

77. Johnson P, Samsioe G, Gustafsson A: Studies in cholestasis of pregnancy with special reference to clinical aspects and liver function tests, *Acta Obstet Gynecol Scand* 54 (suppl):77, 1975.

78. Johnson WG, Baskett TF: Obstetric cholestasis: a 14-year review, *Am J Obstet Gynecol* 143:299, 1979.

79. Katz M: Randomized controlled trials of home uterine activity monitoring: a review and critique (letter), *Obstet Gynecol* 79:1051-1052, 1992.

80. Katz M, Gill PJ, Newman RB: Detection of preterm labor by ambulatory monitoring of uterine activity: a preliminary report, *Obstet Gynecol* 68:773, 1986.

81. Katz M, Robertson PA, Creasy RK: Cardiovascular complications associated with terbutaline treatment for premature labor, *Am J Obstet Gynecol* 139:605, 1981.

82. Katz M, Robertson PA, Creasy RK: Cardiovascular complications associated with terbutaline treatment for preterm labor, *Am J Obstet Gynecol* 146:916-924, 1983.

83. Kohl SG, Casey G: Twin gestation, *Mt Sinai J Med* 42:523-539, 1975.

84. Kovacs BW, Kirschbaum TH, Paul RH: Twin gestations. I. Antenatal care and complications, *Obstet Gynecol* 74:313-317, 1989.

85. Kurtz GR, Keating WJ, Loftus JB: Twin pregnancy and delivery: analysis of 500 twin pregnancies, *Obstet Gynecol* 6:370-278, 1955.

86. Laatikinen T: Effect of cholestyramine and phenobarbital on pruritus and serum bile and acid levels in cholestasis of pregnancy, *Am J Obstet Gynecol* 132:501, 1978.

87. Landy HJ, Weingold AB: Management of a multiple gestation complicated by an antepartum fetal demise, *Obstet Gynecol Surv* 44:171, 1989.

88. Lavin JP et al: Vaginal delivery in patients with a prior cesarean section, *Obstet Gynecol* 59:135-148, 1982.

89. Leuschner U et al: Ursodeoxycholic acid in primary biliary cirrhosis: results of a controlled double-blind trial, *Gastroenterology* 97:1268-1274, 1989.

90. Lipitz S et al: High-order multifetal gestation: management and outcome, *Obstet Gynecol* 76:215-218, 1990.

91. Mabie WC et al: Pulmonary edema induced by betamimetic drugs, *South Med J* 76:1354-1357, 1983.

92. Mabie WC et al: Computed tomography in acute fatty liver of pregnancy, *Am J Obstet Gynecol* 158:142, 1988.

93. Macgillivray I: *Labour in multiple pregnancies*. In MacGillivray I, Nylander PPS, editors: *Human multiple reproduction*, London, 1975, W.B. Saunders.

94. Marmol JG et al: Maternal death and high-risk pregnancy: an analysis of 40 maternal deaths in the collaborative project, *Obstet Gynecol* 30:816-820, 1967.

95. Marteau P et al: Effect of chronic administration of ursodeoxycholic acid on the ileal absorption of endogenous bile acids in man, *Hepatology* 12:1206-1208, 1990.

96. Martin MR: Maternal deaths in South Australia, 1970 to 1975, *Med J Aust* 1:310-313, 1979.

97. May WJ, Greiss FC Jr: Maternal mortality in North Carolina: a 40-year experience, *Am J Obstet Gynecol* 161:555-560, 1989.

98. McFarlane A, Scott JS: Pre-eclampsia/eclampsia in twin pregnancies, *J Med Genetics* 13:208-211, 1976.

99. McMullan PF, Norman RJ, Marivate M: Pregnancy-induced hypertension in twin pregnancy, *Br J Obstet Gynaecol* 91:240-243, 1984.

100. McNeely MDD et al: Creatine kinase and its isoenzymes in the serum of women during pregnancy and the peripartum period, *Clin Chem* 23:1878-1880, 1977.

101. Moise KJ, Shah DM: Acute fatty liver of pregnancy: etiology of fetal distress and fetal wastage, *Obstet Gynecol* 69:482-485, 1987.

102. Morton ME et al: Neonatal complications after the administration of indomethacin for preterm labor, *N Engl J Med* 329:1602-1607, 1993.

103. Mou SM et al: Multicenter randomized clinical trial of home uterine activity monitoring for detection of preterm labor, *Am J Obstet Gynecol* 165:858-66, 1991.

104. Munnell EW, Taylor HC: Complications and fetal mortality in 136 cases of multiple pregnancy, *Am J Obstet Gynecol* 52:588-597, 1946.

105. National institutes of health consensus development conference statement: Effect of corticosteroids for fetal maturation on perinatal outcomes, *Am J Obstet Gynecol* 173:246-252, 1995.

106. Neibyl JR et al: The inhibition of premature labor with indomethacin, *Am J Obstet Gynecol* 136:1014-1018, 1980.

107. Newman RB, Hamer C, Miller MC. Outpatient triplet management: a contemporary review, *Am J Obstet Gynecol* 161:547-555, 1989.

108. Nylander PPS, MacGillivray I: *Complications of twin pregnancy*. In MacGillivray I, Nylander PPS editors: *Human multiple reproduction*, London, 1975, W.B. Saunders.

109. Ober WB, LeCompte PM: Acute fatty metamorphosis of the liver associated with pregnancy: a distinctive lesion, *Am J Med* 19:743, 1955.

110. O'Brien C et al: Ursodeoxycholic acid treatment produces marked clinical and biochemical amelioration of primary sclerosing cholangitis, *Gastroenterology* 96:A640, 1989.

111. O'Connor MC, Murphy H, Dalrymple IJ: Double blind trial of ritodrine and placebo in twin pregnancy, *Br J Obstet Gynaecol* 86:706, 1979.

112. Palma J et al: Effects of ursodeoxycholic acid in patients with intrahepatic cholestasis of pregnancy, *Hepatology* 15:1043-1047, 1992.

113. Papiernik E: Proposal for a programmed prevention policy of preterm births, *Clin Obstet Gynecol* 27:613-630, 1984.

114. Pockros PJ, Peters RL, Reynolds TB: Idiopathic fatty liver of pregnancy: findings in ten cases, *Medicine* 63:1-11, 1984.

115. Podda M et al: Effects of ursodeoxycholic acid and taurine on serum liver enzymes and bile acids in chronic hepatitis, *Gastroenterology* 98:1044-1050, 1990.

116. Potter EL, Crunden AB: Twin pregnancies in the service of the Chicago Lying-In Hospital, *Am J Obstet Gynecol* 42:870-878, 1941.

117. Pryde PG et al: Triply discordant triplets: probability management options and risks, *Am J Med Genet* 44:361-364, 1992.

118. Purdie JM, Walters BN: Acute fatty liver of pregnancy: clinical features and diagnosis, *Aust N Z J Obstet Gynaecol* 28:62, 1988.

119. Rayburn W, Piehl E, Schork MA: Intravenous ritodrine therapy: a comparison between twin and singleton gestations, *Obstet Gynecol* 67:243, 1986.

120. Read MD, Wellby DE: The use of a calcium antagonist (nifedipine) to suppress preterm labor, *Br J Obstet Gynaecol* 93:933-938, 1986.

121. Rencoret R, Aste H: Jaundice during pregnancy, *Med J Aust* 1:167, 1973.

122. Reyes H et al: Prevalence of intrahepatic cholestasis of pregnancy in Chile, *Ann Internal Med* 88:487, 1978.

123. Roberts JM: *Pregnancy-related hypertension*. In Creasy RK, Resnik R, editors: *Maternal fetal medicine: principles and practice*, ed 3, Philadelphia Pa., 1994, W.B. Saunders.

124. Roberts R: Where, oh where has the MB gone? *N Engl J Med* 313:1081-1083, 1985.

125. Robertson PA et al: Maternal morbidity associated with isoxsuprine and terbutaline tocolysis, *Eur J Obstet Gynecol Reprod Biol* 11:371-378, 1981.

126. Rolfes DB, Ishak KG: Acute fatty liver in pregnancy: a clinicopathologic study of 35 cases, *Hepatology* 5:1149, 1985.

127. Romero R et al: Prolongation of a preterm pregnancy complicated by death of a single twin in utero and disseminated intravascular coagulation: effects of treatment with heparin, *N Engl J Med* 310:772, 1984.

128. Ron-El R et al: Triplet and quadruplet pregnancies and management, *Obstet Gynecol* 57:458-463, 1981.

129. Ross RC, Philpott NW: Five year survey of multiple pregnancies, *Can Med Assoc J* 69:370-378, 1953.

130. Russell JK: Maternal and fetal hazards associated with twin pregnancy, *J Obstet Gynaecol Br Emp* 59:208-213, 1952.

131. Sachs BP et al: Maternal mortality in Massachusetts: trends and prevention, *N Engl J Med* 316:667-672, 1987.

132. Samuels P, Cohen AW: Pregnancies complicated by liver disease and liver function, *Obstet Gynecol Clin N Am* 19:745-763, 1992.

133. Sassoon DA et al: Perinatal outcome in triplet versus twin gestations, *Obstet Gynecol* 75:817-820, 1990.

134. Saunders MC et al: The effects of hospital admission for bedrest on the duration of twin pregnancy: a randomised trial, *Lancet* ii:793-795, 1985.

135. Schoeman MN, Batey RG, Wilcken B: Recurrent acute fatty liver of pregnancy associated with a fatty-acid oxidation defect in the offspring, *Gastroenterology* 100:544, 1991.

136. Seoud MAF et al: Outcome of twin, triplet, and quadruplet in vitro fertilization pregnan-

cies: the Norfolk experience, *Fertil Steril* 57:825-834, 1992.

137. Shaffer EA: Liver disease in pregnancy, *Curr Probl Obstet Gynecol* 7:15, 1984.

138. Sheehan HL: The pathology of acute yellow atrophy and delayed chloroform poisoning, *J Obstet Gynaecol Br Emp* 47:49, 1940.

139. Sibai BM: Eclampsia. VI. Maternal-perinatal outcome in 254 consecutive cases, *Am J Obstet Gynecol* 163:1049-1054, 1990.

140. Skaerris J, Aberg A: Prevention of prematurity in twin pregnancy by orally administered terbutaline, *Acta Obstet Gynecol Scand (Suppl)* 108:39, 1982.

141. Spellacy WN, Handler A, Ferre CD: A case-control study of 1253 twin pregnancies from a 1982-1987 perinatal data base, *Obstet Gynecol* 75:168-171, 1990.

142. Stiehl A, Raedsch R, Rudolph G: Acute effects of ursodeoxycholic and chenodeoxycholic acid on the small intestinal absorption of bile acids, *Gastroenterology* 98:424-428, 1990.

143. Strong TH et al: Vaginal birth after cesarean delivery in the twin gestation, *Am J Obstet Gynecol* 161:29-32, 1989.

144. Suonio S, Huttunen M: Puerperal endometri-
tis after abdominal twin delivery, *Acta Obstet Gynecol Scand* 7:26-27, 1994.

145. Syrop CH, Varner MW: Triplet gestation: maternal and neonatal implications, *Acta Genet Med Gemellol (Roma)* 34:81-88, 1985.

146. Thompson SA, Lyons TL, Makowski EL: Outcomes of twin gestations at the University of Colorado Health Sciences Center, 1973-1983, *J Reprod Med* 32:328-339, 1987.

147. Usta IM et al: Acute fatty liver of pregnancy: an experience in the diagnosis and management of fourteen cases, *Am J Obstet Gynecol* 171:1342-1347, 1994.

148. Varner MW: Maternal mortality in Iowa from 1952 to 1986, *Surg Gynecol Obstet* 168:555-562, 1989.

149. Wittmann BK et al: Maternal mortality in British Columbia in 1971-1986, *Can Med Assoc J* 139:37-40, 1988.

150. Wojcicka-Jagodzinska J et al: Carbohydrate metabolism in the course of intrahepatic cholestasis in pregnancy, *Am J Obstet Gynecol* 161:959, 1989.

151. Yeh J et al: Results of in vitro fertilization pregnancies: experience at Boston's Beth Israel Hospital, *Int J Fertil* 35:116-119, 1990.

8 Fetal Complications

Jonathan W. Weeks

Multiple gestations are becoming more common. Although spontaneous twinning rates in the United States have remained constant at approximately 1% to 1.5% of pregnancies; multiple birth rates among couples enrolled in infertility services have increased to as high as 20%. Consequently, the incidence of multiple gestation in larger referral centers is approaching those of several common obstetric maladies such as gestational diabetes and preeclampsia.

Fetal Death

Multiple gestations are often complicated by the loss of one or more fetuses. The fetal death rate is 3 to 10 times that of singletons. Fetal loss may result from uteroplacental dysfunction or conditions intrinsic to either fetus. This chapter provides the reader with an overview of the most vexing fetal complications of multiple gestation. Although therapeutic interventions for many of these conditions have enjoyed limited success, a clear understanding of the epidemiology of fetal morbidity and mortality in multiple gestations will assist the reader with future counseling, diagnosis, and timely referral.

VANISHING TWINS

High resolution real-time sonography and transvaginal sonography have become relatively inexpensive and widely available in most developed countries. Since the development of these technologies, many reports of multiple gestations with subsequent dissolution of one or more gestational sacs have appeared in the literature. Because of the rarity of higher-order multiple gestations, this phenomenon is often referred to as "the vanishing twin phenomenon," but early dissolution of multiple sacs has also been reported.[38] When two fetuses are identified in the first trimester, 20% to 50% of cases ultimately result in singleton births.[22,44,25] When the diagnosis of twins is made before identification of the fetal pole, an even greater proportion of pregnancies undergo spontaneous reduction to singletons. Nakamura et al.[30] noted a 33% incidence of vanishing twins in cases where two fetuses were identified. When cases with two gestational sacs but only one fetal pole were included, 70% of twin gestations were affected by the vanishing twin phenomenon.

The occurrence of a vanishing fetus or sac is not associated with adverse effects on the mother or surviving twins. A careful inspection of the placenta may reveal

TABLE 8-1

Stillbirth* Rates in Twins, Triplets, and Quadruplets

AUTHOR	TWINS	TRIPLETS	QUADRUPLETS
Ron-El et al.[35a]	—	36 (37)†	0 (7)
Gonen et al.[17a]	27.8 (24)	0 (5)	0 (1)
Elster, Bleyl, and Craven[15a]	—	27.2 (1138)	—
Jonas and Lumley[18c]	—	68 (133)	83 (6)
Seoud et al.[38]	22.7 (115)	0 (15)	0 (4)
Millar, Wadhera, and Nimrod[27b]‡	20.8 (19070)	41.7 (323)	61.1 (23)
Elliott, Urig, and Clewell[15]	—	—	0 (10)
Collins and Bleyl[8a]	—	—	29 (71)

*fetal deaths ≥20 weeks per 1000 total births; †the number of sets of each type of multiple gestation appears in parentheses; ‡summary of authors data from 1986-1990.

remnants of the collapsed sac and flattened fetus (fetus papyraceus).

STILLBIRTH

Perinatal mortality rates in multiple gestations are 3 to 10 times higher than they are in singleton pregnancies. Neonatal deaths are responsible for the greatest portion of perinatal deaths in multiple gestations. Stillbirth, defined as fetal death beyond 20 weeks' gestation, is 3 to 5 times more common in multiple gestations. High stillbirth rates are related to higher incidences of congenital anomalies, intrauterine growth restriction, and fetal anomalies. Stillbirth rates do not appear to increase dramatically with increasing fetal numbers (Table 8-1). Most investigators have reported stillbirth rates of 2% to 3% in twins. Stillbirths occur in 0% to 7% of triplets and in 0% to 8% quadruplets. The surprisingly low fetal death rates in supergestations may be the result of fewer monochorionic placentas. Of the pregnancies reported in Table 8-1, 60% to 100% resulted from ovulation induction (OI), gamete intrafallopian transfer (GIFT), or in vitro fertilization (IVF). Clearly these pregnancies are benefited by more favorable placentation (see Chapter 2), early prenatal care, good nutrition, and high levels of parental education.

SINGLE FETAL DEMISE

A single antepartum fetal demise complicates 0.5% to 6.8% of all multifetal pregnancies. Several authors have noted the incidence of a single intrauterine fetal demise to be especially high in monochorionic gestations. Litshgi and Stucki[26] reported 13 cases of single intrauterine demise, 7 of which were from monochorionic gestations. In 1984 D'Alton, Newton, and Cetrulo[10] noted that 11/15 single intrauterine fetal demises were associated with monochorionic placentation.

Fetal death in monochorionic gestations is attributed to the high incidence of placental vascular anastamoses and twin-twin transfusion syndrome (TTS), which are discussed later in this chapter. Fetal death in dichorionic gestations has been associated with vascular thrombosis, intrauterine growth retardation (IUGR), abruptio placentae, and preeclampsia. Cord accidents and velamentous cord insertions have been described in single demises associated with both dichorionic and monochorionic placentation. Benirschke[2] found velamentous insertions in 23% of monochorionic-diamniotic placentas and in 13% of dichorionic-diamniotic placentas. Livnat et al.[27] reported three cases of twin gestations complicated by fetus papyraceus in which placental examination revealed velamentous cord insertions.

SINGLE FETAL DEMISE AND CO-TWIN MORBIDITY

When one fetus from a multiple gestation dies in utero the mother and her medical team are compelled to consider whether the surviving fetus will be adversely affected. Will the surviving fetus die? If so, when? Might the survivor experience a greater incidence of major morbidity? Is early delivery of the survivor associated with improved outcome?

In 1961 Benirschke[2] reported his research on placentation in a large series of twin gestations. He described one monoamniotic twin gestation with a single antepartum demise in which the surviving twin experienced respiratory distress syndrome (RDS), seizures, and muscle rigidity. Autopsy revealed central nervous system (CNS), renal, and splenic infarction. Benirschke[2] inferred that embolization from the demised twin to the surviving twin had occurred. Since then a number of investigators have postulated that thromboplastin-like substances pass from the dead twin to the survivor and instigate intrauterine disseminated intravascular coagulation (DIC).

Kilby, Govind, and O'Brien[20] reported on 342 twins delivered after more than 20 weeks' gestation over 5 years. Twenty gestations (5.85%) were complicated by a single fetal demise during the antepartum period. All of the cases with preterm single demises were managed conservatively. Five of the fetal demises were associated with major fetal anomalies, including two neural tube defects (NTDs), one bilateral multicytic dysplastic kidney, one thanatophoric dwarf, and one fetus with pulmonary stenosis. All five of the twins affected by major anomalies had dichorionic placentation. Three of the surviving twins were noted to have significant short-term morbidity; there was one case of TTS, one neonate with periventricular leukomalacia, and one infant with hypoxic encephalopathy. The periventricular leukomalacia was detected in utero when the single demise was diagnosed. The hypoxic encephalopathy was felt to be secondary to intrapartum complications. Although the authors stated that gross and histopathologic placental studies were performed in 17 of the cases complicated by a single demise, the reason for the demise was unexplained in the majority of cases.

Carlson and Towers[5] studied all multiple pregnancies complicated by a fetal death for 7 years at a large perinatal referral center in southern California. They reported three twin gestations in which both fetuses died and 17 cases of a single fetal death among 642 multiple pregnancies. The three cases in which both fetuses succumbed all had monochorionic placentas. Among the 17 multiple gestations with one dead fetus, nine were associated with monochorionic placentation and 8 had dichorionic placentation. One of the surviving twins had neurologic abnormalities;

delivery had been affected on the same day that the single fetal demise was detected. High resolution head ultrasound showed evidence of multicystic encephalomalacia. One year later the infant was noted to have hypertonicity and developmental delay.

Szymonowicz, Preston, and Yu[41] reviewed all monochorionic twin gestations with a single fetal demise over 10 years at the Queen Victoria Medical Center in Melbourne Australia. Six such cases were identified. The fetal deaths occurred 1 to 11 weeks before delivery of the surviving twins, and in no instance was the cause of the fetal demise discerned. Four of the surviving twins died in the neonatal period, and two survived with cerebral palsy and mental deficiency. All of the surviving twins had necropsy or radiologic evidence of intracranial infarcts. Three survivors suffered lung infarcts, and three had renal, splenic, or liver infarcts. As a result of three necropsies, the authors also noted fresh thrombi, organized thrombi, and sclerotic changes all in the same fetus. These cases provide strong support for Benirschke's theory[2] of an ongoing process of embolization from the demised fetus to the survivor via placental anastamoses.

Sherer was able to sonographically document a case of suspected intracranial embolic insult in the surviving twin of a monochorionic gestation affected by a single fetal demise.[39] Serial ultrasonography revealed evidence of intraventricular hemorrhage, mild ventriculomegaly, and subsequent microcephaly. A neonatal computed tomography (CT) scan confirmed the microcephaly and demonstrated marked cortical atrophy with an increase in cerebrospinal fluid.

Szymonowicz, Preston, and Yu[41] also pooled data from 16 previous reports on single fetal demise, published from 1932 to 1986, that were associated with monochorionic placentation. The 53 surviving twins were noted to have CNS infarcts in 72% of cases. The incidences of gastrointestinal, renal, and pulmonary infarcts were 19%, 15%, and 8%, respectively. Enbom's review of the literature[16] concluded that there is a high incidence of unfavorable outcomes among survivors of affected monochorionic gestations; 46% of survivors in his review suffered death or major morbidity. Both reviews have likely overestimated the magnitude of risk, since most of the published case reports were retrospective and did not review all multiple gestations managed at the authors' institutions during the study period. If an analysis is restricted to reports that document a review of all cases of monochorionic gestation with single intrauterine demise at the author's institution, the risk of morbidity or death in the surviving twin appears to be 17% (Table 8-2).

What has been consistent throughout 60 years of reports on single fetal demise in monochorionic twins is that when morbidity does occur in the surviving twin, there is a propensity for CNS involvement. When one considers that the most commonly proposed mechanism of injury to the survivor is embolization from the dead twin and that the fetal circulation preferentially shunts umbilical venous blood towards the carotid artery, the commonality of CNS injury in this condition is not suprising (Figure 8-1).

In recent years, some investigators have speculated that the genesis of morbidity in surviving twins may be severe anemia and hypotension coincident with acute hemorrhage from the survivor to the dead twin.

TABLE 8-2

Major Morbidity and Mortality in Monochorionic Gestations Complicated by a Fetal Death

AUTHOR	NUMBER OF CASES	OUTCOME IN SURVIVORS
Kilby, Govind, and O'Brien[20]	7	Leukomalacia (1)
Carlson and Towers[5]	9	Encephalomalacia (1)
Hagay et al.[18a]	4	Twin demise (2)
D'Alton, Newton, and Cetrulo[9]	10	Encephalomalacia (1)
Melnic[27a]	6	Cerebellar infarct (1)
Total	36	6 (17%)

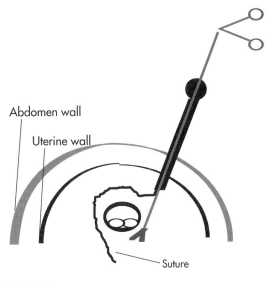

FIGURE 8-1   A forceps is used to drop a flexible, large caliber suture above the umbilical cord. The forceps is then redirected to retrieve the free end.

Okamura et al.[31] used funipuncture to evaluate survivors' hematologic profiles in seven pregnancies complicated by a single twin's demise. Five of the pregnancies were monochorionic. None of the five showed abnormal coagulation times, platelet counts, fibrinogen degradation products, or D-dimer concentrations. In contrast, all of these fetuses had low hemoglobin concentrations. One surviving recipient twin underwent serial sampling. Its hemoglobin concentration fell from 54% initially to 31% by funipuncture 26 hours later; at delivery 1 hour later it was 31%. Abnormal findings on head CT or sonography were seen in three of five monochorionic pregnancies. The absence of laboratory evidence of DIC and the uniform presence of anemia (sometimes progressive) in surviving twins presents a strong challenge to the commonly held theory of DIC resulting from thromboplastin embolization.

SINGLE FETAL DEMISE AND MATERNAL MORBIDITY

In 1955 Pritchard and Ratnoff[31a] reported the occurrence of DIC in singleton pregnancies with intrauterine fetal demise and delayed delivery. The risk of DIC was increased when the interval from fetal death to delivery exceeded 5 weeks. Since this report, the possibility of maternal coagulopathy has been a concern when expectant management is undertaken in multiple gestations complicated by the death of a single fetus. This concern is not entirely theoretical, since "fetal death syndrome" has been reported in multiple gestations.[40,35] Skelly et al.[40] described a triplet gestation complicated by DIC following a single fetal demise. At approximately 24 weeks' gestation the patient experienced an antepartum hemorrhage. Intravenous heparin therapy produced a reversal of the coagulopathy and allowed delivery to be delayed by approximately 10 weeks. Romero et al.[35] reported a similar experience in a twin pregnancy. DIC developed approximately 3½ weeks after the fetal demise. Heparin therapy corrected the coagulopathy, allowing delivery to be delayed until 25 days later when an amniocentesis revealed a lecithin/sphingomyelin (L/S) ratio of 4:1. Notwithstanding these two case reports, the occurrence of DIC after a fetal demise in a twin or triplet gestation appears to be rare. None of the subjects in the two largest series to date experienced maternal coagulopathy. Carlson and Towers,[5] in their series of 17 affected pregnancies, noted a mean interval from diagnosis to delivery of only 16 days. However, seven patients were delivered on the day of diagnosis, yielding a mean diagnosis to delivery interval of 27 days among the 10 patients who were managed expectantly. Kilby, Govind, and O'Brien[20] reported 20 cases of single intrauterine death. Again, no subjects experienced DIC. The median gestational age at diagnosis was 26.5 weeks, whereas the median gestational age at birth was 36.0 weeks. Neither Carlson nor Kilby reported the proportion of subjects expectantly managed for longer than 4 weeks.

MANAGEMENT AFTER A SINGLE INTRAUTERINE DEMISE

When a multiple gestation is affected by a single fetal death, the surviving twin is at risk for premature delivery, abruptio placentae, intrapartum fetal distress, and major organ system injury resulting from vascular disruption. Maternal transfer to a center with a unit for maternal-fetal medicine and neonatal support is advised.

A careful assessment of the surviving fetus(es) should be performed for the purpose of detecting previously unrecognized congenital anomalies or ultrasonographic evidence of CNS, renal, adrenal or pulmonary infarct. In view of the high incidence of fetal distress among survivors, prudence dictates the liberal use of electronic fetal monitoring. Since fetal distress often occurs within 72 hours of a single demise, patients who are in the third trimester should be hospitalized for a minimum of 12 to 24 hours of continuous monitoring. Signs of fetal jeopardy should prompt immediate delivery.

The timing of damage to surviving monochorionic twins is unclear. In the reports of D'Alton, Newton, and Cetrulo[10] and Carlson,[5] the only neonates with neurologic injury were delivered on the day of diagnosis. However, Szymonowicz, Preston, and Yu[41] presented strong evidence of serial embolization in their series of affected monochorionic gestations.

Inasmuch as the incidence of major morbidity resulting from prematurity in neonates over 33 weeks' gestation is low, delivery should be considered in well-dated monochorionic pregnancies at 34 weeks' gestation or more. Monochorionic pregnancies at 32 to 34 weeks' gestation should be evaluated with amniocentesis to determine fetal lung maturity. A mature foam stability index, L/S ratio, or positive phoshatidyl glycerol level should prompt delivery. The management of affected dichorionic gestations should be individualized after consideration of the maternal medical condition, fetal well being, estimated fetal weight (EFW), and fetal lung maturity status (Figure 8-2). Generally, delivery is also appropriate for dichori-

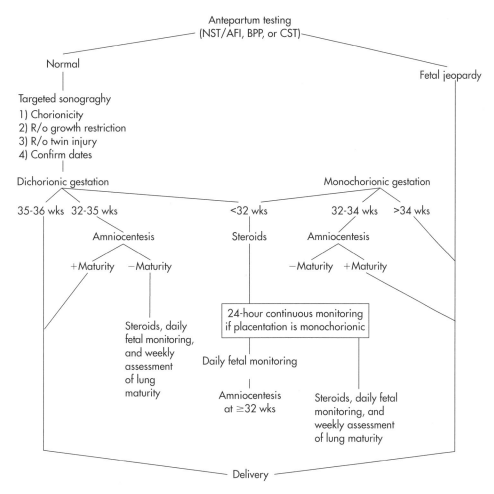

Antepartum testing
(NST/AFI, BPP, or CST)

Normal

Fetal jeopardy

Targeted sonograghy

1) Chorionicity
2) R/o growth restriction
3) R/o twin injury
4) Confirm dates

Dichorionic gestation   Monochorionic gestation

35-36 wks   32-35 wks   <32 wks   32-34 wks   >34 wks

Amniocentesis   Steroids   Amniocentesis

+Maturity   −Maturity   −Maturity   +Maturity

Steroids, daily
fetal monitoring,
and weekly
assessment
of lung
maturity

24-hour continuous monitoring
if placentation is monochorionic

Daily fetal monitoring

Amniocentesis
at ≥32 wks

Steroids, daily fetal
monitoring, and
weekly assessment
of lung maturity

Delivery

FIGURE 8-2   Fetal follow-up after single intrauterine fetal demise. *NST*, nonstress test; *AFI*, amniotic fluid volume; *BPP*, biophysical profile; *CST*, contraction stress test; R/o, rule out.

onic gestations advanced to the thirty-sixth week.

Surviving twins should receive careful postnatal observation, even in cases of documented lung maturity and normal Apgars scores. If the reason for the single demise remains undetermined, a circumspect evaluation of the survivor is fitting. Serologic studies to rule out congenital infection, a careful examination for anomalies, and karyotyping should be considered. Baseline cranial and renal sonogra-phy and a chest X-ray may also be helpful.

Twin-Twin Transfusion Syndrome

The occurrence of interfetus vascular anastomoses in multiple gestations has been recognized for several centuries. As early as the 1600s, physicians described the exsanguination of the undelivered twin when the delivered twin's umbilical cord was cut and left unoccluded.[1] In the early

1940s Herlitz[18b] described a twin pregnancy complicated by anemia in one twin and polycythemia in the other. This was the first report of the complication that has come to be known as TTS. TTS complicates 2% to 12% of monochorionic twin gestations. Although it is a relatively uncommon condition, TTS has received a great deal of attention in the recent medical literature. Unfortunately this scrutiny has not produced a significant diminution in perinatal mortality rates, which typically range from 60% to 85%.

PATHOPHYSIOLOGY OF TTS

Intertwin vascular anastomosis has been demonstrated in over 80% of monochorionic gestations, but it is exceedingly rare in multichorionic gestations. Robertson and Neer[33] found intertwin vascular anastamoses in 55/56 (98%) of monochorionic placentas, compared with 1/58 (1.7%) of fused dichorionic placentas. Hence TTS is primarily a problem of monochorionicity, affecting 2% to 12% of such pregnancies.[1,32] A 1991 placental registry found that of 373 twin sets with vascular anastamoses in which both twins survived, 5% had clinical evidence of TTS; of 107 monochorionic twins studied at autopsy, TTS was diagnosed in 45%.[1] The lethality of this disorder is underscored by the exceedingly high incidence of TTS among stillborn compared with liveborn monochorionic twins.

Intertwin vascular anastamoses may consist of balanced or unbalanced vascular communications. Balanced anastamoses are the result of shared circulation via like vessels (for example, artery to artery or vein to vein) or when an arteriovenous anastamosis is compensated by a reciprocal venoarterial shunt. Unbalanced vascular communications result from shared circulation across unlike vessels (for example, artery to vein) or when a previously balanced anastamosis becomes unbalanced because of a discordant change in fetal health or perfusion pressure.

The manifestations of TTS may occur within a short time (acute TTS) or over an extended period (chronic TTS). Acute TTS occurs after a rapid, large intertwin transfusion. The diagnosis is usually made retrospectively. The syndrome is characterized by a lack of growth discordance antenatally, but whereas one twin is plethoric and the other is pale, there is little hemoglobin or hematocrit discordance. With continued survival, fluid shifts occur and unmask the donor's anemia and the recipient's polycythemia. Serial hematologic studies eventually reveal reticulocytosis in the donor and hyperbilirubinemia in the recipient.

Smaller shunts produce growth discordance or a third trimester hydramnios and oligohydramnios sequence. In such a case a chronic, unbalanced vascular shunt results in an anemic donor and a hypervolemic, hypertensive recipient. The recipient then develops hypertrophy within the media of the pulmonary and renal vessels. Compensatory cardiomegaly ensues, as do polyuria and hydramnios. High renal perfusion pressures causes glomerular injury and profound proteinuria, which then result in a progressive decrease in plasma colloid oncotic pressure. Eventually the hypervolemia and hypoproteinemia produce hydropic changes and death. In utero demise of the donor twin may occur secondary to the progressive hypovolemia, hypertension, and malnutrition.

Nageotte et al.[29] studied cord blood levels of the mammalian diuretic hormone, atriopeptin, in two cases of TTS. Atriopeptin levels from the recipients were markedly elevated above those of the donors. Diuresis in the recipient twin is known to be responsible for the hydramnios seen in TTS. Therefore atriopeptin appears to play a role in the maintenance of the hydramnios and oligohydramnios that are seen in TTS, and it may play a role in the genesis of this syndrome.

POSTNATAL DIAGNOSIS

A definitive diagnosis of TTS requires a thorough placental evaluation. The first step is a gross inspection. The placenta should reveal a single placental plate. Generally there is a distinct contrast in the appearance of the cotelydons. The donor side appears pale, edematous, or atrophied, and the recipient side appears congested, plethoric, and hypertrophied. Inspection of the fetal side may reveal a marked disparity in sac size as well as the requisite thin dividing membrane composed of two amnions without an intervening chorion. On rare occasions one may find surface vessels that demonstrate vascular shunting, but the most common shunts involve deep transvillous anastamoses that can only be demonstrated with injection studies. Among the most simple techniques is the injection of sterile milk into the vein of the recipient cord. The donor cord is left unclamped, and the surface vessels are inspected for emerging white vessels. Robertson and Neer[33] described a much more elaborate method that demonstrated vascular anastamoses in 90% of instances (Box 8-1).

Before the advent of sonography, intertwin hemoglobin and birth weight differences were used to diagnose TTS (Table 8-3). A hemoglobin disparity of 5 gm/dl or

BOX 8-1

Placental Injection Technique for Detection of Vascular Shunts

1. Cannulate both arteries and the vein.[33]
2. Remove blood by flushing the vein for 30 minutes with a dextran solution plus heparin that is suspended 100 cm above the placenta.
3. Warm the placenta to 37° C in a water bath.
4. Perfuse the vessels on both sides using a colloid solution and different colored dyes.
5. Inspect the surface vessels for transplacental shunts.

more accompanied by birth weight discordance of greater than or equal to 15% to 20% was felt to be diagnostic. However, Danskin and Neilson[11] have recently reported that these criteria are often met in dichorionic gestations. Indeed, of the four sets of twins in their study that had hemoglobin differences greater than 5 gm/dl and weight differences greater than 20%, three were dichorionic. Clearly the criteria for diagnosis of TTS based on purely neonatal findings is inadequate. Blickstein[3] has proposed a new set of criteria that includes antenatal sonographic findings, neonatal evaluation, and placental findings (Table 8-4).

NONINVASIVE ANTENATAL DIAGNOSIS

TTS should be suspected whenever patients with known multiple gestations have complaints of excessively rapid increases in abdominal girth, symptoms of preterm labor, or a perception of decreased fetal movement. However, careful sonographic follow-up for multiple gestations should al-

TABLE 8-3

Diagnosis of TTS

ANTEPARTUM DIAGNOSIS

Criteria	Suggested cut-off values
Sonography	Monochorionic, like-sex gestation, and inter-twin AC* difference of >18 mm or EFW difference of >15% or hydramnios/ oligohydramnios
Umbilical artery Doppler	Intertwin difference in S/D† ratio or PI‡ of >0.4

NEONATAL DIAGNOSIS

Placenta	Monochorionic and evidence of shunt with injection of dye or milk
Birth weight	Difference of >15%
Hemoglobin	Inter-twin difference >5 g/dl

AC, abdominal circumference; †*S/D*, systolic/diastolic; ‡*PI*, pulsatility index.

TABLE 8-4

Composite Definition of the Twin-twin Transfusion Syndrome*

CRITERIA	FINDINGS

MINOR CRITERIA

Sonographic	Intertwin abdominal circumference difference >18 mm, hydramnios/ oligohydramnios, and signs of monozygosity
Umbilical artery Dopplers	Intertwin difference in S/D ratio >0.4

MAJOR CRITERIA

Placenta	Evidence of transplacental shunt
Birth weight	Intertwin difference >15%
Hemoglobin	Intertwin difference >5 gm/dl

*TTS is defined as the existence of two major or one minor and one major criteria.
Modified from Blickstein I: Obstet Gynecol 76:714, 1990.

low detection before the appearance of clinical signs and symptoms. Since TTS is a disorder of monochorionic gestations, the sonographic findings include the following: (1) a single placenta, (2) isosexual fetuses, and (3) growth discordance with hydramnios and oligohydramnios. Evidence of hydrops in one twin may also be present (Box 8-1). As discussed in Chapter 6, the most severe form of hydramnios and oligohydramnios culminates in the "stuck twin syndrome." Even when these criteria are met, the diagnosis of TTS may be erroneous. Hydramnios and oligohydramnios may also be caused by

discordant uteroplacental function, structural anomalies (such as one twin with renal agenesis), or congenital viral infections with discordant effects.

Umbilical artery Doppler studies have not proven to be useful for the diagnosis of TTS. Although several investigators have reported systolic to diastolic (S/D) ratio and pulsatility index (PI) discordance in many affected twin pairs, the differences have been small (0.5 to 1.0 units).

INVASIVE ANTENATAL DIAGNOSIS

Fisk et al.[17] were the first to report a series of pregnancies with "fetofetal transfusion" syndrome that were evaluated with percutaneous umbilical blood sampling. Five mid-trimester pregnancies and one third-trimester pregnancy comprised the series. TTS was suspected on the basis of discordant fetal growth and amniotic fluid volume, concordant gender, and sonographic evidence of monochorionic placentation. An interfetal hemoglobin disparity of more than 5 gm/dl was present in only one case, a third trimester gestation. Erythroblastemia and a weight discordance of more than 20% were detected in all fetuses. In two cases, donor fetuses were given an intravascular transfusion of 6 to 18 ml of O-negative, CMV-negative adult red blood cells. Kliehauer-Betke smears of recipient blood obtained by cordocentesis 16 to 25 minutes later showed 7% to 14% adult cells.

Weiner[46] recently reported his experience with an aggressive approach to antenatal diagnosis of TTS at less than 25 weeks' gestation that included amniocentesis for amniotic fluid reduction followed by serial cordocentesis. He used the initial amnioreduction to improve patient comfort, to facilitate sonographic evaluation by allowing for the use of a higher frequency transducer, and to facilitate the subsequent cordocentesis. At the initial cordocentesis both twins in a pregnancy were sampled for hemoglobin concentration, karyotype, and evidence of viral infection (such as torch titers and liver enzymes). When the initial hematologic studies were consistent with TTS (that is, an intertwin hemoglobin difference of greater than 5 gm/dl), 15 to 20 ml of adult O-negative blood was transfused into the presumed donor. This was followed by cordocentesis of the recipient 12 to 24 hours later. Weiner considered the ab-

sence of passage of adult red blood cells to effectively exclude TTS as a cause for the hydramnios and oligohydramnios and size discordance.

Bruner and Rosemond[4] have also used cordocentesis and transfusion of the donor fetus to assess the adequacy of currently accepted criteria for the diagnosis of TTS. Of nine twin gestations with sonographic evidence of monochorionic placentation, like sex, hydramnios and oligohydramnios, and growth discordance, cordocentesis was attempted in seven pregnancies. Six procedures were successful. The mean gestational age at the time of cordocentesis was 23 ± 2.6 weeks. The passage of adult, O-negative red blood cells from the donor to the recipient was demonstrated in only four of six cases (66%). An intertwin (fetal) hemoglobin difference of more than 5 gm/dl was present in only one of the four cases of TTS documented by passage of adult red blood cells (in that case the recipient was anemic) The authors concluded that currently accepted criteria for the diagnosis of TTS are inadequate and that true TTS represents only a subset of monochorionic, like-sex twins with the hydramnios and oligohydramnios sequence.

Other investigators have not found interfetal hemoglobin differences or the immediate passage of adult red blood cells to be adequate diagnostic discriminators. D'Alton[9] was among the first to express a loss of enthusiasm for cordocentesis and interfetal hemoglobin comparison in suspected TTS. She recently described a case involving a monochorionic gestation with a 1000-gm fetal weight disparity, similar hematocrit levels, and normal karyotypes. The twins were delivered 6 weeks later with all of the classic postnatal findings of

TTS. Ryan et al.[36] described a 22-week-old monochorionic gestation with suspected TTS in which adult red blood cells were given to an anemic, hydropic Twin A. After 30 minutes Twin B remained active, and a cordocentesis specimen did not reveal adult cells on the Kleihauer-Betke smear. The twins were delivered at 28 weeks' gestation because of preterm labor. Twin A weighed 750 gm and was hydropic with a hemoglobin level of 9 gm/dl, and Twin B weighed 1100 gm and had a hemoglobin level of 22.4 gm/dl. Kleihauer-Betke tests with cord blood demonstrated 7% and 8% adult cells in Twins A and B, respectively. The placenta proved to be monochorionic, and injection studies revealed a patent vascular anastamosis.

The conclusion that can be drawn from early experiences with cordocentesis for evaluation of apparent TTS is that the lack of in vivo hemoglobin differences of more than 5 gm/dl does not exclude the possibility of TTS. Future research protocols that incorporate donor infusion with adult red blood cells or medications such as pancuronium or atracurium should not exclude twins with concordant hemoglobin concentrations. Passage of markers from donor to recipient appears to clearly represent true twin-to-twin transfusion. Further research is needed to determine why some monochorionic gestations with apparent TTS do not demonstrate the passage of red blood cells in spite of demonstrable anastamoses during placental injection studies. Such cases may be related to intermittent obstruction at velamentous insertions, or they may simply be examples of an anastomosis that is balanced in vivo but is artificially unbalanced during in vitro studies.

TREATMENT AND OUTCOME

The medical literature has shown high perinatal mortality rates among multiple gestations complicated by TTS. Prognosis is particularly poor under the following circumstances: (1) the condition occurs in the second trimester; (2) hydrops is present in one or both twins; or (3) hydramnios is severe enough to cause bona fide preterm labor. When all of these conditions are present, perinatal mortality approaches 100%. Several treatment approaches have been proposed, including selective fetocide, therapeutic amniocentesis, laser occlusion of placental vessels, and medical therapies. The variety of therapeutic approaches and the radical nature of several of them underscores the lethality of TTS.

THERAPEUTIC AMNIOCENTESIS

Amniocentesis for the purpose of reducing amniotic fluid volume was first described in the British literature in 1961.[3] Several anecdotal reports appeared in the medical literature over the next 3 decades, but Urig, Clewell, and Elliott[43] were the first to compare patients managed by therapeutic amniocentesis with those managed expectantly. They noted a 0% perinatal survival rate among five cases of TTS diagnosed at 18 to 22 weeks' gestation that were managed expectantly. This was in marked contrast to the 60% survival rate of 5 patients who had their first therapeutic amniocentesis at 21 to 25 weeks, before any signs of preterm labor developed. The authors concluded that the intrauterine milieu could be "normalized" in TTS if therapeutic amniocentesis is employed early in the course of the disease. Based on this retrospective study, Elliott began utilizing therapeutic amniocentesis (TA) on all patients with TTS. They subsequently reported on 17 cases of TTS that were diagnosed at 16 to 28 weeks' gestation.[15] In all cases the donor twin had an amniotic fluid pocket of at least 8 cm and the donor had oligohydramnios that was severe enough to produce the appearance of a monoamniotic gestation (stuck twin syndrome). The mean number of therapeutic amniocenteses was four (ranging from 1 to 10), and an average of 1.6 L was removed per amniocentesis. All patients eventually achieved normalization of amniotic fluid in both sacs. Repeated aggressive amniocentesis was associated with an 80- ± 33-day interval from diagnosis to delivery. Seventy-nine percent of infants survived and were discharged from the nursery. Moreover, spontaneous regression of hydrops was observed in three of five cases, and four of five pairs with a single hydropic fetus survived. There were no cases of infectious morbidity or placental abruption. Two patients had spontaneous amniorrhexis within a day of their therapeutic taps. One was at 30 weeks' gestation, and the other was at 32 weeks' gestation. All four of the infants survived.

Reisner et al.[32] published their experience with 37 cases of TTS. Twenty-seven cases were treated with TA, 5 patients choose to terminate their pregnancies, and 5 patients choose expectant management. The amniocentesis patients had between 1 and 6 taps done, with an average of 1700 ml of fluid withdrawn per procedure. Normalization of amniotic fluid volume occurred in all oligohydramniotic twins. The mean interval from TA to delivery was 8 weeks, as opposed to 5 weeks in the patients who were managed expectantly. The TA group had nearly a twofold increase in overall perinatal survival. Thirty-nine of 54 infants (72%) survived from the TA group, compared with only 4 of 10 (40%) in those not undergoing amniocentesis. However, prognosis was significantly affected by gestational age at diagnosis. When TTS was diagnosed after 20 weeks' gestation, TA was associated with survival in 78% of patients as opposed to only 33% in the no-amniocentesis group. TTS diagnosed at less than 20 weeks was associated with survival rates of 57% and 50% in the TA and no-TA groups, respectively. Complications from serial amniocentesis were limited to three cases of rupture of the intraamniotic membrane (1 to 3 weeks before delivery), resulting in iatrogenic monoamniotic twins. There was no increase in premature amniorrhexis or abruptio placentae.

Other investigators have reported perinatal survival rates of less than 40% despite utilization of TA. Saunders, Snijders, and Nicolaides[37] treated 19 TTS pregnancies with TA. The mean gestational age at initial examination was 21 weeks and 5 days (ranging from 17 to 25 weeks). Only 14/38 fetuses survived. Gonsoulin et al.[18] noted an overal survival rate of only 18% when decompression amniocentesis was used to treat TTS. In both of these studies, the decision to perform either the initial or repeat therapeutic amniocentesis was based on the presence of symptoms. Contradistinctively, Elliott obtained daily ultrasonography and procedures were repeated in the face of hydramnios (the deepest pocket was greater than or equal to 8 cm) even in the absence of symptoms.

Although TA for TTS has not been subjected to the scrutiny of a prospective randomized trial, several investigators have reported an extension in diagnosis to delivery interval and improved perinatal survival with the use of this simple technique. TA appears to be most effective in cases where TTS is diagnosed between 20 and 30 weeks' gestation. When the condition is diagnosed at less than 20 weeks' gestation, prognosis is poor; spontaneous abortion and early preterm delivery are common. Cases diagnosed beyond 30 weeks' gestation have a reduced burden of prematurity and therefore improved perinatal survival, regardless of management approach. Larger series are needed to determine whether TA is capable of further improving survival or significantly reducing neonatal morbidity at later gestational ages. Given the high incidence of neonatal morbidity at less than 32 weeks' gestation and the relative safety of TA, continuation of therapeutic taps until 32 weeks seems sensible.

SELECTIVE FETOCIDE

Selective fetocide has been considered for the management of severe TTS for the following reasons: (1) it represents the most direct approach to interruption of the twin-to-twin shunt, and (2) the spontaneous death of one twin with subsequent resolution of hydramnios and twin survival has been reported. In 1963 Benirschke and Driscoll proposed selective fetocide by umbilical cord occlusion in a severe case of TTS.[2] Their first attempt failed as a result of an anterior placenta. Since then, several investigators have continued to view selective fetocide as a viable therapeutic option. Selective fetocide must produce death in the selected twin without transference of the lethal or noxious sub-

stance to the surviving twin. Several approaches have been described. Chitkara et al.[8] described fetal cardiac puncture with iatrogenic trauma to produce cardiac tamponade or exsanguination in an anomalous twin.

Wittmann et al.[47] reported the use of selective fetocide at 25 weeks' gestation in a severe case of TTS with associated maternal respiratory embarrassment. A number 17 Touhy needle was advanced into the fetal chest with the assistance of continuous sonographic guidance. The donor twin received a pericardial injection of saline. Cardiac activity ceased 2 hours later. The mothers preterm contractions abated 24 hours after the procedure, and her amniotic fluid normalized in 2 weeks. She ultimately delivered a 2900-gm, normal infant after 37 weeks' gestation.

Chescheir and Seeds[7] have reported selective fetocide by inducing massive hydrothorax via a percutaneous ultrasound-guided injection of saline into the oligohydramniotic twin. Serial ultrasonography showed fivefold reduction in bladder filling and urinary output in surviving twin. However, hydramnios persisted and 2 weeks after the procedure at 23 weeks' gestation, preterm amniorrhexis and preterm delivery occurred.

Lemery et al.[24] described a successful fetal umbilical cord ligation under ultrasound guidance in a case of severe TTS. At 27 weeks' gestation, the recipient was noted to be hydropic, both twins had abnormal fetal heart rate tracings, and biophysical profile (BPP) scores were 2 and 4 for the recipient and donor, respectively. A 5-ml endoscopic cannula was positioned just above the umbilical cord under ultrasound guidance. A chorionic villus biopsy forceps was then used to pass one end of a monofilament suture through the scope. The suture was released above the cord. The free end was retrieved from the underside of the cord with the biopsy forceps and pulled out of the cannula (see Figure 8-1). The procedure was accomplished in 60 minutes. Over the next several days, the BPP of remaining fetus improved. Preterm labor ensued 2 weeks after the procedure. A 1170-gm female infant with Apgar scores of 3, 4, and 6 at 1, 5, and 10 minutes, respectively, was delivered. The infant's head magnetic resonance imaging (MRI) studies were normal at birth and at 3 months of age. The infant was noted to be developmentally normal at 1 year of age.

Clearly, selective fetocide can be accomplished by surgical and nonsurgical methods. However, this approach to the management of severe TTS has the following practical and theoretical disadvantages:

1. The requisite expertise for the necessary ultrasound-guided or surgical approaches is limited to few obstetric centers.
2. The nature of the procedure limits perinatal survival to 50% at best.
3. Techniques other than cord occlusion are likely to result in the same high incidences of severe twin morbidity that are seen in spontaneous single intrauterine fetal demise (such as cerebral, renal, pulmonary, or limb infarcts).
4. Since not all cases of twin discordance with hydramnios and oligohydramnios are the result of true TTS, selective fetocide may not confer a true pathophysiologic benefit in some cases.

FETOSCOPIC LASER ABLATION OF VASCULAR ANASTOMOSES

The feasibility of fetoscopically directed occlusion of sheep placental surface vessels with neodymium: yttrium-aluminum-garnet (Nd:YAG) laser was demonstrated by DeLia in 1985.[12] Several years later he reported his experience with this technique in humans. A hysterotomy incision was used for placement of a 10-mm trocar and cannula. Intrauterine ablation of vascular communications between the fetoplacental circulations with a fetoscopic laser was performed in three cases of TTS that were diagnosed by 18 to 22 weeks' gestation. There was no perioperative maternal or fetal morbidity. Two patients, at 27 and 34 weeks' gestation, were delivered of their infants after preterm premature amniorrhexis. Their procedures to delivery intervals were 8 and 12 weeks, respectively. The third patient was delivered of her infants at 29 weeks' gestation with severe preeclampsia. There were two neonatal deaths, one from the 27-week delivery and one from the 29-week delivery. In each case, the neonatal deaths resulted from complications of prematurity.

DeLia et al.[13] presented an update of their experience with fetoscopic laser occlusion of chorioangiopagus (FLOC) in severe TTS at the 1993 meeting of the Society of Perinatal Obstetricians. Twenty two patients with sonographic findings of TTS, gestations of less than 25 weeks, and posterior placentas were treated with FLOC. The procedure was aborted in three patients because prior amniocenteses or the FLOC hysterotomy incision resulted in bloody fluid and poor visualization. Nineteen patients underwent the entire procedure. The amniotic fluid normalized, and symptoms were alleviated in all cases after FLOC. Both twins survived in six patients, eight patients had one survivor (fetal or neonatal death), four patients had no survivors, and one patient was still pregnant at the time of the report. The 14 women with one or more survivors were delivered of their infants at an average of 12 weeks after the procedure, and their fetuses achieved a mean gestational age of 32 weeks. Overall, 20/38 fetuses (56%) who completed the entire procedure survived.

If DeLia's analysis had included the three cases in which the procedure could not be completed, the fetal and neonatal survival rate would have been lowered to 45%. An "intent-to-treat analysis" would have been most appropriate, since all of the patients had already been subjected to the morbidity of anesthesia and hysterotomy.

Ville et al.[45] reported their preliminary experience with endoscopic laser coagulation. After patients had been given a local anesthestic, the procedure was performed with a 2.7-mm trocar and cannula that was introduced percutaneously under ultrasound guidance. They used a 2-mm fetoscope along with a 400-μm Nd:YAG laser fiber to treat 45 cases of severe TTS at 15 to 28 weeks' gestation. The investigators successfully coagulated the communicating vessels in all cases, including 18 cases in which the placentas were located anteriorly. Overall, 53% of fetuses survived to delivery, and 50% survived both the perinatal and neonatal periods. Neither twin survived in 13 cases, both survived to delivery in 16 cases (there were 3 subsequent neonatal deaths), and 16 cases were complicated by a single intrauterine fetal demise. Although the authors concluded that TTS can be treated effectively with this technique, their overall survival rate was not significantly greater than what has been described with serial amniocentesis. The enthusiasm of the investigators was at least in part a consequence of their findings of developmental normalcy in all survivors at 12 months of age.

MEDICAL THERAPIES

Researchers in several large clinical trials of prostaglandin synthetase inhibitors for suppression of preterm labor have reported the onset of oligohydramnios, especially with prolonged use. Dunn and Zambraski[14] have shown prostaglandins to play a role in maintenance of renal blood flow and renin production. These findings prompted investigations of the efficacy of indomethacin for reduction of amniotic fluid volume in twin gestations complicated by hydramnios. Lange et al.[23] studied six twin gestations complicated by hydramnios and premature labor. Indomethacin was initially given as a 100-mg suppository followed by 50 mg orally every 6 hours. Treatment was continued until 32 weeks' gestation was achieved or until the amniotic fluid volume normalized (with the deepest pocket less than 8 cm). All subjects entered the study at less than 31 weeks' gestation and were treated for 10 to 44 days. The investigators noted a significant decrease in amniotic fluid volume in all cases. Normalization of fluid volume was achieved in 4 to 20 days, and the interval from initiation of therapy to delivery was 12 to 101 days. There were no adverse maternal side effects. There was one case of iatrogenic oligohydramnios that resolved after discontinuation of therapy. Although these results were encouraging, there was little to no discussion of the cause of hydramnios in the six subjects.

The authors were appropriately cautious in their conclusions and stated that further study was needed.

Kirshon, Mari, and Moise[21] used indomethacin in 8 gravidas with symptomatic hydramnios, three of whom had monochorionic twin gestations. Serial sonography showed decreased fetal urine production and amniotic fluid volume in all cases. However, three of the four fetuses in the monochorionic gestations were stillborn.

Jones et al.[19] used indomethacin in three cases of severe TTS. All patients had symptoms at 22 weeks' gestation or less. They used the same regimen as Lange. In no case did they demonstrate a reduction in amniotic fluid volume. Two cases were complicated by a single fetal demise within 72 hours of initiating therapy. One patient delivered at 25 weeks as a result of preterm labor; neither twin survived. The perinatal mortality rate was 66%, and one of the two survivors has multicystic encephalomalacia.

Although experience with indomethacin for treatment of TTS is limited, it does not appear to be effective in reducing perinatal mortality. Moreover, this approach may acutely compromise the donor twin by further reducing urine output and amniotic fluid volume.

SUMMARY

TTS is a serious complication of multiple gestations, particularly when it appears in the second trimester. Expectant management with or without tocolytics is associated with perinatal survival in less than one third of cases. Of the current treatment options, serial TA has been the most commonly studied and used. It is clearly the simplest, most widely available, least morbid procedure. Studies to date suggest

that perinatal survival rates may be as high as 70% when taps are performed before the onset of maternal symptoms and when liberal quantities of amniotic fluid are removed often. Although FLOC appears to be efficacious in restoring normal amniotic fluid volumes and improving survival, the procedure requires transport to a capable fetoscopist, expensive equipment, and a potentially morbid hysterotomy incision. Patients with anterior placentas or bloody amniotic fluid are not suitable candidates. Moreover, experience with this procedure is limited to a few investigators. The theoretical advantages of FLOC include the ability to effect a cure with a single procedure without sacrificing one twin and the ability to prevent shunting of thromboplastins or blood in the event that one twin succumbs despite all therapeutic measures. Further study is needed to determine if FLOC is associated with greater survival rates in pregnancies where a single fetal demise occurs. Selective fetocide may be best used in cases where there is a single fetus with a major anomaly or when there is evidence of severe, progressive disease despite the use of serial amniocentesis. In such desperate situations, umbilical cord occlusion appears to be the technique of choice.

Monoamniotic Gestations

Monoamniotic twinning occurs in 1% of twin gestations and in 2/10,000 pregnancies overall. Despite its rarity, the high fetal death rate associated with monoamniotic twinning is well known. Fully 60% of fetuses sharing a single sac succumb to death during the antepartum period, most typically because of cord entanglement, which leads to occlusion and asphyxia. In the past, monoamniotic twins were not diagnosed until after delivery. The proliferation of inexpensive high resolution ultrasonography has allowed prenatal detection of most cases of monoamniotic gestations; hence a management dilemma has emerged. Should delivery be affected once an antenatal diagnosis has been made? Rodis et al.[34] recommended intensive antepartum surveillance and early delivery to avoid antepartum loss. However, two recent series have shown that fetal deaths are most likely to occur early in gestion. Carr, Aronson, and Coustan[6] reported no fetal losses beyond 32 weeks' gestation. Tessen and Zlatnik[42] reported no fetal deaths among seven sets of monoamniotic twins advanced beyond 32 weeks' gestation.[42] However, in an addendum to their manuscript, the authors described a double fetal death at 35 weeks' gestation in a subsequent monoamniotic pregnancy (a 12% incidence of double fetal loss between 32 and 35 weeks).

Most clinicians have chosen to deliver known monoamniotic gestations by cesarean section to avoid the possibility of intrapartum cord accidents. In both of the aforementioned series of monoamniotic twins, over half of the patients were delivered vaginally. However, the authors did not report the proportion that were delivered before viability. In some cases a single antenatal death had already occurred.

Given the rarity of monoamniotic gestations, collaborative studies are needed to determine optimal management. Inasmuch as neonatal mortality or major morbidity is rare with documented pulmonary maturity beyond 34 weeks' gestation, early delivery in such instances seems justified.

Acardiac Twinning

Acardiac twinning occurs when one "pump" fetus perfuses a second nonviable twin without a head, heart, or upper torso. Perinatal mortality in such pregnancies exceeds 50% owing to the high incidence of pump-twin congestive heart failure and severe hydramnios with premature labor. Moore, Gale, and Benirschke[28] published a report on the largest single series of pregnancies complicated by acardiac twinning. They found that preterm delivery was strongly associated with the development of hydramnios or pump-twin congestive heart failure. They also found that a greater acardiac to pump twin weight ratio was associated with earlier delivery and increased pump mortality. Conversely, an acardiac to pump ratio of less than 25% was felt to indicate a prognosis good enough to allow conservative management. The dimensions and weights of 23 acardiac twins were used to create a regression equation that was predictive of acardiac weight (weight in gm $= -1.66 \times$ length $+ 1.21 \times$ length^2). This formula may allow better selection of cases for such interventions as endoscopic umbilical occlusion or selective hysterotomy.

References

1. Baldwin V: *Pathology of multiple pregnancy*, New York, 1993, Springer-Verlag.
2. Benirschke K: Twin pregnancy in perinatal mortality, *NY State J Med* 61:1499, 1961.
3. Blickstein I: The twin-twin transfusion syndrome, *Obstet Gynecol* 76:714-722, 1990.
4. Bruner J, Rosemond R: Twin-to-twin transfusion syndrome: a subset of the twin oligohydramnios-polyhydramnios sequence, *Am J Obstet Gynecol* 169:925-930, 1993.
5. Carlson N, and Towers C: Multiple gestation complicated by the death of one fetus, *Obstet Gynecol* 73:685-689, 1989.

6. Carr S, Aronson M, Coustan D: Survival rates of monoamniotic twins do not decrease after 30 weeks gestation, *Am J Obstet Gynecol* 163:719-722, 1990.

7. Chescheir N, Seeds J: Polyhydramnios and oligohydramnios in twin gestations, *Obstet Gynecol* 71:882-884.

8. Chitkara U et al: Selective second-trimester termination of the anomalous fetus in twin pregnancies, *Obstet Gynecol Surv* 73:690-694, 1989.

8a. Collins M, Bleyl J: Seventy-one quadruplet pregnancies: management and outcome, *Am J Obstet Gynecol* 162:1384-1392, 1990.

9. D'Alton M: *Ultrasonography for antenatal management of twin gestation. In Ultrasound in obstetrics and gynecology*, Boston, 1993, Little, Brown & Co.

10. D'Alton M, Newton E, Cetrulo C: Intrauterine fetal demise in multiple gestation, *Acta Genet Med Gemellol* 33:43-49, 1984.

11. Danskin F, Neilson J: Twin-to-twin transfusion syndrome: what are appropriate diagnostic criteria? *Am J Obstet Gynecol* 161:365-369, 1989.

12. DeLia J, Rogers J, Dixon J: Treatment of placental vasculature with neodynium-ytrium-aluminum-garnet laser via fetoscopy, *Am J Obstet Gynecol* 151:1126, 1127, 1985.

13. DeLia J et al: Twin-twin transfusion syndrome treated by fetoscopic neodynium: YAG laser occlusion of chorioangiopagus, *Am J Obstet Gynecol* 168:308, 1993.

14. Dunn M and Zambraski E: Renal affects of drugs that inhibit prostaglandin synthesis, *Kidney Int* 18:609-622, 1984.

15. Elliott J, Urig M, Clewell W: Aggressive therapeutic amniocentesis for treatment of twin-twin transfusion syndrome, *Obstet Gynecol* 77:537-540, 1991.

15a. Elster A, Bleyl J, Craven T: Birth weight standards for triplets under modern obstetric care in the United States, 1984-1989, *Obstet and Gynecol* 77:387-393, 1991.

16. Enbom J: Twin pregnancy with intrauterine death of one twin, *Am J Obstet Gynecol* 152:424-429, 1985.

17. Fisk N et al: Fetofetal transfusion syndrome: do the neonatal criteria apply in utero? *Arch Dis Child* 65:657-661, 1990.

17a. Gonen R et al: The outcome of triplet, quadruplet and quintuplet pregnancies managed in a perinatal unit: obstetric, neonatal and follow-up data, *Am J Obstet Gynecol* 162:454-459, 1990.

18. Gonsoulin W et al: Outcome of twin-twin transfusion diagnosed before 28 weeks of gestation, *Obstet Gynecol* 75:214-216, 1990.

18a. Hagay Z et al: Management and outcome of multiple pregnancies complicated by the antenatal death of one fetus, *J Reprod Med* 31:717-720, 1986.

18b. Herlitz G: Zur Kenntnis der anamischen und polyzytanilachen Zustande bei Neugeborenen, sowie des Icterus gravis neonatorum, *Acta Pediatrica* 29:211, 1941.

18c. Jonas H, Lumley J: Triplets and quadruplets born in Victoria between 1982 and 1990: the impact of IVF and GIFT on rising birthrates, *Med J Aust* 158:659-663, 1993.

19. Jones J et al: Indomethacin in severe twin-twin transfusion syndrome, *Am J Perinat* 10:24-26, 1993.

20. Kilby M, Govind A, O'Brien P: Outcome of twin pregnancies complicated by a single intrauterine death: a comparison with viable twin pregnancies, *Obstet Gynecol* 84:107-109, 1994.

21. Kirshon B, Mari G, Moise K: Indomethacin therapy in the treatment of symptomatic polyhydramnios, *Obstet Gynecol* 75:202-205, 1990.

22. Landy H et al: The vanishing twin: ultrasonographic assessment of fetal disappearance in the first trimester, *Am J Obstet Gynecol* 155:14-19, 1986.

23. Lange I et al: Twin with hydramnios: treating premature labor at the source, *Am J Obstet Gynecol* 160:552-557, 1989.

24. Lemery D et al: Fetal umbilical cord ligation under ultrasound guidance, *Ultrasound Obstet Gynecol* 4:399-401, 1994.

25. Levi S: Ultrasonic assessment of the high rate of human multiple pregnancy in the first trimester, *J Clin Ultrasound* 4:3-5, 1976.

26. Litschgi M, Stucki D: Course of twin pregnancy after fetal death in utero, *Geburtshilfe Perinatol* 184:227, 1980.

27. Livnat E et al: Fetus papyraceus in twin pregnancy, *Obstet Gynecol* 51:41S, 1978.

27a. Melnic M: Brain damage in survivor after in utero death in monozygous co-twin, *Lancet* 2:128, 1977.

27b. Millar W, Wadhera S, Nimrod C: Multiple births: trends and patterns in Canada, 1974-1990, *Health Reports* 4:223-250, 1992.

28. Moore T, Gale S, Benirschke K: Perinatal outcome of forty-nine pregnancies complicated by acardiac twinning, *Am J Obstet Gynecol* 163:907-912, 1990.

29. Nageotte M et al: Atiopeptin in the twin transfusion syndrome, *Obstet Gynecol* 73:867, 1989.

30. Nakamura I et al: Seasonality in early loss of one fetus among twin pregnancies, *Acta Genet Med Gemellol (Roma)* 39:339-344, 1990.

31. Okamura K et al: Funipucture for evaluation of hematologic and coagulation indices in the surviving twin following co-twin's death, *Obstet and Gynecol* 83:975-978, 1994.

31a. Pritchard J, Ratnoff O: Studies of fibrinogen and other hemostatic factors in women with intrauterine death and delayed delivery, *Surg Gynecol Obstet*, 1955.

32. Reisner D et al: stuck twin syndrome: outcome in thirty-seven consecutive cases, *Am J Obstet Gynecol* 169:991-995, 1993.

33. Robertson E, Neer K: Placental injection studies in twin gestation, *Am J Obstet Gynecol* 147:170-173, 1983.

34. Rodis J et al: Antenatal diagnosis and management of monoamniotic twins, *Am J Obstet Gynecol* 157:1255-1257, 1987.

35. Romero R et al: Prolongation of a preterm pregnancy complicated by death of a single twin in utero and disseminated intravascular coagulation, *N Engl J Med* 310:772-774, 1984.

35a. Ron-El R et al: Triplet, quadruplet and quintuplet pregnancies: management and outcome, *Acta Obstet Gynecol Scand* 71:347-350, 1992.

36. Ryan G et al: Misleading tests in the diagnosis of twin-twin transfusion syndrome, *Am J Obstet Gynecol* 170:399, 1994.

37. Saunders N, Snijders R, Nicolaides K: Therapeutic amniocentesis in twin-twin transfusion syndrome appearing in the second trimester of pregnancy, *Am J Obstet Gynecol* 166:820-824, 1992.

38. Seoud M et al: Outcome of twin, triplet, and quadruplet in vitro fertilization pregnancies: the Norfolk experience, *Fertil Steril* 57:825-834, 1992.

39. Sherer D et al: Twin-twin transfusion with abrupt onset of microcephaly in the surviving recipient following spontaneous death of the donor twin, *Am J Obstet Gynecol* 169:85-88, 1993.

40. Skelly H et al: Consumptive coagulopathy following fetal death in a triplet pregnancy, *Am J Obstet Gynecol* 142:595-596, 1982.

41. Szymonowicz W, Preston H, Yu V: The surviving monozygotic twin, *Arch Dis Child* 61:454-458, 1986.

42. Tessen J, Zlatnik F: Monoamniotic twins: a retrospective controlled study, *Obstet Gynecol* 77:832-834, 1991.

43. Urig M, Clewell W, and Elliott J: Twin-twin transfusion syndrome, *Am J Obstet Gynecol* 163:1522-1526, 1990.

44. Varma T: Ultrasound evidence of early pregnancy failure in patients with multiple conceptions, *Br J Obstet Gynecol* 86:290-292, 1979.

45. Ville Y et al: Preliminary experience with endoscopic laser surgery for severe twin-twin transfusion syndrome, *N Engl J Med* 332:224-227.

46. Weiner C: Challenge of twin-twin transfusion syndrome, *Contemp Ob/Gyn* 37:83-104, 1992.

47. Wittman B et al: The role of fetocide in the management of severe twin transfusion syndrome, *Am J Obstet Gynecol* 155:1023-1026.

9 Intrapartum Management

Suneet P. Chauhan and William E. Roberts

Although conventional medical wisdom accepts the premise that the patient with a multiple gestation is at increased risk for adverse pregnancy outcome, the magnitude of the risk is much worse than expected. In the United States, twin gestations account for 2.09% of live births yet are responsible for 11.2% of neonatal deaths and 8.4% of infant deaths.[69] Furthermore, although uncommon, twin gestations are responsible for 14% of low-birth-weight (LBW) infants and 16% of very-low-birth-weight (VLBW) infants in this country. Compared to singletons, a twin pregnancy has relative risks of 10.3 and 9.6 for the delivery of LBW and VLBW infants, respectively.[53] Thus twin gestations are commonly associated with delivery of LBW infants (50.1%) and VLBW infants (10.1%). This is of particular importance to those involved in perinatal medicine, because most of the morbidity and mortality associated with a twin pregnancy is attributable to preterm delivery and complications associated with the care of small neonates.

Recent reproductive outcome statistics for twin gestations are of concern because they represent no significant improvement in the perinatal mortality from earlier epidemiologic studies.[59] Furthermore, during the past 3 decades, the incidence of twin births in the United States increased at twice the rate of singleton births, and the rate of triplet and higher-order multiple gestations increased at 7 times the rate of singleton gestations.[54] The reason for the increase in both the number and proportion of multiple births in the United States is multifactorial. One responsible factor is the trend toward a delay in maternal age at childbirth, since multiple births occur with greater frequency among older patients. The percentage of all births to women age 30 and older increased from 20% in 1980 to 25% just 5 years later.[62] Another reason for the increase in multiple pregnancies is the widespread use of ovulation-induction (OI) agents. The medical induction of ovulation with fertility agents increases the risk of multiple births.[58,81] However, the exact magnitude of this contribution is unknown, because the U.S. Standard Certification of Live Birth does not differentiate between spontaneous and induced pregnancies.[55] Finally, because of the legal complexity of embryo disposal and cryopreservation, most in vitro fertilization programs in the United States have implemented a policy of multiple embryo transfers. The impact of such a policy on the overall increase in multiple pregnancies is difficult to assess because of the lack of national information regarding both the extent and outcome of infertility treatment in this country.

Although the primary cause of perinatal morbidity and mortality in twin gestations is preterm delivery, other established contributors include congenital anomalies, fetal growth restriction, placental abnormalities (previa, vasa previa, abruption, and accreta), preeclampsia, and prolapse of the umbilical cord. Some of these factors associated with morbidity and mortality are unique to the intrapartum period and suggest that appropriate management of the patient coupled with close fetal surveillance would improve the overall outcome of the twin gestation.

The purpose of this chapter is to comprehensively review the obstetric literature and the experience at the University of Mississippi Medical Center in regard to the intrapartum management of patients with multiple gestations. Although overall guidelines and suggestions are formulated with support from the obstetric literature, it is important to recognize the dynamic nature of obstetrics and the problems imposed by the relative rarity of the multiple pregnancy. This, in conjunction with the medicolegal environment, mandates that any approach to the problem of twin delivery be flexible. Therefore the recommendations in this chapter are directives that not only can but should be modified in certain circumstances and are predicated on the skill and experience of the obstetrician and the availability of anesthetic and neonatal services, as well as the level of sophistication of the hospital facilities.

Preparations for Delivery

With the widespread availability of ultrasound equipment and a liberal policy to justify antenatal sonographic examinations, most patients with multiple pregnancies have had the benefit of antenatal diagnosis. Hopefully, the diagnosis of a twin gestation has been made in the early second trimester of pregnancy to allow sufficient time for the initiation of comprehensive prenatal care, as well as ongoing fetal assessments. At the time of admission to the labor and delivery suite, preparations for birth become paramount.

Multiple pregnancies are often complicated by malpresentation with an increased need for operative abdominal or vaginal delivery. This necessitates early anasthesia consultation. Although conduction anesthesia is generally preferred in the twin pregnancy during labor, personnel must be skilled in the administration of all types of anesthetics. Because of the potential need for neonatal resuscitation resulting from prematurity and low Apgar scores, pediatric or neonatal consultation is also required for the immediate, specialized care of newborn infants. Adequate obstetric personnel should include one clinician for each infant. Additionally, that clinician must be competent in both operative abdominal and vaginal deliveries. A summary of necessary personnel is shown in Box 9-1. Because of the large number of personnel required to respond to an unexpected complication, most multiple pregnancies are best served by delivery in large regional or tertiary perinatal units where people experienced in multifetal deliveries are readily available 24 hours a day.

After admission, intravenous access with a large-bore indwelling catheter should be initiated with infusion of an isotonic electrolyte solution. A complete blood cell (CBC) count with a type evalu-

Necessary Personnel Attending the Delivery of a Multiple Pregnancy

Obstetric: one provider proficient in operative abdominal and vaginal deliveries for each fetus.
Labor and delivery: sufficient number to allow performance of an immediate cesarean section as well as a vaginal delivery.
Pediatric/neonatal: pediatrician/neonatologist, 2 nurses, and one respiratory technician for each fetus.
Anesthesia: individual skilled in administering all types of anesthetic.

ation and screen should be routine. Care should be exercised in positioning the patient during labor to prevent aortocaval compression. For reasons noted later in this chapter, an intrapartum ultrasound examination should be performed with special emphasis on determination of the position and estimated of weight of each fetus. Electronic fetal heart rate monitoring should be routinely used, preferably with a dual channel monitor. This allows the simultaneous recording of both fetal heart rates and simplifies the task of dual, concurrent twin assessment. Finally, because of the increased likelihood of emergency delivery when the patient is under general anesthesia, clear, nonparticulate antacids should be administered routinely to all patients when they are admitted and every 4 hours during labor.

After preterm labor, preeclampsia is the next most common complication of the multiple gestation and occurs in over 14% of twin pregnancies.[41] Because of the in-

creased fetal and maternal risk associated with eclampsia, most patients with definite clinical signs and symptoms of preeclampsia receive anticonvulsant therapy and seizure precautions. At the University of Mississippi Medical Center, treatment of patients with multiple pregnancies who have preeclampsia is the same as that for similarly affected patients with singleton gestations (that is, they are given magnesium sulfate as a bolus of 4 to 6 gm intravenously followed by 1 to 2 gm/hr intravenously with close monitoring of maternal urine output).

Regardless of the anticipated mode of delivery, the actual birthing process should take place in an operating room replete with personnel and equipment for emergency cesarean delivery. Delivery of multiple fetuses in a birthing center is not advised. Additionally, extra supplies for cord clamping, infant identification, cord bloods, and immediate care, as well as possible resuscitation, of each infant should be in the immediate area. Finally, a portable ultrasound unit is essential and should be readily available to clinicians to allow them to monitor the heart rate of the second twin and to assist in obstetric manipulations such as external cephalic version, internal podalic version, and breech extraction.

Intrapartum Sonographic Evaluation

Ultrasound examination is pivotal to the intrapartum management of the patient with a multiple gestation. The position and estimated fetal weight (EFW) of each fetus must be determined. Another reason to justify an ultrasound machine in the labor and delivery area is its importance as an adjunct to assist the clinician during delivery of the second twin. Even if a sonogram has been performed recently, it should be repeated in the labor and delivery area, since the fetal positions and the amniotic fluid volume associated with each twin could have changed after the onset of labor. Furthermore, as reported by Divon et al.,[28] a fetal malpresentation often resolves before the onset of parturition. These investigators prospectively performed ultrasound examinations on 119 twin gestations at 2-week intervals. The rate of spontaneous version, which they define as a change from one clinically important presentation to another (that is, breech to transverse or vertex to breech), decreased with advancing gestational age from a 60% spontaneous version rate around 28 to 30 weeks' gestation to a lower 30% spontaneous version rate at term. They also observed that the spontaneous version rate was lowest for a vertex-vertex twin presentation (6.8%) but, in contrast, was universally seen in mothers with a transverse-transverse twin presentation (100%).

Although there are 10 possible fetal presentation combinations for a twin gestation (Figure 9-1), they can be simplified into the following three clinically important groups: (1) both fetuses in vertex presentation (vertex-vertex), (2) Twin A in vertex presentation and Twin B in nonvertex presentation (vertex-nonvertex), and (3) Twin A in nonvertex presentation and Twin B in other presentation modes (nonvertex-other). A summary of 7 published reports, as well as the experience at the University of Mississippi Medical Center, is presented in Table 9-1. If the factor of gestational age is discarded, the vertex-

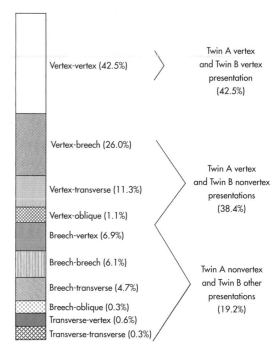

FIGURE 9-1   Type and frequency of intrapartum twin presentations. Occurrence of intrapartum presentations for 362 twin gestations. *(Modified from Chervenak et al: Obstet Gynecol 65:119-124, 1985).*

vertex combination is the most common presentation encountered during the intrapartum period; it is followed closely by the vertex-nonvertex presentation. The nonvertex-other presentation is the least common. Finally, of the 4057 twin sets in labor, Twin A was in the vertex position in over 75% of cases. As can be seen in Table 9-1, the experience at the University of Mississippi Medical Center differs from that of the other published series, since at this institution the vertex-nonvertex presentation is the most common intrapartum presentation. This is probably secondary to earlier gestational age, since the mean gestational age in the Mississippi series is 33 weeks, compared with 36 to 37 weeks' gestation in the other series.

TABLE 9-1

The Intrapartum Presentations Among Twin Gestations

STUDY	N	VERTEX-VERTEX	VERTEX-NONVERTEX	NONVERTEX-OTHER
Divon et al.[29]	119	50 (42.0%)	54 (45.4%)	15 (12.6%)
Chervenak et al.[24]	362	154 (42.5%)	139 (38.4%)	69 (19.1%)
Laros and Dattel[50]	174	76 (43.7%)	63 (36.2%)	35 (20.1%)
Caspersen[18]	213	96 (45.1%)	75 (35.2%)	42 (19.7%)
Thompson, Lyons, and Makowski[85]	341	131 (38.4%)	114 (33.4%)	96 (28.2%)
Kelsick and Minkoff[46]	2364	1118 (47.3%)	796 (33.7%)	450 (19.0%)
Crawford JS[26]	200	88 (44.0%)	57 (28.5%)	55 (27.5%)
University of Mississippi	284	87 (30.6%)	112 (39.4%)	85 (29.9%)
Total	4057	1800 (44.3%)	1410 (34.8%)	847 (20.9%)

In addition to an evaluation of both fetal positions, the intrapartum ultrasound examination should include an assessment of fetal parameters that allow the physician to calculate an EFW for each fetus. In spite of the limitation posed by the 12% to 15% error associated with the sonographic EFW in the third trimester of pregnancy, this exercise provides useful information for the overall management of a multiple gestation. First, the prediction of the neonatal weight helps the clinician better counsel the patient in regard to the morbidity and mortality associated with preterm multiple birth. Recall that the weight-specific neonatal morbidity and mortality for twins is not the same as that for singleton gestations. This disparity has been described recently in an epidemiologic review of 746,792 single births and 16,378 twin deliveries in New York City from 1978 to 1984.[48] Based on birth weight alone, the author made the following observations: (1) twins suffer a higher neonatal mortality rate than singletons for birth weights less than 1250 gm, (2) twins have a lower neonatal mortality rate than

singletons at birth weights between 1250 gm and 2500 gm, and (3) the neonatal mortality rate for twins increases markedly at birth weights exceeding 3000 gm when compared with singleton gestations (Figure 9-2). In fact, at birth weights over 3000 gm, the perinatal mortality is 70% higher for the twin neonate compared with a singleton.

Because twinning occurs more commonly in blacks, Fowler et al.[36] hypothesized that some of the increase in the weight-specific morbidity and mortality rates for twins could be related to race. Using the United States Linked Birth/Infant Death Data set from 1983 and 1984, investigators evaluated the twin mortality among 41,554 white and 10,062 black live births. These data provide an evaluation of weight-specific mortality in regard not only to twin versus singleton gestations but also as a comparison of mortality by race. Black twins with birth weights below 1500 gm have an increased survival rate compared with white twin newborns with similar birth weights. The lowest infant mortality among white twins occurs at a birth

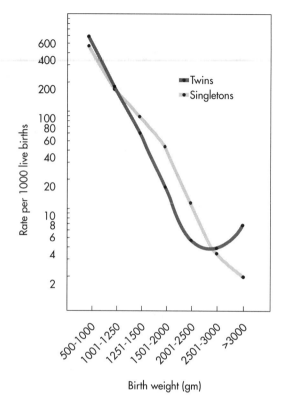

FIGURE 9-2 Birth-specific neonatal mortality rates for twins and singletons, New York City, 1978 to 1984. *(Modified from: Kiely JL: Bull N Y Acad Med 66:618-637, 1990).*

weight of 3250 gm compared with 2250 gm for black twin neonates. However, even at this optimal birth weight, the infant mortality for a black twin is nearly 4 times that of a white twin (12/1000 live births versus 3.2/1000 live births). These data also confirm the finding of the New York City epidemiologic study that the infant mortality for white twins increases after 3250 gm, with a near exponential rise in mortality after 3500 gm.

Another epidemiologic study, conducted at the University of Illinois from 1982 through 1986, compared neonatal morbidity among twin and singleton gestations.[37] These investigators retrospec-

tively reviewed the perinatal outcome of 998 twin and 80,906 singleton pregnancies and compared the incidence of hyaline membrane disease (HMD) and other respiratory disorders, as well as the incidence of neonatal seizures within birth weight ranges of 500 to 1499 gm, 1500 to 2999 gm, and greater than 3000 gm. Twin neonates have significantly higher rates of HMD and other respiratory disorders than do singleton neonates at birth weights of 1500 gm and over. On the other hand, the incidence of neonatal seizure activity is no different between twin and singleton neonates at all birth weight ranges studied, provided gestational age was controlled.

The second reason for obtaining an EFW of each twin during labor is that it could aid in the delivery management of twins in a vertex-nonvertex presentation. Recall that this is the second most common intrapartum twin presentation and occurs in over one third of twin sets (see Table 9-1). Some investigators consider that the route of delivery for the second malpresenting twin should be based in part on the calculated birth weight.[1,2,8,23,38] Because there is increased morbidity and mortality associated with breech delivery of the preterm singleton fetus weighing less than 1500 gm, the avoidance of breech extraction is advocated for Twin B if the EFW is below this limit. However, this approach is based in part on an assumption that the sonographic calculation of EFW for twin fetuses in labor is as accurate as the process for singleton pregnancy. Although numerous investigators have confirmed the accuracy of sonographically calculated EFW among singleton gestations, there is little information regarding its efficacy to help the clinician accurately predict the birth weight in multiple gestations. This concern is further disconcerting because of studies among singleton pregnancies that suggest that the accuracy of sonographic calculated EFW is compromised in malpresenting and LBW infants, and these two conditions are commonly encountered in multiple pregnancies.[8]

Despite these concerns and the potential limitations of the sonographically calculated EFW, a group of investigators recently reported that the prediction of birth weight using certain parameters is reliable in twin pregnancies in which the mother is in labor. Chauhan et al.[19] retrospectively identified 78 twins gestations in which a sonographic EFW was obtained within 72 hours of delivery. The sonographic accuracy of predicting the actual birth weight was similar in twin and singleton gestations. The mean standardized absolute error was similar for both fetuses regardless of whether the presentation was vertex-vertex, vertex-nonvertex, or nonvertex-other. Moreover, they observed that the accuracy for Twin A and Twin B EFWs were similar regardless of whether the actual birth weight was less than or over 1500 gm. Finally, it was noted that among the 30 vertex-nonvertex twin gestations, there were 12 pregnancies in which Twin B weighed less than 1500 gm. All had a calculated sonographic EFW below 1700 gm.

In the singleton gestation, the accuracy of the sonographic EFW generally improves as additional fetal measurements are used in the calculation.[86] Therefore it is reasonable to assume that the accuracy of the sonographic EFW will improve in the twin gestation if three or more fetal measurements are used to calculate the EFW rather than only one or two. Chauhan et al.[20] compared the accuracy of

eight different sonographic models in 181 twin gestations during early labor and observed that the standardized absolute error is greatest when predictions are based on only one fetal value (abdominal circumference [AC] or femur length [FL]). However, unlike the results in singleton pregnancies, the accuracy of the sonographic EFW in twins did not differ significantly if the estimate of actual birth weight was derived from a combination of two, three, or four fetal parameters. This paradox is true for both fetuses, regardless of presentation and whether the actual weight is less than or more than 1500 gm. Therefore the sonographic EFW based on the combination of two fetal measurements, rather than more cumbersome multiple measurements, is reliable and sufficient in the twin gestation.

In the same report, Chauhan et al.[20] confirmed their earlier observation of the critical sonographically calculated EFW that would consistently identify the nonvertex Twin B with an actual birth weight of less than 1500 gm. Using a relative operating characteristic curve, the authors noted that an EFW (based on biparietal diameter [BPD] plus AC or AC and FL) less than or equal to 1700 gm can be used to consistently (100% true positive rate) identify the nonvertex Twin B fetus with an actual birth weight below 1500 gm. Specifically, the authors noted that in the 49 vertex-nonvertex twin presentations, there were 21 cases where the actual birth weight of the second twin was less than or equal to 1500 gm, and all were correctly identified with a sonographic estimate of birth weight less than 1700 gm. Clinicians from other institutions are encouraged to determine their own sonographic calculated EFW threshold that identifies the nonvertex presenting Twin B with a birth weight below 1500 gm. Before one determines a personal threshold, it seems reasonable to use the more conservative sonographic EFW of less than or equal to 2000 gm as the critical EFW to ensure that the nonvertex Twin B weighing less than 1500 gm is not a candidate for elective vaginal delivery.

The third advantage of an intrapartum EFW is the identification of discordant growth among twins. Serial antenatal ultrasound examinations usually detect most patients with this complication that is unique to the multiple pregnancy. However, perhaps because of noncompliance or because the abnormal growth might not become evident until late in pregnancy, discordant growth may not be diagnosed until the intrapartum period. In the series studied by Divon et al.,[28] discordant growth was defined as an actual birth weight difference of 15% or more (larger minus the smaller divided by the larger and multiplied by 100). In their series, sonographic examination within 14 days of delivery was associated with sensitivity, specificity, and positive and negative predictive values of 47%, 81%, 74%, and 56%. In the series of Chauhan et al.,[19] where discordant growth was similarly defined, use of the intrapartum sonographic examination achieved a sensitivity, specificity, and positive and negative predictive values of 50%, 85%, 83%, and 53%, respectively.

Finally, perhaps the most important role of ultrasound in the management of a twin gestation occurs after the delivery of Twin A. Regardless of the presentation of Twin B, the sonographic evaluation of the fetal heart rate is helpful in the assessment of fetal well being. Until the fetal heart electrode can be safely applied, ultrasound provides a simple method to monitor the fetal heart rate. If Twin B is in a nonvertex position, the ultrasound is critical for the performance of obstetric procedures such as external cephalic version and internal podalic version.[22,73,74]

Intrapartum Management

After establishing that the patient with a the multiple pregnancy is in labor, several intrapartum principles need implementation. Continuous monitoring of both fetuses throughout labor is crucial, since multiple gestations are at increased risk for fetal stress with resultant hypoxemia and intrapartum or neonatal death. Kiely,[48] in his extensive epidemiologic review of the morbidity and mortality associated with twin pregnancy, noted that twins have an incidence of intrapartum death that is 3 times higher (6.1/1000 live births) than singletons (2.0/1000 live births). However, if the birth weight of twin neonates is below 2500 gm, the intrapartum death rate is actually less than that of the singletons (relative risk=0.43). On the other hand, newborns of multiple gestations that have birth weights exceeding 2500 gm have a much higher likelihood of intrapartum fetal death (relative risk=3.54). As mentioned earlier in this chapter, as well as in the American College of Obstetricians and Gynecologists (ACOG) Technical Bulletin,[4] anesthesia and pediatric personnel should be notified of the admission of all patients in labor with multiple gestations. Because of the increased need for operative delivery, blood should be sent for type and screen tests, and intravenous access should be established.

Clinically, the various twin presentations can be simplified into three groups. The purpose of the division is founded on traditional concepts regarding mode of delivery based on the presentation and gestational age of the fetuses. In spite of some recent data to repudiate such a grouping of twin pregnancies,[27] this review complies with tradition and pragmatically presents data and delivery options according to the following three groups: (1) Twin A vertex and Twin B vertex, (2) Twin A vertex and Twin B nonvertex, and (3) Twin A nonvertex and Twin B other.

TWIN A VERTEX AND TWIN B VERTEX PRESENTATION

As shown in Table 9-1, the Twin A vertex and Twin B vertex is the most common intrapartum presentation for twin gestations and occurs in 44.3% of cases. The results of two studies, as well as the experience at the University of Mississippi, of the route of delivery for patients with this presentation are summarized in Table 9-2. Most reports on the intrapartum management of twin gestations with the Twin A vertex and Twin B vertex presentation do not describe the outcome of labor in sufficient detail to critically analyze the method of

delivery.[26,29,46,85] This lack of information is probably because there is little disagreement regarding the route of delivery for fetuses in vertex presentation. Twins with this presentation are generally considered candidates for vaginal delivery and undergo successful vaginal delivery in 63% to 77% of cases. As in singleton pregnancies, there may be obstetric or medical indications that preclude an attempt at vaginal delivery. Most series have a 20% to 25% incidence of abdominal delivery in patients with this type of twin presentation.

The review of the mode of delivery for the 372 patients with Twin A vertex and Twin B vertex presentations that is summarized in Table 9-2 is noteworthy for two reasons. First, although both twins are in vertex presentation during labor, Twin B may need to be delivered by breech extraction. Even though this is uncommon and occurred in only 0.8% to 3.9% of cases reviewed, the clinician must anticipate and be prepared to manage a malpresentation of Twin B. The second area of concern noted in Table 9-2 is the need for an abdominal delivery of Twin B after Twin A has undergone successful vaginal delivery. Generally, this occurs as a result of fetal malpresentation, an intolerance of

TABLE 9-2

The Route of Delivery Among Twins Gestations with Vertex-Vertex Presentation					
STUDY	N	V VD-A AND B*	V VD-A; BVD-B	V VD-A; CS-B	CS-A; CS-B
Chervenak et al.[24]	154	119 (77.3%)	6 (3.9%)	2 (1.3%)	27 (17.5%)
Thompson, Lyons, and Makowski[85]	131	96 (73.3%)	1 (0.8%)	8 (6.1%)	26 (19.8%)
University of Mississippi	87	55 (63.2%)	1 (1.1%)	9 (10.3%)	22 (25.3%)
Total	372	270 (72.6%)	8 (2.2%)	19 (5.1%)	75 (20.2%)

*VVD, vertex vaginal delivery; BVD, breech vaginal delivery; CS, cesarean section.

labor by Twin B, umbilical cord prolapse, or an arrest of labor. In the series reviewed by Chervenak et al.,[24] one cesarean delivery was undertaken for fetal distress and the other for failure of the vertex to engage after an hour of labor. The reason for abdominal delivery in the eight cases in Thompson, Lyons, and Makowski's series was not mentioned.[85] At the University of Mississippi, abdominal delivery was undertaken for Twin B after vaginal delivery for Twin A in nine cases. The reasons for the cesarean deliveries were umbilical cord prolapse (n=3), abnormal fetal heart rate tracing (n=3), malpresentation (n=2), and an arrest disorder of labor (n=1). Because of the extremes in the incidence of vaginal delivery of Twin A with cesarean delivery of the second twin (that is, 1.3% to 10.3%), one must wonder whether other factors such as discordant fetal weight and preterm gestation might be responsible.

The time interval between the delivery of twins has recently undergone critical review. Early data suggested that the interval between the delivery of Twin A and Twin B should not exceed 30 minutes. Potential complications correlated with prolonged time intervals between the delivery of the first and second twin include uteroplacental insufficiency (UPI), abnormal fetal presentation, and umbilical cord prolapse with associated conditions of hypoxia with birth asphyxia and death. Now, with ultrasonographic and electronic fetal heart rate monitoring techniques to assess fetal well being, such an arbitrary time limit between the delivery of twins is no longer advocated, provided Twin B has no evidence of fetal compromise. Rayburn and associates were the first to report that the incidence of low Apgar scores, trau-matic delivery, and neonatal morbidity and mortality were no different for term and near-term twins for delivery intervals of less than 15 minutes, 16 to 30 minutes, and more than 30 minutes.[75] Since that pilot study, other authors have confirmed these findings.[2,24,50,85] As mentioned in the ACOG Technical Bulletin on multiple gestation, if Twin B has not been delivered within a reasonable time, oxytocin augmentation of labor should be considered. As with the administration of any uterotonic agent in either the multiple or the singleton gestation, prerequisites include a hypotonic contraction pattern as the cause of the arrest of labor and no evidence of fetal compromise with continuous monitoring of the fetal heart.

TWIN A VERTEX AND TWIN B NONVERTEX PRESENTATION

Most obstetricians agree that vaginal delivery for the vertex presenting Twin A is safe, regardless of gestational age. However, there is no consensus with regard to the mode of delivery for the malpresenting Twin B. The confusion about appropriate perinatal management centers on three as of yet unresolved issues. First, is there increased morbidity for the term or near-term malpresenting second twin if vaginal delivery is undertaken instead of an abdominal delivery? Second, can external cephalic version (ECV) be reliably performed, and if so, how does the morbidity associated with the procedure compare with vaginal and cesarean delivery? Furthermore, if a difference in morbidity is apparent with ECV, is it dependent on gestational age? Finally, regardless of gestational age or birth weight, can Twin B be safely delivered vaginally? In an attempt to present meaningful data in an unbiased fashion, the obstetric literature is reviewed in terms of not only the outcome parameters but also the primary mode of management of the Twin A vertex and Twin B nonvertex presentation. In other words, data from institutions where clinicians have greater experience and expertise in certain obstetric maneuvers, such as external cephalic version or breech extraction, is probably more reflective and pertinent with regard to outcome for that mode of management.

Table 9-3 summarizes the mode of delivery for the Twin A vertex and Twin B nonvertex presentation at four institutions and the University of Mississippi Medical Center. Although there are numerous other studies in the obstetric literature describing the mode of delivery for this type of twin presentation, they are not included in this analysis because they compared outcome parameters of Twin B with those of cohort Twin A. This is of paramount importance and a probable source of error and misinformation in these studies, since fetal growth restriction, fetal anomalies, and abnormal placentation occur more commonly in Twin B fetuses.[71] There is re-

markable variability among the series listed in Table 9-3 regarding to the incidence of abdominal delivery for both fetuses (7.7% to 50.9%), breech extraction for Twin B (20.5% to 92.3%), and a combination of vaginal delivery for Twin A and abdominal delivery for Twin B (3.3% to 19.6%). However, the incidence of vaginal delivery for both fetuses in a vertex presentation was similar (8.9% to 14.0%). Possible explanations for the variation in the route of delivery include the period of the study, difference in gestational age at delivery, possible discordant growth among the twins, whether an external cephalic version was attempted, and whether clinicians were proficient in breech extraction procedures.

Earlier studies suggested that abdominal delivery was associated with less morbidity for the malpresenting Twin B fetus. In a 1981 review, Evrard and Gold[32] reported on nine cases where cesarean delivery was needed for Twin B after successful vaginal delivery of Twin A. In these nine cases, there were two perinatal deaths. The authors felt these deaths were the result of birth trauma or perinatal asphyxia and could have been prevented by

TABLE 9-3

The Route of Delivery Among Twins Gestations with Vertex-Nonvertex Presentation					
STUDY	N	CS-A AND B*	V VD-A; BVD-B	V VD-A AND B	V VD-A; CS-B
Chervenak et al.[23]	135	36 (26.7%)	76 (56.3%)	18 (13.3%)	5 (3.7%)
Blickstein et al.[11]	39	3 (7.7%)	36 (92.3%)	—	—
Gocke et al.[38]	136	40 (29.4%)	59 (43.4%)	19 (14.0%)	18 (13.2%)
Adam, Allen, and Baskett[2]	120	19 (15.8%)	86 (71.7%)	11 (9.2%)	4 (3.3%)
University of Mississippi	112	57 (50.9%)	23 (20.5%)	10 (8.9%)	22 (19.6%)
Total	542	155 (28.6%)	280 (51.7%)	58 (10.7%)	49 (9.0%)

*CS, Cesarean Section; VVD, Vertex Vaginal Delivery; BVD, Breech Vaginal Delivery.

the initial performance of a cesarean section rather than vaginal delivery of Twin A followed by obstetric maneuvers to attempt vaginal delivery of Twin B. The authors did caution readers of the retrospective nature of their review and the small sample size. In fact, recent data collected prospectively and with larger numbers of patients indicate that vaginal delivery of Twin B is safe under certain conditions.[27]

In 1982, Acker et al.[1] prospectively compared the 5-minute Apgar score and neonatal outcome variables in nonvertex Twin B fetuses delivered abdominally (n=76) versus those delivered vaginally (n=74). All neonates weighed over 1500 gm. There were no deaths in either group, and the incidence of neonatal depression was similar (11/76 versus 7/74, p=0.24). In a more recent analysis of the mode of delivery in Twin A vertex and Twin B nonvertex presentations, Adam et al.[2] reported no difference in the incidence of significant (grade 3 or 4) intraventricular hemorrhage (IVH) or in the incidence of respiratory distress in Twin B infants delivered vaginally compared with those delivered abdominally, provided the birth weight exceeded 1500 gm. Morales et al.[61] performed a multivariate analysis of their prospectively collected data of Twin A vertex and Twin B nonvertex presentations. These investigators concluded that all clinically significant neonatal morbidity, not just IVH, was tightly associated with gestational age and birth weight but was not associated with the mode of delivery. Finally, Greig et al.[40] have reported that the mean umbilical arterial pH values are not different among second malpresenting twins delivered vaginally compared with those delivered by cesarean section. In summary, for larger, prospective studies

where the well-being of the malpresenting Twin B fetus is continuously assessed, there is no clinically significant difference in morbidity or mortality with regard to mode of delivery, provided the fetus weighs over 1500 gm.

A second area of controversy of Twin A vertex and Twin B nonvertex presentations involves ECV. After experience with singleton pregnancies complicated by fetal malpresentation verified that ECV was successful in the majority of cases and without untoward perinatal outcome, it was reasonable to consider its performance for the malpresenting Twin B fetus.[33,80] In 1983, Chervenak et al.[22] reported their experience with ECV of second twins. They were able to successfully turn 20/25 malpresenting second twins (80%), with 18 undergoing successful vaginal delivery (90%). The indication for abdominal delivery in the two patients who were successfully turned was failure to descend. Because of their overall success with ECV and with no apparent perinatal complications, the ACOG Technical Bulletin on multiple gestation recommends ECV for the second twin of a Twin A vertex and Twin B nonvertex presentation.[4] Subsequent studies by Adam et al.[2] as well as Greig et al.[40] confirmed a high success rate for ECV without apparent complications.

However, Gocke et al.[38] were unable to achieve as high a success rate of ECV (Table 9-4). In only 25/41 cases (61%) were these investigators able to convert a breech or transverse twin B to a vertex presentation. Of the 25 patients who underwent successful ECV, abdominal delivery was required in six, making the overall successful vertex vaginal delivery rate only 19/41, or 46.3%. Of even more concern in the series of Gocke et al.[38] was the

TABLE 9-4

External Cephalic Version of Nonvertex Twin B and Route of Delivery

STUDY	N	SUCCESSFUL AND VAGINAL	SUCCESSFUL AND CESAREAN	UNSUCCESSFUL AND VAGINAL	UNSUCCESSFUL AND CESAREAN	COMPLICATIONS
Chervenak et al.[22]	25	18 (72.0%)	2 (8.0%)	2 (8.0%)	3 (12.0%)	1 Cord prolapse 1 Abruption
Gocke et al.[38]	41	19 (46.3%)	6 (14.6%)	6 (14.6%)	10 (24.3%)	3 Cord prolapse 2 Fetal distress 1 Compound presentation
Adam et al.[2]	15	12 (80.0%)	—	3 (20.0%)	—	—
Greig et al.[40]	16	10 (62.6%)	—	3 (18.7%)	3 (18.7%)	—
University of Mississippi	21	10 (47.6%)	—	1 (4.8%)	10 (47.6%)	2 Fetal distress 2 Cord prolapse
Total	118	69 (58.5%)	8 (6.8%)	15 (12.7%)	26 (22.0%)	12 (10.2%)

disturbingly high rate of complications associated with ECV. In the 16 patients where ECV was attempted but was unsuccessful, five required emergent abdominal delivery. Three of the five Twin B fetuses suffered umbilical cord prolapse, and two others had surgical intervention for fetal distress. Thus 5/41, or 12.2% of patients undergoing ECV, had an immediate procedure-related complication requiring emergent obstetric intervention. The experience at the University of Mississippi Medical Center has been similar to that of Gocke et al. Of the 21 patients for whom ECV was attempted, 10 patients (47.6%) were successfully turned and delivered vaginally. In 10 other patients, the ECV was unsuccessful and abdominal delivery was required. One patient who had an unsuccessful ECV attempt underwent breech extraction for Twin B. If one combines the data from the five institutions listed in Table 9-4, successful ECV followed by vaginal delivery occurred in 69/118 patients,

or 58.5% of cases. The overall abdominal delivery rate for Twin B was 34/118 patients, or 28.8% and includes both unsuccessful ECV attempts as well as successful ECVs that required cesarean delivery. Finally, when one combines the studies, an alarming rate of complications associated with ECV is again demonstrated (12/118 patients, or 10.2%). Even in the series reported by Chervenak et al.,[22] who pioneered the technique and established the safety of intrapartum ECV, the incidence of obstetric complications associated with ECV and requiring immediate obstetric intervention was 8.0% (2/25 patients).

Perhaps a review of the maternal and fetal complications associated with ECV in the singleton gestation would be informative and provide insight into the ECV-related complications seen in twin pregnancies. Zhang, Bowes, and Fortney[87] have reviewed all the published series of ECV in singleton pregnancies from the English literature. These authors define fetal complications as procedure-related events that require either emergent abdominal delivery or immediate labor induction. They also include any version attempt that was discontinued because of fetal distress and all cases of postprocedure fetal death as fetal complications. Maternal complications include cessation of the ECV as a result of severe pain, abruptio placentae, version-related bleeding, immediate fetal membrane rupture, and the sudden onset of labor. In the analysis of Zhang et al.,[87] the range of fetal complications among the studies was 0.2% to 1.4% and 0.7% to 1.2% for maternal complications. The overall success rate for ECV in the singleton pregnancy is 64.5% (range 49% to 79%). The conclusion of these reviewers, as well as the majority of obstetricians, is that ECV in the singleton gestation is successful in the majority of cases and has a low and acceptable rate of fetal and maternal complications. Thus ECV appears to be a reasonable option for the term, singleton, malpresenting fetus. On the other hand, data on ECVs in the multiple pregnancy is limited but appears to have a higher complication rate. The higher complication rate of ECV in twin pregnancies is probably because the procedure is performed in labor and only after there has been a sudden decompression of the gravid uterus with possible disruption of uteroplacental blood flow. However, if a provider is opposed to the performance of a breech extraction and abdominal delivery is the only alternative in the Twin A vertex and Twin B nonvertex presentation, then ECV appears to have value. As with intrauterine and intravaginal manipulative procedures used in breech extractions, it is important to initiate the ECV immediately after the delivery of Twin A and before the onset of uterine contractions. On average an ECV allows vaginal delivery for Twin B in one half of patients, but one must be cognizant of the high complication rate of ECV in the twin pregnancy and prepared for immediate obstetric intervention. Finally, it would appear worthwhile for each institution to address this area of controversy, review its own data, and determine whether ECV is a reasonable option at their obstetric facility.

For those providers and institutions where ECV is practical for a malpresenting Twin B fetus, several principles of management need review. Box 9-2 shows a protocol that includes suggestions made by several authors experienced with ECV

BOX 9-2

Guidelines for ECV of Nonvertex Twin B

1. Obtain sonographic estimation of the birth weight of both fetuses.
2. Avoid ECV if there is a weight discrepancy of 500 gm or more between the two fetuses.
3. Epidural anesthesia is the preferred method of pain relief and should be placed before delivery of the first twin.
4. Gentle pressure with the transducer may be sufficient to guide the vertex into the pelvic inlet (Figure 9-3).
5. The initial attempt at version should be in the direction of the shortest arc between the vertex and pelvic inlet.
6. Assess fetal heart rate and ensure fetal well being throughout the ECV.
7. Be prepared for performance of breech extraction or rapid abdominal delivery necessitated by complications of umbilical cord prolapse or fetal distress.

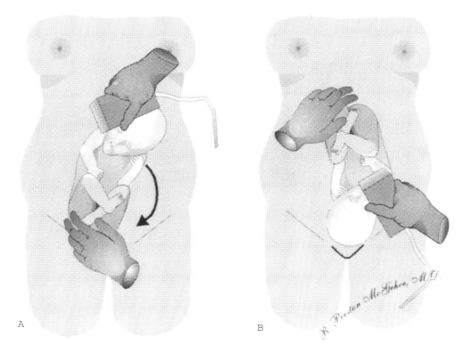

FIGURE 9-3   Using the ultrasound transducer to aid in ECV. A, Gentle pressure with the transducer is
applied to guide the vertex into the pelvis. B, The initial attempt at version should be in the shortest
arc between the vertex and the pelvic inlet.

of Twin B. In the series reviewed by Chervenak et al.,[22] ECV was never successful when the birth weight of the second twin was 500 gm or more than the birth weight of the first, vaginally delivered twin. No prospective, randomized study has been performed to objectively determine the likelihood of success with ECV if twin A is 500 gm or more than the estimated weight of Twin B. However, common sense would dictate extreme caution in such situations of growth discordance, because the uteroplacental blood flow to Twin B is already compromised. Therefore the sonographic estimation of weight and the position of each twin are pivotal in the management of the Twin A vertex and Twin B nonvertex presentation, and one should avoid ECV in situations where there is a disparity of 500 gm or more between the estimated weights of each twin.

Although the type of anesthetic used and its relationship to the success or failure of ECV has not been analyzed in twin pregnancies, epidural anesthetic is associated with a higher success rate for ECV in the singleton gestation.[17] Therefore in hopes of achieving a higher rate of success for ECV along with other beneficial reasons enumerated later on p. 266. An epidural is the preferred anesthetic for the parturient in labor with a twin gestation. The remaining practical guidelines in the protocol for ECV are self-explanatory. Finally, because of the high rate of complications with ECV and the not uncommon requirement for immediate abdominal delivery, an operating room with the necessary personnel must be readily available.

A third area of controversy in the management of the Twin A vertex and Twin B nonvertex presentation is whether the malpresenting twin can be safely delivered vaginally as a breech and, if so, whether it is dependent on gestational age. In situations where ECV is either unsuccessful or was not attempted, the second twin may present as a spontaneous breech delivery. However, if the fetus is in a transverse or oblique presentation, an internal podalic version or breech extraction needs to be performed. These specialized and often difficult obstetric maneuvers should only be attempted when fetal well being is continuously assessed and when they are performed or supervised by someone experienced in the procedure. Otherwise, abdominal delivery should be undertaken

because of the expected increase in fetal and maternal morbidity that is associated with inexperience with the procedure.

Guidelines for an internal podalic version (IPV) are listed in Box 9-3, and the technique is illustrated in Figures 9-4 through 9-7. An IPV is generally performed when the fetus is in a transverse position. The goals of an IPV are to align the fetus in a longitudinal lie with the back in an anterior position along with the delivery of the lower extremities through the cervix. These goals are best accomplished with a back-up position of the fetus but can also be attempted with the fetus in the back-down position. The IPV procedure should be initiated shortly after delivery of the first twin, before uterine contractions have resumed and while the cervix remains fully dilated. Because amniotic

BOX 9-3

Guidelines for IPV

A. Prerequisites for attempted IPV
 1. Ensure that the uterus is relaxed and the cervix is fully dilated.
 2. Proceed immediately with IPV after delivery of the first twin.
 3. Do not rupture the fetal membranes until the feet are secured (see below).
B. Scapula or acromion posterior position (back-up transverse lie)
 1. Grasp both feet by the ankles and gently bring them through the cervix (Figure 9-4).
 2. Simultaneously lift the head of the fetus and direct it toward the uterine fundus (Figure 9-4).
 3. If both feet cannot be grasped, then the anterior foot should be grasped.
 4. After the foot or feet are secured, slowly deliver the lower extremity

through the introitus (Figure 9-5). The membranes can now safely be ruptured and the fetus can be delivered by total breech extraction.
C. Scapula or acromion anterior position (back-down transverse lie)
 1. Insert the hand through the vagina and behind the body of the fetus and grasp the posterior foot, or preferably, both feet (Figure 9-6).
 2. Gentle pressure is applied against the vertex of the fetus to assist in rotation of the back longitudinally and anteriorly (Figure 9-7).
 3. Once the feet are at or beyond the introitus, the membranes can safely be ruptured and the fetus can be delivered by total breech extraction.

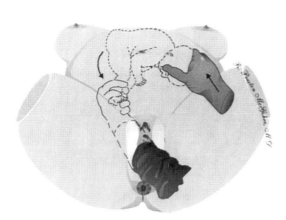

FIGURE 9-4 Scapula or acromion posterior position (back-up transverse lie). The anterior foot or preferably both feet are grasped through intact fetal membranes. At the same time the fetal vertex is transabdominally directed toward the uterine fundus.

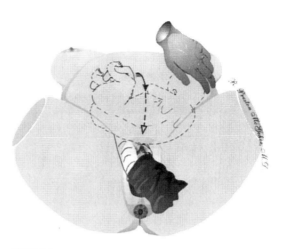

FIGURE 9-6 Scapula or acromion anterior position (back-down transverse lie). The hand is inserted behind the fetal body to grasp the posterior foot, or preferably both feet, through intact fetal membranes.

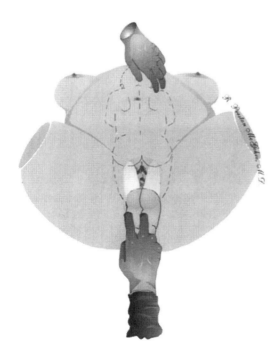

FIGURE 9-5 Scapula or acromion posterior position (back-up transverse lie). After the feet are secured, they are brought through the introitus. If the membranes have not already ruptured, they can be safely ruptured at this time.

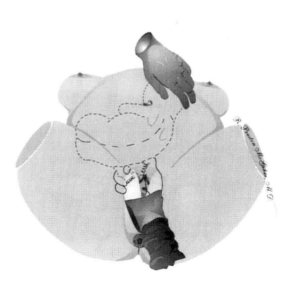

FIGURE 9-7 Scapula or acromion anterior position (back-down transverse lie). The posterior leg or legs are brought into the vagina while the abdominal hand directs the fetal head toward the uterine fundus. After both feet are secured and through the introitus, the membranes can safely be ruptured.

fluid assists in fetal rotation, the feet should be grasped through the intact membranes. Once the feet are secured and have been delivered through the cervix, the membranes can be ruptured. Downward traction is continued and, along with maternal expulsive efforts, a total breech extraction is accomplished.

Because it is associated with decreased fetal morbidity, an assisted breech delivery is the preferred method of manage-

ment of a singleton breech presentation. If the breech twin spontaneously enters or can be easily guided into the pelvis after the delivery of the first twin, then the membranes should be ruptured and the patient allowed to push. The maneuvers for an assisted breech delivery are outlined in Box 9-4.

Total breech extraction is the most common internal vaginal maneuver used to deliver a nonvertex-presenting second twin.

BOX 9-4

Technique of Total Breech Extraction

A. Double footling breech
  1. The operator vaginally inserts a hand and grasps a foot, or preferably both feet, of the fetus.
  2. After the feet are securely grasped, they are slowly delivered through the introitus.
  3. Once the feet are at the introitus, the membranes can be safely ruptured and downward traction is continued until the scapulae are visible at the vaginal outlet.
  4. The remainder of delivery is as in an assisted breech delivery, Steps 4 and 5.
B. Assisted breech delivery
  1. The patient is encouraged to push with contractions to aid in the expulsion of the fetus. Because of the decreased morbidity with an assisted breech delivery, the infant should be allowed to be delivered spontaneously to the umbilicus. This fixes the fetal arms in the maternal pelvis and prevents extension (that is, nuchal arms) with downward traction.
  2. If the legs are not spontaneously delivered once the umbilicus is at the vaginal outlet, the Pinard maneuver should be performed to deliver the lower extremities (Figure 9-8). With this ma-

neuver one or two fingers are placed on the medial aspect of the leg and parallel to the femur. The leg is then externally rotated at the hip. This brings the fetal foot against the operator's hand so it can be delivered. The procedure is then repeated on the other side.
  3. Once the legs are delivered, the fetal trunk should be wrapped with a towel to improve handling and traction. With the thumbs on the sacroiliac synchondroses, gentle downward traction is applied until the axillae are visible.
  4. When the scapulae appear at the vaginal outlet, two fingers are slipped over the fetal shoulder and parallel to the humerus. Lateral motion achieves rotation of the arm at the shoulder and the arm moves across the chest and is delivered at the posterior vagina (Figure 9-9). The fetal trunk is gently rotated to expose the other scapula and a similar maneuver is performed for delivery of that upper extremity.
  5. Once the head is at the pelvic floor, delivery can be accomplished by performance of the Mauriceau-Smellie-Veit maneuver, the Wigand maneuver, or Piper forceps to the aftercoming head.

Sometimes, an IPV is followed by a total breech extraction and becomes one continuous maneuver. Once the feet and lower extremities are delivered through the introitus to the level of the umbilicus, the remainder of the fetus is delivered as it is in an assisted breech extraction.

There are three methods to safely deliver the aftercoming head. The Mauriceau-Smellie-Veit (MSV) maneuver has been

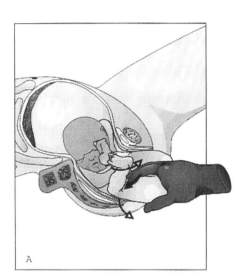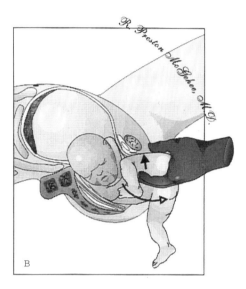

FIGURE 9-8 Pinard maneuver (lower extremities). A, After spontaneous delivery of the breech, one or two fingers are placed along the medial aspect of the leg and parallel to the femur. The leg is then externally rotated, bringing the fetal foot against the operator's hand and allowing for easy delivery. B, A similar procedure is performed on the other extremity.

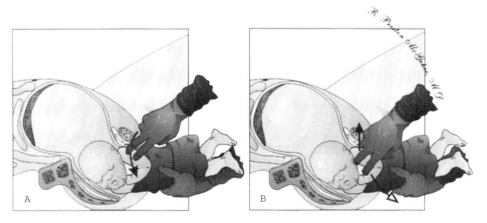

FIGURE 9-9 Pinard maneuver (upper extremities). A, When the scapulae appear at the introitus, one or two fingers are slipped over the anterior fetal shoulder and parallel to the humerus. Lateral motion rotates the arm bringing the fetal hand in proximity to the operator's hand for delivery. B, After gentle rotation of the fetal trunk, the procedure is repeated for delivery of the other arm.

used in breech deliveries for centuries and remains popular today as a testament to its value and safety (Figure 9-10). The MSV maneuver involves placing the index and the third finger of one hand externally along the malar eminences. The index and usually the fourth finger of the opposite hand are placed dorsally on either side of the shoulders. The head is delivered by flexion. The second maneuver to deliver the fetal head and maintain flexion is known as the Wigand maneuver (Figure 9-11). With this maneuver, an assistant maintains suprapubic pressure while the operator has two fingers of one hand in the mouth of the fetus to maintain gentle flexion. However, because of fear of disarticulation of the fetal jaw or damage to the tongue of the fetus, the Wigard maneuver

is no longer recommended for delivery of the aftercoming head in a breech presentation. The third most commonly employed maneuver to deliver the head is the application of a Piper forceps (Figure 9-12). The cardinal principles of an obstetric forceps delivery also apply to the application of forceps to the aftercoming head in a breech presentation. Namely, the general architecture of the maternal pelvis is known, the position of the fetal head within the maternal pelvis is known, the cervix is fully dilated, and the membranes are ruptured. While the clinician is in a kneeling position, an assistant slightly elevates the body of the fetus, exercising care not to hyperextend the head of the fetus and maintaining the body in a horizontal position to the floor. With the

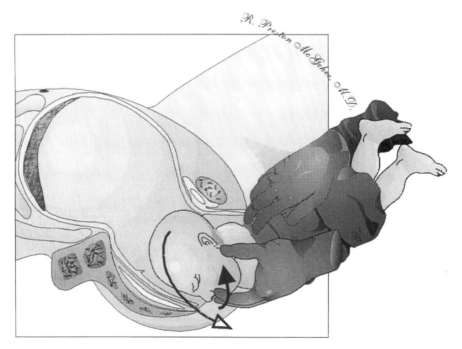

FIGURE 9-10   Mauriceau-Smellie-Veit maneuver. The index and third finger of one hand are placed externally along the malar eminences the fetal maxilla. Upward pressure *(dark arrow)* with this hand maintains flexion of the fetal vertex.

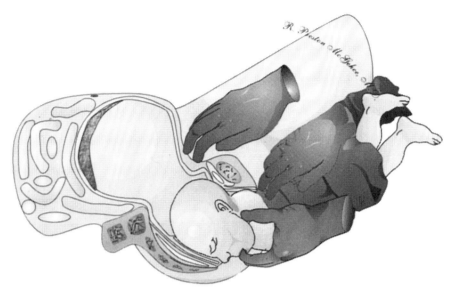

FIGURE 9-11 Wigand maneuver. While suprapubic pressure is being applied by an assistant or with one hand, two fingers of the other hand of the operator are placed in the mouth of the fetus. Upper pressure with this hand maintains flexion of the fetal vertex.

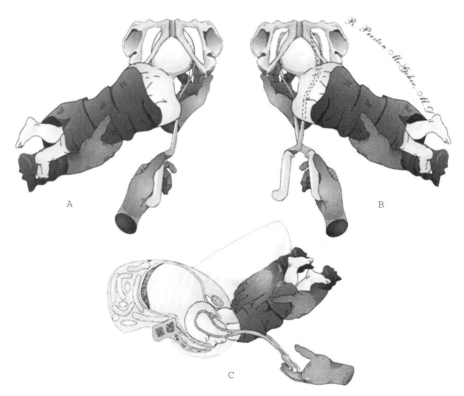

FIGURE 9-12 Piper forceps to the aftercoming head. A, An assistant slightly elevates the body of the fetus, maintaining a horizontal plane to the floor. With the fetus displaced slightly to the maternal right, the right forceps blade is inserted along the occipitomental plane. B, After placement of the right forceps blade, the fetus is displaced slightly to the maternal left with placement of the left forceps blade along the occipitomental plane. C, The forceps blades are locked inferior to the plane of the fetus and then elevated to allow the body of the fetus to saddle the forceps. This technique flexes the fetal vertex. Delivery is accomplished with downward traction.

back of the fetus anterior, the right forceps blade is inserted first along the occipital-mental plane, and it is followed by the insertion of the left blade. The blades are locked along a plane inferior to that of the body of the fetus and then elevated to allow the body of the fetus to straddle the shank of the forceps. This technique for locking the forceps results in flexion of the fetal head. The two main complications encountered with total breech extractions include nuchal arms and entrapment of the aftercoming head. Both complications are discussed in detail later in this chapter.

Table 9-5 list the results of several recent series where the second twin had a malpresentation. Only studies involving the Twin A vertex and Twin B nonvertex presentation and second twins delivered by an IPV or by an assisted or total breech extraction were included. Furthermore, each study included the neonatal outcome statistics of all infants. Two important concepts are apparent after this analysis. First, in infants weighing more than 1500 gm at birth, the overall complication rate of breech delivery was low (1.4%). This is of particular importance when compared with the overall complication rate of ECV of 10.2% (see Table 9-4). A second observation is that in the obstetric literature there is limited experience of operative internal vaginal maneuvers followed by

TABLE 9-5

Breech Extraction of the Nonvertex Second Twin

AUTHORS	TOTAL N	ACTUAL BW* ≤1500 GM	MORBIDITY	RECOMMEND BREECH EXTRACTION IF BW ≤1500 GM
Acker et al.[1]	76	2	None	No
Chervenak et al.[23]	76	16	1 Fractured clavicle and humerus (BW 3420 gm)	No
Rabinovici et al.[73]	19	3	2 Fetal distress 2 Cord prolapse	No
Blickstein et al.[11]	39	9	None	No
Rabinovici et al.[74]	11	0	None	No
Gocke et al.[38]	53	—	2 Cesarean sections for failed extraction	No
Adam et al.[2]	41	7	1 Fractured humerus (BW 3300 gm)	No
Davison et al.[27]	54	—	None	Yes
Greig et al.[40]	63	9	1 Fractured humerus (BW not available)	No
Fishman, Grubb, and Kovacs[34]	183	15	None	No
University of Mississippi	23	1	None	No
Total	638	62	9 (1.4%)	

*BW, birth weight.

breech delivery of VLBW infants (1500 g or less). Even so, most investigators do not advocate vaginal delivery of VLBW infants with a persistent malpresentation. However, in the series of Davison et al.,[27] there was no demonstrable increase in either neonatal morbidity or mortality in VLBW infants delivered vaginally in breech presentation. Although it was a retrospective analysis, these investigators compared the neonatal course of 54 Twin B neonates delivered by breech extraction with 43 Twin B infants delivered abdominally because of malpresentation. The range of birth weight for each group was 750 to 2000 gm, and the mean birth weight in each group was similar. There was no significant difference in either the incidence or in the severity of respiratory distress syndrome (RDS), necrotizing enterocolitis, and severe IVH between the two groups.

When the incidence and type of complications associated with breech extraction of the 10 published series and the experience at the University of Mississippi Medical Center are reviewed (see Table 9-5), one additional and striking finding is noted. In the summary of the entire series, there are no reported cases of nuchal arms or head entrapment. One might speculate that the three cases of fracture of the humerus were the result of maneuvers to relieve a nuchal arm. Even if this is the case, the overall incidence remains low (3/638 or 0.5%). In a review by Cheng and Hannah[21] of published series of breech deliveries in singleton pregnancies, the incidence of extended or nuchal arms ranged from 0 to 5.6%, and the range of incidence of difficulty of the aftercoming head was 0 to 8.5%. Maneuvers to relieve nuchal arms were associated with high morbidity

and mortality, 25% and 22%, respectively. Additionally, complications associated with techniques to assist in delivery of an entrapped head had a 45% rate of complications. Therefore even if these complications are underreported in the twin series, they must not occur as often as they do in singleton breech deliveries; otherwise this would be reflected in an increase in neonatal morbidity. The probable reason for the decrease in these complications in the twin pregnancy is the usually smaller size of the second twin compared with first twin, as well as the fact that the cervix has recently been fully dilated with vaginal delivery of the vertex first twin. However, the decrease in these complications may also be the result of small sample size of the series and perhaps because of appropriate patient selection. If so, with an increase in the emphasis on vaginal delivery of the Twin A vertex and Twin B nonvertex presentation, these complications may be encountered more often in the future. Therefore the clinician must be prepared to manage these obstetric complications associated with breech delivery.

If the clinician notes that either arm of the fetus is in a nuchal position (that is, extended above the head), the first decision must be whether to proceed with a vaginal delivery or perform a cesarean section. This decision should be predicated on the skill and experience of the clinician, the status of the fetus, the capability to perform an abdominal delivery, and factors that may contribute to the nuchal arms. Factors associated with nuchal arms include a uterine constriction ring, an incompletely dilated cervix, too-rapid breech extraction, deflexion of the fetal head, fetal anomalies, and uterine abnormalities such as septal changes or leiomyomata. Anesthesia personnel who are skilled in monitoring rapid-sequence general anesthesia must be present, since general anesthesia may be necessary to allow a complete intravaginal and intrauterine examination of the situation. Only then can one reliably determine whether delivery of the nuchal arm is possible or if perhaps a safer option would be to proceed with an abdominal delivery. Nuchal arms are best reduced by rotating the fetus in the direction of the fetal hand (Figure 9-13). With this maneuver, the soft tissue of the birth canal provides enough resistance to bring the hand anterior to the head of the fetus. The Pinard maneuver can then be performed to deliver the upper extremity (see Figure 9-9). If entrapment of the head occurs after delivery of the fetal body, Dührssen's incisions will probably be required to expedite delivery of the head. To perform Dührssen's incisions, the cervix must be adequately exposed by the placement of a pair of ring forceps at the 10 o'clock and 2 o'clock positions (Figure 9-14). Between the pair of ring forceps, a 1 to 2-cm incision is made with scissors. If these two incisions do not relieve the entrapment of the head, a third incision can be performed at the 6 o'clock position. After delivery, the incisions are closed with interrupted, absorbable suture. Because of the associated complications of extension of the incision with uterine vessel laceration or entry into the rectum or bladder, Dührssen's incisions are not performed often in modern obstetrics. However, the technique should be known and reviewed by all obstetricians, since Dührssen's incisions may be a life-saving procedure when head en-

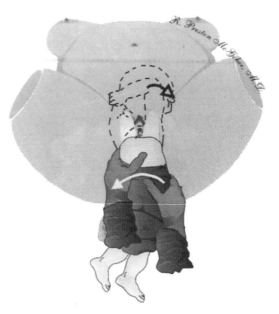

FIGURE 9-13   Nuchal arms. Rotation of body toward the fetal hand provides resistance and brings the arm or hand in front of the fetal head. A Pinard maneuver can then be performed to deliver the upper extremity.

trapment is encountered in a breech delivery and abdominal delivery is no longer an option.

In summary, there is no mandate that all Twin A vertex and Twin B nonvertex presentations be delivered abdominally. The consensus is that either abdominal delivery should be primarily performed or an ECV should be attempted for the second twin when the gestational age is 32 weeks or younger or when the estimated birth weight of each of the concordant twins is 1500 gm or less. On the other hand, for gestational ages exceeding 32 weeks and concordant twins with EFWs between 1500 gm and 3500 gm, breech extraction with or without a preceding IPV can not only be safely performed but is associated with fewer complications than attempted ECV of the second twin. Other mandates for vaginal delivery besides con-

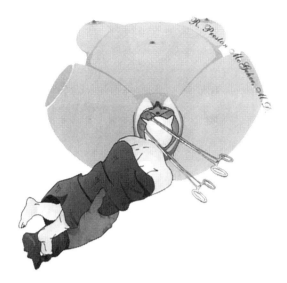

FIGURE 9-14 Dührssen's incisions. The cervix is grasped with a pair of ring forceps and a 1 to 2-cm incision is made with scissors. The incision is closed with interrupted absorbable sutures.

cordant fetal growth in the 1500 to 3500 gm range include a flexed head for the second twin, an absence of fetal anomalies, a relaxed uterus, an operator present with skill and experience in intravaginal and intrauterine manipulative procedures, and an operating team ready to perform a rapid abdominal delivery. These necessary prerequisites are not possible in many private practice settings. Furthermore, acquiring and maintaining the necessary skills for IPV, breech extraction, and other intravaginal and intrauterine maneuvers may not be possible for a general obstetrician in private practice. Most consider a busy obstetric practice one in which 15 deliveries per partner are performed each month, or 180 deliveries per partner annually. If one assumes a 1/75 incidence of twin pregnancy, then the busy obstetrician will see between 2 and 3 sets of twins each year. Because the Twin A vertex and Twin B nonvertex presentation

occurs in only 1 of 3 sets of twins, a provider would encounter the need to perform the necessary procedures to safely deliver the malpresenting second twin no more than once annually. One might wonder whether such a limited experience and such a rare opportunity to practice and maintain skills is sufficient for even the busy obstetrician. Because most obstetricians perform many more abdominal deliveries than intravaginal and intrauterine manipulative procedures for fetal malpresentations, the Twin A vertex and Twin B nonvertex presentation is probably best managed in most private practice settings by primary cesarean delivery.

TWIN A NONVERTEX AND TWIN B OTHER PRESENTATION

Twin A nonvertex and Twin B other presentation is the least common intrapartum twin presentation and occurs in approximately 20% of patients (see Table 9-1). The rationale for not considering the presentation of the second twin is that intrapartum management is primarily dictated by the presentation of Twin A, and that of Twin B does not influence the mode of delivery. Since an ECV is not considered a reasonable option for the management of the malpresenting Twin A, the only alternative to cesarean section is a vaginal breech delivery. Compared with other intrapartum presentations, fetuses in a Twin A nonvertex and Twin B other presentation are at significantly higher risk for entanglement if vaginal delivery is attempted.

As thoroughly described by Nissen,[66] there are four types of entanglements encountered with attempted vaginal delivery of the Twin A nonvertex and Twin B other presentation. The following entanglements are possible: (1) *collision*, defined as contact between different parts of the two fetuses that prevents descent and engagement of either fetus; (2) *impaction*, the partial engagement of both fetuses despite some contact between them; (3) *compaction*, which occurs when the presenting parts of each fetus enter the true pelvis at the same time and prevents further descent; and (4) *interlocking*, described as the direct contact of the chins of the two fetuses that can occur both above and below the level of the true pelvis. Because of the significant morbidity and mortality associated with fetal entanglement, a review of the diagnosis, management, and associated risks is warranted.

In 1958, Nissen[66] analyzed 69 published cases of fetal entanglement described in the world's literature over 69 years (1887-1957). Of the 69 cases, 45% to 65% of the twin sets that entangled were in a Twin A breech and Twin B vertex presentation. Both fetuses in vertex presentation were noted in 25% of the cases (17/69). A vertex Twin A with a transverse Twin B presentation occurred in 7% of cases (5/69), and the Twin A breech and Twin B breech presentation was responsible for only 2 cases of fetal entanglement, or 3% of the total. The total perinatal loss from complications of fetal entanglement was 43% (60/138). Of the 60 perinatal deaths, 44, or over 73%, were the Twin A fetus. Over 45% (28/60) of the perinatal deaths were the result of embryotomy. Of all the presentations, the one associated with the highest neonatal wastage was the Twin A breech and Twin B vertex presentation, where 50% of vaginally delivered cases experienced a perinatal loss (45/90). In another review by Khunda,[47] 37 additional cases occurring between 1960 and 1970 were analyzed. He substantiated the claim by Nissen of a high fetal mortality rate associated with fetal entanglement (31%, or 23/74). He also reported that the majority of the losses occurred in Twin A (65%, or 15/23).

An analysis of 41 cases of fetal entanglement that occurred in Sweden between 1961 and 1987 was conducted by Rydhstrom and Cullberg.[77] During the 26 years of review, the incidence of interlocking twins was 1/645 twin births (41/26,428). The authors noted that interlocking occurred significantly more often with the Twin A breech and Twin B vertex presentation (1/91) compared with other intrapartum presentations (1/1982, p<0.001). Furthermore, the author noted that besides the Twin A breech and Twin B vertex presentation, other contributory factors included intrauterine fetal growth restriction, an actual birth weight below 2000 gm, and the antenatal death of the first twin. In fact, the highest rate of twin entanglement (1/16) occurred in situations of antepartum death of one twin in the Twin A breech and Twin B vertex presentation. A final conclusion of the analysis was the significantly higher rate of neonatal loss if entrapment occurred in the Twin A breech and Twin B vertex presentation as opposed to another intrapartum presentation (38.9% versus 8.3%, respectively).

In 1993, Blickstein et al.[12] published the largest study from a single institution that compared the neonatal outcome of Twin A breech and Twin B vertex presentations that delivered vaginally (n=24) with those delivered abdominally (n=35). The perinatal outcome was similar in both groups. Specifically, the incidence of birth asphyxia, RDS, neonatal jaundice, birth trauma, and perinatal mortality was the same in each group. Based on their experience, Blickstein et al.[12] recommend a prospective, randomized, clinical trial to determine the optimal mode of delivery when Twin A is in a nonvertex position. At present, vaginal delivery of the Twin A nonvertex and Twin B other presentation should be considered investigational and undertaken only if there are personnel present who are skilled in the management of this type of delivery and adept in maneuvers to decompress interlocking twins.

If for some reason there is a delay in the diagnosis of fetal entanglement and interlocking of the chins is encountered during the second stage of labor, the following steps are undertaken to avoid fetal loss. While preparation is underway for abdominal delivery, the heart rates of both fetuses are continuously monitored to ensure viability and fetal well being. Because downward traction of the first fetus compounds the problem and makes disengagement more difficult, all attempts at vaginal delivery or disengagement of viable twins should be abandoned. Although techniques such as the Kimball-Rand maneuver are described in the obstetric literature (Figure 9-15),[66] they should only be performed in situations where abdominal delivery is not available or in situations of extreme fetal prematurity. In the Kimball-Rand maneuver the first twin is delivered to the neck, and while downward traction is applied by an assistant, a Piper forceps is applied to the vertex of the second twin. Both fetuses are then delivered vaginally while simultaneously applying extension and traction to the first

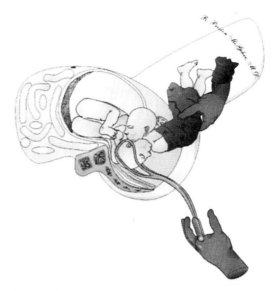

FIGURE 9-15 The Kimball-Rand maneuver. A, Twin A is hyperextended with Piper forceps application to the vertex of Twin B. B, Simultaneous traction is applied to Twin A and Twin B.

breech twin and traction and extension on the second vertex cohort.

Another reported but obviously not studied technique used in the management of locked twins is the Zavanelli maneuver.[42,84] As described in handling other types of obstructed delivery, the Zavanelli maneuver involves placing the partially delivered Twin A in the vagina and proceeding with an abdominal delivery. In the two cases cited, it appears the Zavanelli maneuver was life-saving in potentially catastrophic situations of locked twins.

In summary, because of the inability to either predict or prevent fetal entanglement and the high morbidity and mortality associated with fetal entanglement, the ACOG considers abdominal delivery the preferred route of delivery for all twins in the Twin A nonvertex and Twin B other presentation. Only in extreme circumstances should one attempt a vaginal delivery for this intrapartum presentation.

The Postdate Twin Pregnancy

"The postmature infant has stayed too long in intrauterine surroundings; he has remained so long in utero that his difficulty is to be born with safety to himself and his mother. The problem of the postmature infant in intranatal." These remarks by Ballantyne in 1902[6] eloquently describe the postmature infant. In this manuscript, Ballantyne not only discusses the incidence but also the risks associated with fetal dysmaturity. By definition, postterm pregnancy is a gestation of 42 weeks or more and has a reported incidence of 3% to 12%.[4] The clinical importance of postdate pregnancy is its association with placental insufficiency and the resultant increase in poor pregnancy outcome.

By 37 weeks of gestation, the tertiary villous structure of the placenta is complete with an 11-m^2 surface area available for exchange of gases and nutrients.[3] However by 42 weeks of gestation, as a result of continued placental maturation with a progressive decline in the surface area for exchange, placental dysfunction develops with a decreased ability to nutritionally support the fetus. A series of events, known collectively as fetal dysmaturity, develops and is initially characterized by a decrease in amniotic fluid volume caused by a decline in fetal urine production. The loss of amniotic fluid volume places the umbilical cord at increased risk for compression, which causes acute fetal hypoxemia and sudden death. Additionally, meconium passage in utero often accompanies the postdate pregnancy and is the result of maturation of the fetal gastrointestinal tract.[30] This may result in either in utero or peripartal aspiration of meconium with respiratory distress at birth and can result in the neonatal meconium aspiration syndrome. Finally, failure of intrauterine growth becomes noticeable. The dysmature infant has parchment-like skin secondary to the loss of subcutaneous fat and dehydration. The extremities are long and thin with no vernix or lanugo hair. Furthermore, the skin is often macerated and discolored. These findings associated with fetal dysmaturity are more the result of placental dysfunction than a prolonged pregnancy. One wonders whether fetal dysmaturity resulting from continued placental maturation arises in the multiple pregnancy and if so, whether it occurs at either an increased rate or earlier in gestation.

It is well known that twins contribute disproportionately to perinatal mortality. In a recent review the neonatal mortality for twin gestations was 41 to 42 deaths per 1000 live births, a rate 7 times the 5.86 neonatal mortality rate for a singleton pregnancy.[69] Although most of the excess in perinatal mortality in twin gestations is secondary to preterm delivery, some of the increase in mortality is related to placental dysfunction with fetal growth restriction in apparently uncomplicated but prolonged twin gestations. The average length of gestation for a twin pregnancy is 36.8 weeks, compared with 39.5 weeks for a singleton pregnancy.[48] This corresponds to an average birth weight of 2380 gm for a twin neonate in contrast to 3249 gm for a singleton neonate. Even so, the average birth weight for twins compares favorably with the nadir in neonatal mortality (see Figure 9-2). Furthermore, unlike the singleton pregnancy, an increase in birth weight within the normal range does not correlate with a continued decline in neonatal mortality in the twin pregnancy. An increase in birth weight above 3000 gm is associated with an exponential rise in neonatal mortality. This observation has been noted by other investigators.[13,36,49,56,69] Because this rise in neonatal mortality after 37 weeks of gestation is associated with an increase in birth weight, responsible factors are not just uteroplacental insufficiency (UPI) and resultant fetal growth restriction.

In addition to a difference in mortality rates related to birth weight, there is also a maturational difference between twin and singleton gestations. Histologic changes consistent with "aging" of the placenta are seen as early as 31 weeks of gestation in the twin pregnancy, in contrast to 39 to 40 weeks of gestation in the singleton pregnancy.[10] Advanced sonographic maturation of the twin placenta (that is, grade III) is also noted as early as 29 to 31 weeks of gestation, 6 to 8 weeks before such findings are visualized in the normal singleton pregnancy.[67] Because the grading system used to describe placental maturation is correlated with fetal pulmonary maturity, it is no surprise that documented fetal pulmonary maturity occurs several weeks earlier in the twin pregnancy than in the singleton gestation.[44,52,68] Thus maturational differences in various organ systems of the fetus, in addition to observational differences in mortality rates for twin and singleton neonates, support the contention that the postmaturity state not only does occur in the twin pregnancy but occurs earlier in gestation. This line of reasoning explains the increase in mortality as well as the higher incidence of low Apgar scores,

respiratory disorders, and seizures in larger twins.[37,48] At present there is a mounting body of evidence to suggest a full-term twin gestation is achieved earlier than a singleton gestation. Based on histologic and physiologic changes, a full-term twin pregnancy coincides with the average length of gestation, namely 36 to 37 weeks. Furthermore, a postterm twin pregnancy develops at 39 to 41 weeks of gestation and is associated with a greatly increased risk for adverse pregnancy outcome.[48] If this definition of postterm twin pregnancy is adopted, between 10% and 15% of twin gestations would be prolonged.[36,56] This incidence of postterm twin pregnancy is similar to that seen in singleton pregnancies.

Uterotonic Agents

Because twin labor is associated with a higher incidence of dysfunctional labor, there is an increased likelihood that oxytocin will be required for a woman with a twin gestation. Even so, there appears to be a reluctance by many obstetricians to initiate an oxytocin infusion because of the fear of uterine rupture caused by overdistention. However, such a fear appears unfounded, provided oxytocin is used appropriately. In their review of uterine ruptures, Golan, Sandbank, and Rubin[39] found that the majority of ruptures occurred in cases of neglected cephalopelvic disproportion or in high-order multiple gestations. Leroy[51] reviewed the labor course of 483 consecutive twin deliveries and found no cases of uterine rupture. In this series, 30% of cases required oxytocin infusion for treatment of hypotonic labor. In the group of patients receiving oxytocin, the neonatal mortality was significantly lower than in the group not receiving oxytocin. Analysis of the categoric data revealed that the difference in neonatal mortality was probably because of the higher incidence of preterm deliveries that occurred in the nonperfused group. Once gestational age and birth weight were taken into account, there was no significant difference in neonatal mortality in the group that did versus the group that did not receive oxytocin. Nonetheless, there was no increase in maternal or neonatal untoward outcomes attributable to the use of oxytocin to augment labor.

In Leroy's review of twin deliveries,[51] 13% of patients received oxytocin only after the delivery of the first twin. There was no difference in the perinatal mortality rate between those who did and those who did not receive oxytocin after delivery of Twin A. However, even though the incidence of transverse presentations for Twin B was similar in the two groups, more IPV procedures (11.7% versus 5.8%, p=0.055) were performed on second twins in the group that did not receive oxytocin. One can speculate and anecdotally review personal experience as to whether the initiation of oxytocin after delivery of the first twin might restore uterine tonus, result in an increase in the incidence of longitudinal lies, and thereby avoid intrauterine manipulative procedures. Regardless, there was no increase in either fetal or maternal adverse outcomes with oxytocin administration after delivery of the first twin.

Because of an increase in the incidence of preeclampsia, placental abnormalities, and discordant fetal growth in the twin gestation, induction of labor may become necessary. If the clinician is confronted with an unfavorable cervix and if time permits, low-dose prostaglandin E_2 and $F_{2\alpha}$ vaginal gel has demonstrated both efficacy and safety in the twin gestation.[37] After 4 to 6 hours of placement of the intravaginal prostaglandin, an amniotomy can usually be performed and followed by an infusion of oxytocin. As mentioned, fetal heart rate monitoring is a prerequisite for any laboring twin pregnancy and if oxytocin is used, an intrauterine pressure catheter is advised.

Vaginal Birth after Cesarean Delivery

Nearly one fourth of births in the United States are cesarean deliveries, and one in three of these are repeat cesarean sections.[63] In an attempt to safely lower the incidence of repeat cesarean deliveries, the National Institute of Child Health and Development Conference in Childbirth in 1980 reviewed the issue of elective repeat cesarean section. The consensus of the conference was that vaginal birth after cesarean delivery (VBAC) is an acceptable alternative to routine elective repeat cesarean section.[64] Since 1980, the practice of VBAC has been actively pursued in the United States, and current data indicate that a trial of labor is successful in 60% to 80% of patients with prior low transverse uterine incisions who are offered VBAC in subsequent pregnancies.[15,35] Twin pregnancies were excluded from early VBAC protocols because of fear of catastrophic uterine rupture resulting from uterine overdistension. However, as experience with the procedure increased, data indicating that a VBAC was associated with lower maternal morbidity and no significant difference in maternal or fetal mortality continued to accumulate. As a result, some centers broadened the acceptance criteria for VBAC to include women with multiple prior cesarean deliveries, prior low vertical uterine incisions, breech presentations, and twin gestations.

The incidence of uterine scar disruption after a prior cesarean delivery is not increased in singleton pregnancies by a trial of labor. Additionally, most uterine scar disruptions are asymptomatic, occur in upwards of 2% of patients with prior cesarean deliveries, and occur equally in patients with prior low transverse or low vertical uterine incisions.[72,76] The most common sign of uterine rupture is fetal stress manifested by bradycardia or a prolonged fetal heart rate deceleration.[70] Other signs of overt uterine rupture include vaginal bleeding, a sudden change in uterine activity, a decrease in the station of the fetus, or an abrupt change in fetal position. Because none of these early signs of uterine rupture are related to a change in the intensity or perception of pain, epidural anesthesia does not delay the diagnosis of uterine rupture and is not contraindicated for patients who desire a VBAC.

In a review of 23 sets of twins undergoing VBAC during the early 1960s, there were no cases of uterine scar disruption or uterine rupture and all patients achieved vaginal delivery.[14] In a retrospective analysis of 31 patients with twin gestations who underwent a VBAC, Strong et al.[82] reported a 72% successful vaginal delivery rate with one uterine scar disruption, resulting in a 3% uterine dehiscence rate. However, there were no cases of uterine rupture in the series. The authors noted that the single patient with the scar disruption received oxytocin augmentation during labor, underwent midforceps delivery for both Twin A and Twin B, and had previously had multiple cesarean sections. One can speculate whether these factors contributed to the uterine dehiscence. Even so, the authors felt that their experience supported a policy of VBAC in properly selected patients with twin gestations. Selection criteria should include only patients in whom Twin A is in a vertex presentation and both twins can be satisfactorily monitored throughout the course of labor. Such suggestions seem prudent and would allow the majority of patients with twin gestations and a prior cesarean delivery the opportunity to undergo a trial of labor with minimal maternal and fetal risk. Furthermore, the judicious use of oxytocin for labor augmentation or induction appears safe, but no data exist regarding the use of cervical ripening agents such as prostaglandin E_2 in patients with twin pregnancies and prior cesarean sections.

Anesthesia Considerations

Much of the improvement in perinatal morbidity and mortality in the multiple pregnancy is the result of comprehensive prenatal care, the development of techniques for ongoing fetal surveillance, and advances in neonatal medicine. Even so, expert intrapartum care of the patient with a multiple pregnancy remains an important aspect of overall obstetric management. Although Chapter 10 in this book is devoted to the management of anesthesia in the multiple pregnancy, no discussion of the intrapartum care of the multiple pregnancy would be complete without some mention of the various techniques for the relief of pain during labor.

The need for analgesia and anesthesia during labor is greater for the patient with a twin gestation than the patient with a singleton pregnancy because of the increased rate of instrumental and operative maneuvers. As in other areas of prenatal care and intrapartum management, controversy exists in regard to the safest, most effective form of analgesia or anesthesia for labor in the twin gestation. Some of the confusion is the result of the understandable reluctance of clinicians to participate in a prospective, randomized trial involving intrapartum management protocols that may differ from their personal preference. In spite of these limitations, published reports of the experience of others are available for review and consideration.

In a prospective study of 200 consecutive twin pregnancies, Crawford[26] analyzed the intrapartum course with particular emphasis on the techniques of analgesia and anesthesia that were provided during labor and delivery.[26] There was no significant difference in the Apgar scores or umbilical cord blood determinants of Twin A and Twin B in patients undergoing elective cesarean delivery under epidural versus general anesthesia. Furthermore, the uterine-incision–to–delivery time for Twin A and Twin B was not significantly different with regard to the type of anesthesia used for delivery. Maternal hypotension is also a concern, as pregnancy is known to cause a higher cephalad spread of conduction anesthetics.[43] Additionally, there is an increased sensitivity of nerve fibers to local anesthetics during pregnancy caused by elevated levels of progesterone.[16] These factors combined would

appear to place women with twin gestations who undergo epidural anesthesia at increased risk for the development of hypotension and potential fetal compromise. It is reassuring that Crawford's study showed there was no greater incidence of hypotension in the women undergoing epidural anesthesia compared with those undergoing general anesthesia.

In patients undergoing emergency cesarean delivery under general anesthesia, Twin A was born with significantly higher Apgar scores and better umbilical cord blood gas determinants than Twin B. This difference in the birth status of Twin A and Twin B was not seen in women undergoing emergency cesarean delivery under epidural anesthesia. The difference in Apgar scores and umbilical cord blood assessments may be the result of the indication for emergency delivery (such as fetal distress, placental abruption, or umbilical cord prolapse) rather than the type of anesthetic used for delivery. Regardless, Crawford's data suggest that epidural anesthesia is not associated with either an increase in the incidence of fetal distress or a tendency toward lower Apgar scores and birth asphyxia.

The most salient findings in Crawford's prospective study of the intrapartum management of twin deliveries was in the group of patients delivered vaginally. One important finding was the number of cases in which Twin A was delivered vaginally and Twin B was delivered by cesarean section. This occurred in 3.3% of patients who were given an epidural anesthetic in labor but in 6.8% of patients for whom no epidural was provided. Although this difference did not achieve statistical significance (p=0.06), it probably represents a type II error. Only 138 patients were available for comparison in Crawford's review. A power analysis indicates 700 patients are needed for evaluation to achieve the statistical power of 80% necessary to detect a difference of the magnitude found in Crawford's review.

Another important clinical finding of the study was the strong association that the provision of an epidural anesthetic for vaginal delivery is markedly beneficial to the second twin. The biochemical status of Twin B delivered vaginally from women under epidural anesthesia was significantly better than it was in second twins delivered vaginally from women without epidural anesthesia. This supports the conclusions of other investigators that regardless of whether infants are delivered vertex or breech, second twins delivered when the mother is under epidural anesthesia are in significantly better condition than those delivered without an epidural.[31] Finally, although the provision of an epidural in labor was associated with a longer second stage of labor and a higher incidence of operative vaginal delivery, the overall incidence of cesarean delivery was the same. Additionally, in spite of the increased need for operative vaginal intervention, the condition of both twins was superior in women provided with epidural anesthesia during labor to that of twins delivered from mothers who had not received an epidural. In summary, the data suggest that epidural anesthesia for either a cesarean or vaginal delivery is safe in the multiple pregnancy and offers several distinct advantages over other forms of pain relief for labor and delivery.

Intrapartum Management of Monoamniotic Twins

A monoamniotic twin gestation is uncommon, occurs in only 1/10,000 deliveries, and represents only 1% to 3% of twin pregnancies.[9] Even so, perinatal personnel must be vigilant in their attempt to diagnose the monoamniotic twin pregnancy because perinatal death occurs in up to 68% of cases.[79] Umbilical cord accidents, including twisting, intertwining, and knotting of the two cords, are extremely common, occur in 60% to 70% of cases, and are the most common cause of death (72% of cases).[60] The twin-twin transfusion syndrome (TTS) is often encountered, and along with the ever present complication of preterm birth, it contributes to the high rates of perinatal morbidity and mortality associated with monoamniotic twinning.

An antenatal diagnosis of a monoamniotic twin pregnancy is either made or suspected by the nonvisualization of a separating membrane between twins on repeated ultrasound examinations. One should also suspect monoamniotic twinning when cord entanglement is observed during an ultrasound examination. Other sonographic findings in the monoamniotic twin pregnancy include a single fused placenta, fetuses of the same sex, adequate amniotic fluid surrounding both fetuses, and both fetuses moving freely within the uterine cavity. Because some false positive diagnoses occur even when these sonographic guidelines are followed, some clinicians advocate confirmation of the monoamniotic twin pregnancy with a sequential amniocentesis and amniography.[83] Once the diagnosis of a monoamniotic gestation is confirmed, most clinicians recommend amniocentesis at 32 to 36 weeks of gestation, with delivery on documentation of fetal lung maturity. Because of the ever-present danger of entanglement or entrapment of the umbilical cord with the intrapartum descent of the first twin, the preferred mode of delivery is by the abdominal route.

Conjoined Twins

This usually lethal anomaly of the twinning process is fortunately rare and occurs in only 1/50,000 pregnancies or 1/400 pairs of monoamniotic twins. Conjoined twins are the result of imperfect division of the embryo after formation of the embryonic disk. Potential survival of one or both conjoined twins depends on gestational age at delivery, the site of union, the degree of separation, the type and magnitude of shared organs, and the presence of other anomalies.[78] Because of the widespread availability and use of ultrasound, most cases are now diagnosed antenatally.[7] If the diagnosis has been made antenatally, cesarean section is the preferred route of delivery. If the diagnosis was not made before the onset of labor and if a vaginal delivery is attempted, an obstructed labor generally develops and requires surgical intervention in the form of abdominal delivery.

Delivery of Triplet and Higher-Order Multiple Gestations

The often-quoted natural occurrence of triplet and quadruplet pregnancies is the incidence of twin gestations raised to the second and third power, respectively. If one accepts a twin pregnancy incidence in the United States of 1/50, this results in the natural probability of a triplet pregnancy of $1/50^2$, or 1/2500 pregnancies, and a quadruplet pregnancy of $1/50^3$, or 1/125,000 pregnancies.[69] However, for reasons cited earlier in this chapter, the incidence of triplet and higher-order multiple gestations are on the rise in this country. Between 1979 and 1989, the incidence of triplet and higher-order multiple pregnancies increased by 133%.[53] In 1989 there were 2798 triplet or higher-order multiple gestations recorded in the United States, for a rate of 1/1411 pregnancies. This rate shows almost twice as many high-order multiple gestations as one would predict from the natural occurrence formula. In spite of the recent and dramatic rise in high-order multiple gestations in this country, no institution, much less any individual, has enough experience to perform a randomized clinical trial of the intrapartum management of these unusual yet highly complicated pregnancies. Therefore much of data in the obstetric literature is replete with retrospective analyses of small sample sizes, and one must exercise care in extrapolating outcome parameters because a single untoward maternal or fetal outcome parameter can give rise to inaccurate and misleading conclusions.

Because most high-order multiple gestations are complicated by one or more fetal malpresentations, cesarean section is the preferred mode of delivery in this country.[25,65] In the review by Newman, Hamer, and Miller,[65] 186/198 patients (93.9%) were delivered of their infants abdominally. In the 12 patients with triplet gestations where vaginal delivery was attempted, three patients underwent emergent abdominal delivery after vaginal delivery of the first triplet. This data suggests that even in expert hands an inordinately high abdominal delivery rate occurs and that a high complication rate can be anticipated if vaginal delivery is attempted. Therefore the usual practice is to deliver all potentially viable triplet and higher-order multiple gestations by cesarean section. Finally, because of probable preterm infants with specialized needs for skilled teams of neonatologists and numerous other support personnel, these deliveries should be performed at tertiary medical facilities.

Conclusion

The extremely high perinatal morbidity and mortality rates associated with multiple pregnancy are a testament to its high risk condition. It is estimated that 75% of the increase in perinatal mortality in multiple pregnancy is related to preterm birth.[48] Therefore one wonders whether anything meaningful can be done to decrease the rate of perinatal wastage in the multiple pregnancy. Because the exact mechanisms of parturition are not entirely understood, there is presently no therapy capable of preventing preterm labor and delivery. The techniques and methods outlined in this text are aimed at promoting better maternal nutrition, improving uteroplacental blood flow and thus indirectly prolonging gestation. On the other hand, the techniques and procedures reviewed in this chapter are directed at a secondary cause of perinatal morbidity and mortality in the multiple pregnancy, namely that of malpresentation of one or more fetuses. Although an exact estimate

for the magnitude of this secondary cause of perinatal loss is not possible, the results of an extensive review of twin pregnancies over 5 years from 13 hospitals in the Chicago area are alarming.[45] In reviewing the events preceding perinatal loss, the investigators felt 13.9% of deaths were preventable. Furthermore, most of the losses were the result of errors in judgment or technique during the intrapartum period.

Extensive data and analyses have been provided in this chapter to justify the following conclusions: (1) a liberal policy of abdominal delivery for the Twin A vertex and Twin B nonvertex presentation at gestational ages younger than 32 weeks is prudent and is associated with a perinatal mortality comparable to that of a singleton pregnancy of a similar gestational age; (2) the differential morbidity and mortality between the Twin A and Twin B fetus are not increased when intrauterine and intravaginal manipulative procedures are performed by individuals skilled in managing cases of the Twin A vertex and Twin B nonvertex gestation older than 32 weeks' gestation and of concordant fetal growth; (3) all Twin A nonvertex and Twin B other presentations should be delivered abdominally because of the inability to predict and thereby prevent fetal entanglement; (4) cesarean section is the preferred route of delivery for most of the unusual situations encountered in the multiple pregnancy, such as the monoamniotic twin, the conjoined twin pregnancy, and triplet and higher-order multiple gestations; (5) vaginal delivery of twins in the Twin A vertex and Twin B vertex presentation, regardless of gestational age, is reasonable. Finally, the interventions and techniques presented should be thoroughly scrutinized before incorporation into practice. What might be reasonable and justified for one clinician under a certain set of conditions may be ill-advised for another under the same circumstances. The most appropriate intrapartum management for the multiple pregnancy is that based on a critical review and analysis of one's clinical experience and expertise.

Acknowledgments

The authors wish to thank R. Preston McGehee, M.D., for the illustrations used in this chapter.

References

1. Acker D et al: Delivery of the second twin, *Obstet Gynecol* 59:710-711, 1982.
2. Adam C, Allen AC, Baskett TF: Twin delivery: influence of the presentation and method of delivery on the second twin, *Am J Obstet Gynecol* 165:23-27, 1991.
3. Aherne W, Dunnill MS: Morphometry of the human placenta, *Br Med Bull* 22:5-8, 1966.
4. American College of Obstetricians and Gynecologists: Diagnosis and Management of Postterm Pregnancy, *ACOG Technical Bulletin 130*, Washington DC, 1989, author.
5. American College of Obstetricians and Gynecologists: Multiple gestation, *ACOG Technical Bulletin 131*, Washington DC, 1989, author.
6. Ballantyne JW: The problem of the postmature infant, *J Obstet Gynecol Br Emp* 2:36, 1902.
7. Barth RA et al: Conjoined twins: prenatal diagnosis and assessment of associated malformations, *Radiology* 177:201-207, 1990.
8. Benacerraf BR, Gelman R, Frigoletto FD: Sonographically estimated fetal weights: accuracy and limitations, *Am J Obstet Gynecol* 159:1118-1121, 1988.
9. Benirschke K, Kim CK: Multiple pregnancy, *N Engl J Med* 288:1276-1284, 1973.
10. Bleker OP, Breur W, Huidekoper BL: A study of birthweight, placental weight and mortality of twins as compared to singletons, *Br J Obstet Gynaecol* 86:111-118, 1979.
11. Blickstein I et al: Vaginal delivery of the second twin in breech presentation, *Obstet Gynecol* 69:774-776, 1987.
12. Blickstein I et al: Vaginal delivery of breech-vertex twins, *J Reprod Med* 38:879-882, 1993.
13. Botting BJ, MacDonald Davies I, MacFarlane AJ: Recent trends in the incidence of multiple births and associated mortality, *Arch Dis Childhood* 62:941-950, 1987.
14. Brady K, Read JA: Vaginal delivery of twins after previous cesarean section, *N Engl J Med* 319:118-119, 1988.
15. Brody CZ et al: Vaginal birth after cesarean section in Hawaii: experience at Kapiolani Medical Center for Women and Children, *Hawaii Med J* 52:38-42, 1993.
16. Butterworth JF, Walker FO, Lysak SZ: Pregnancy increases median nerve susceptibility to lidocaine, *Anesthesiology* 72:962-965, 1990.
17. Carlan S et al: Epidural anesthesia and external cephalic version (ECV) at term, Abstract No. 165, SPO Meeting, 1994, Las Vegas.
18. Caspersen LS: A discussant to paper by Laros RK, Dattel BJ, *Am J Obstet Gynecol* 158:1334-1336, 1988.
19. Chauhan CP et al: Intrapartum assessment by house staff of birth weight among twins, *Obstet Gynecol* 82:523-526, 1993.
20. Chauhan CP et al: Estimate of birth weight among twins: comparison of eight sonographic models, *J Reprod Med* (In Press).
21. Cheng M, Hannah M: Breech delivery at term: a critical review of the literature, *Obstet Gynecol* 82:605-618, 1993.
22. Chervenak FA et al: Intrapartum external version of the second twin, *Obstet Gynecol* 62:160-165, 1983.
23. Chervenak FA et al: Is routine cesarean section necessary for vertex-breech and vertex-transverse twin gestation? *Am J Obstet Gynecol* 148:1-5, 1984.
24. Chervenak FA et al: Intrapartum management of twin gestation, *Obstet Gynecol* 65:119-124, 1985.
25. Collins MS, Bleyel JA: Seventy-one quadruplet pregnancies: management and outcome, *Am J Obstet Gynecol* 162:1384-1392, 1990.
26. Crawford JS: A prospective study of 200 consecutive twin deliveries, *Anaesthesia* 42:33-43, 1987.
27. Davison L et al: Breech extraction of low-birth-weight second twins: can cesarean section be justified? *Am J Obstet Gynecol* 166:497-502, 1992.
28. Divon MY et al: Discordant twins: a prospective study of the diagnostic value of real-time ultrasonography combined with umbilical ar-

tery velocimetry, *Am J Obstet Gynecol* 161:757-760, 1989.

29. Divon MY et al: Twin gestation: fetal presentation as a function of gestational age, *Am J Obstet Gynecol* 168:1500-1502, 1993.

30. Eden RD et al: Perinatal characteristics of uncomplicated postdate pregnancies, *Obstet Gynecol* 69:296-299, 1987.

31. Eskes TKAB et al: The second twin, *Eur J Obstet Gynecol Reprod Biol* 1985;19:159-166, 1985.

32. Evrard JR, Gold EM: Cesarean section for delivery of the second twin, *Obstet Gynecol* 57:581-583, 1981.

33. Fall O, Nilsson BA: External cephalic version in breech presentation under tocolysis, *Obstet Gynecol* 53:712-715, 1979.

34. Fishman A, Grubb DK, Kovacs BW: Vaginal delivery of the nonvertex second twin, *Am J Obstet Gynecol* 168:861-864, 1993.

35. Flamm BL et al: Vaginal birth after cesarean delivery: results of a 5-year multicenter collaborative study, *Am J Obstet Gynecol* 158:1079-1084, 1988.

36. Fowler MG et al: Double jeopardy: twin infant mortality in the United States, 1983 and 1984, *Am J Obstet Gynecol* 165:15-22, 1991.

37. Ghai V, Vidyasagar D: Morbidity and mortality factors in twins: an epidemiologic approach, *Clin Perinatol* 15:123-140, 1988.

38. Gocke SE et al: Management of the nonvertex second twin: primary cesarean section, external version, or primary breech extraction, *Am J Obstet Gynecol* 161:111-114, 1989.

39. Golan A, Sandbank O, Rubin A: Rupture of the pregnant uterus, *Obstet Gynecol* 56:549-554, 1980.

40. Greig PC et al: The effect of presentation and mode of delivery on neonatal outcome in the second twin, *Am J Obstet Gynecol* 167:901-906, 1992.

41. Herruzo AJ et al: Perinatal morbidity and mortality in twin pregnancies, *Int J Gynecol Obstet* 36:17-22, 1991.

42. Iffy L et al: Abdominal rescue after entrapment of the aftercoming head, *Am J Obstet Gynecol* 154:623-624, 1986.

43. Jawan B et al: Spread of spinal anesthesia for cesarean section in singleton and twin pregnancies, *Br J Anaesth* 1993;70:639-41.

44. Kazzi GM et al: Noninvasive prediction of hyaline membrane disease: an optimized classification of sonographic placental maturation, *Am J Obstet Gynecol* 152:213-219, 1985.

45. Keith L et al: The Northwestern University multihospital twin study. I. A description of 588 twin pregnancies and associated pregnancy loss, 1971 to 1975, *Am J Obstet Gynecol* 138:781-789, 1980.

46. Kelsick F, Minkoff H: Management of the breech second twin, *Am J Obstet Gynecol* 144:783-786, 1982.

47. Khunda S: Locked twins, *Obstet Gynecol* 39:453-459, 1972.

48. Kiely JL: The epidemiology of perinatal mortality in multiple births, *Bull N Y Acad Med* 66:618-637, 1990.

49. Kleinman JC, Fowler MG, Kessel SS: Comparison of infant mortality among twins and singletons: United States, 1960 and 1983, *Am J Epidemiol* 133:133-143, 1991.

50. Laros RK, Dattel BJ: Management of twin pregnancy: the vaginal route is still safe, *Am J Obstet Gynecol* 158:1330-1338, 1988.

51. Leroy F: Oxytocin treatment in twin pregnancy labour, *Acta Genet Med Gemellol (Roma)* 28:303-309, 1979.

52. Leveno KJ et al: Fetal lung maturation in twin gestation, *Am J Obstet Gynecol* 148:405-411, 1984.

53. Luke B, Keith LG: The contribution of singletons, twins and triplets to low birth weight, infant mortality, and handicap in the United States, *J Reprod Med* 37:661-666, 1992.

54. Luke B: The changing pattern of multiple births in the United States: maternal and infant characteristics, 1973 and 1990, *Obstet Gynecol* 84:101-106, 1994.

55. Luke B, Keith LG: The United States Standard Certificate of Live Birth: a critical commentary, *J Reprod Med* 36:587-591, 1991.

56. Luke B et al: The ideal twin pregnancy: patterns of weight gain, discordancy, and length of gestation, *Am J Obstet Gynecol* 169:588-597, 1993.

57. MacLennan AH: Australian clinical trial with prostaglandin E_2 and $F_{2\alpha}$ to induce labor, *Reprod Fertil Dev* 2:557-561, 1990.

58. March CM: Improved pregnancy rate with monitoring of gonodtropin therapy by three modalities, *Am J Obstet Gynecol* 1987 156:1473-1479, 1987.

59. McCarthy BJ et al: The epidemiology of neonatal death in twins, *Am J Obstet Gynecol* 141:252-256, 1981.

60. McLeod FN, McCoy DR: Monoamniotic twins with an unusual cord complication, *Br J Obstet Gynaecol* 88:774-775, 1981.

61. Morales WJ et al: The effect of mode of delivery on the risk of intraventricular hemorrhage in nondiscordant twin gestation under 1500 g, *Obstet Gynecol* 73:107-110, 1989.

62. National Center for Health Statistics: Advance report of final natality statistics, 1985, *Monthly Vital Stat Rep 36 (Suppl)* July 17, 1987.

63. National hospital discharge survey rates of cesarean delivery: United States, 1991, *MMWR* 42:285-289, 1991.

64. National Institutes of Health: Cesarean childbirth, *NIH Publication No. 82-2067*, Washington, DC, 1981, US Government Printing Office.

65. Newman RB, Hamer C, Miller MC: Outpatient triplet management: a contemporary review, *Am J Obstet Gynecol* 161:547-555, 1989.

66. Nissen ED: Twins: collision, impaction, compaction, and interlocking, *Obstet Gynecol* 11:514-526, 1958.

67. Ohel G et al: Advanced ultrasonic placental maturation in twin pregnancies, *Am J Obstet Gynecol* 156:76-78, 1987.

68. Petrucha RA, Golde SH, Platt LD: Real-time ultrasound of the placenta in assessment of fetal pulmonic maturity, *Am J Obstet Gynecol* 142:463-467, 1982.

69. Powers WF, Kiely JL: The risks confronting twins: a national perspective, *Am J Obstet Gynecol* 170:456-461, 1994.

70. Pridjian G: Labor after prior cesarean section, *Clin Obstet Gynecol* 35:445-456, 1992.

71. Prins RP: The second-born twin: can we improve outcomes? *Am J Obstet Gynecol* 170:1649-1657, 1994.

72. Pruett KM, Kirshon B, Cotton DB: Unknown uterine scar and trial of labor, *Am J Obstet Gynecol* 159:807-810, 1988.

73. Rabinovici J et al: Randomized management of the second nonvertex twin: vaginal delivery or cesarean section, *Am J Obstet Gynecol* 156:52-56, 1987.

74. Rabinovici J et al: Internal podalic version with unruptured membranes for the second twin in transverse lie, *Obstet Gynecol* 71:428-430, 1988.

75. Rayburn WF et al: Multiple gestation: time interval between delivery of the first and second twins, *Obstet Gynecol* 63:502-506, 1984.

76. Rosen MG, Dickinson JC: Vaginal birth after cesarean: a meta analysis of indicators for success, *Obstet Gynecol* 76:865-868, 1990.

77. Rydhstrom H, Cullberg G: Pregnancies with growth-retarded twins in breech-vertex presentation at increased risk for entanglement during delivery, *J Perinat Med* 18:45-50, 1990.

78. Sakala EP: Obstetric management of conjoined twins, *Obstet Gynecol (Suppl)* 67:21S-25S, 1986.

79. Salerno LJ: Monoamniotic twinning: a survey of the American literature since 1935 with a report of four new cases, *Obstet Gynecol* 14:205-213, 1959.

80. Saling E, Muller-Holve W: External cephalic version under tocolysis, *J Perinat Med* 3:115-122, 1975.

81. Speroff L, Glass RH, Kase NG: *Clinical gynecologic endocrinology and infertility*, ed 5, Baltimore, 1994, Williams and Wilkins.

82. Strong TH et al: Vaginal birth after cesarean delivery in the twin gestation, *Am J Obstet Gynecol* 161:29-32, 1989.

83. Sutter J, Arab H, Manning FA: Monoamniotic twins: antenatal diagnosis and management, *Am J Obstet Gynecol* 155:836-837, 1986.

84. Swartjes JM, Bleker OP, Schutte MF: The Zavanelli maneuver applied to locked twins, *Am J Obstet Gynecol* 166:532, 1990.

85. Thompson SA, Lyons TJ, Makowski EL: Outcomes of twin gestation at the University of Colorado Health Sciences Center, 1973-1983, *J Reprod Med* 32:328-339, 1987.

86. Vintzileos AM et al: Fetal weight estimation formulas with head, abdominal, femur, and thigh circumference measurements, *Am J Obstet Gynecol* 157:410-414, 1987.

87. Zhang J, Bowes WA, Fortney JA: Efficacy of external cephalic version: a review, *Obstet Gynecol* 82:306-312, 1993.

10 Anesthesia Considerations

William E. Ackerman III

The management of anesthetics in the pregnant patient differs from that of the nonpregnant patient. The pregnant patient may be anemic, may be susceptible to vena caval compression, and may have a decrease in functional residual capacity that occasionally results in hypoxia during induction of general anesthesia for cesarean section. Gastrointestinal changes that occur during pregnancy can make the patient susceptible to aspiration during induction or emergence from general anesthesia. Hormonal changes associated with pregnancy may increase central nervous system (CNS) sensitivity to local anesthetics.

The management of anesthetics in the patient with a multiple gestation can be difficult. Abruptio placentae, anemia, preeclampsia or eclampsia, premature labor, prolonged labor, and antepartum and postpartum hemorrhage are reported to be more common with multiple births than with singleton births. Furthermore, a greater blood loss during delivery, supine hypotension, nausea and vomiting, dyspnea, and lower extremity edema may be encountered with an increased incidence in the patient with multiple gestations. Because of potential maternal complications that may occur, the management of anesthesia in the patient during labor and delivery can play an important role in maternal and neonatal outcome. The purposes of this chapter are to present the basic principles of obstetric anesthesia that are important in the management of the patient with a multiple gestation and to address any controversial issues that may exist.

The management of anesthesia in the patient with a multiple pregnancy can challenge the obstetric anesthesiologist. The anesthesiologist must be aware of potential problems, both maternal and fetal, that can occur during the perinatal period. The anesthesiologist must be aware of the obstetric management of the patient, so a safe anesthetic may be rapidly administered if a maternal or fetal emergency arises. An anesthetic that is administered improperly can contribute to maternal and fetal morbidity and mortality. Therefore the obstetric anesthesiologist must administer an anesthetic with the choice of technique and pharmacologic agents based on the maternal and perinatal status of a patient. Unfortunately there is no ideal anesthetic for a patient with multiple fetuses. The anesthesiologist should be informed when the patient is admitted to the hospital and should become familiar with the patient's medical history. Furthermore, the anesthesiologist should see the patient in consultation before admission to the hospital if the patient has a serious medical condition that may influence the administration of an anesthetic. A history must be taken and a physical examination must be performed before an anesthetic is administered, even in an emergency situation. The anesthesiologist should consult with the patient's obstetrician when the patient is admitted to the labor and delivery area, and the obstetrician should be informed of any potential problems with the anesthetic. The patient should be seen by the obstetric anesthesiologist before the onset of severe labor pain, because she may not be able to give an accurate medical history when she experiences severe pain and may therefore be more difficult to examine. When anesthesia is produced in a high-risk obstetric situation, the anesthesiologist must be physically present in the delivery area on a 24-hour basis.

The patient's family history should include a history of previous problems with anesthetics because some conditions, such as malignant hyperthermia, may be hereditary and could potentially affect the neonate.[17] The patient's surgical history should include any previous airway management problems that occurred during the administration of an anesthetic. The patient's previous anesthetic records should also be reviewed if time permits. In an emergency situation the review of symptoms should include at least the head, neck, and respiratory systems, as well as a history of allergies. The history must include notation concerning limitations in the mouth, jaw, and neck ranges of motion, especially when there is hyperextension, since any of these factors can make airway maintenance difficult. Loose teeth

can be dislodged during intubation and enter a bronchus. Dental appliances can make laryngoscopy or intubation difficult. A history of smoking, asthma, or recent respiratory infection could cause bronchospasm during induction of or emergence from general anesthesia. A careful cardiovascular history must be taken because epidural, spinal, or general anesthesia can affect the heart rate and total peripheral vascular resistance of the patient, which could increase maternal morbidity in the patient with valvular pathology.[18] Regional anesthesia can cause a decrease in the maternal systemic vascular resistance, which could result in maternal hypotension. General anesthesia can also cause increases in the heart rate and peripheral vascular resistance during intubation and on emergence from general anesthesia until the endotracheal tube has been removed. Any significant cardiac history may require consultation with a cardiologist before an anesthetic technique is chosen. Furthermore, invasive monitoring (such as a pulmonary artery catheter or an arterial line) may be indicated before an anesthetic is initiated. The endocrine, hepatic, renal, hematologic, gastrointestinal, musculoskeletal, and psychiatric histories must also be noted if time permits. Patients with a history of diabetes mellitus may have a polyneuropathy, and this entity should be documented on the patient's chart before a regional anesthetic is administered. These patients may also have decreased sympathetic nervous system activity and be more susceptible to hypotension with the administration of a regional or general anesthetic. Patients with hyperthyroidism may have a thyroid crisis during general anesthesia. A patient with hypothyroidism may have a history of paresthesia or hoarseness. It is important to document these findings before administering an anesthetic to avoid potential postpartum legal accusations. A hepatic history is important because amide anesthetics and narcotics are metabolized by the liver. A decrease in clotting factors that can be associated with liver disease could result in an epidural hematoma if an epidural needle or catheter pierced a blood vessel in the epidural canal. The gastrointestinal history should include the time of the patient's last ingestion of food or drink. Recent food or liquid ingestion should be treated with intravenous metoclopramide, and a nonparticulate antacid (such as sodium citrate) should be given before an anesthetic is administered because of the risk of aspiration pneumonitis. A history of vomiting is important because this entity can cause an acute change in the patient's electrolyte status. Hypokalemia can cause an arrhythmia during general anesthesia.[27] Pregnant patients, especially those with multiple gestations, can develop significant changes in posture, such as exaggerated lumbar lordosis, during pregnancy. These patients may have low back pain or sacral iliac joint pain. This complaint may require more extensive physical therapy and occasionally injection of a local anesthetic and steroid into painful areas postpartum. A history of herpes simplex virus labialis is significant because epidural morphine may cause a recurrence of this entity in the postpartum period.[15] A psychiatric history is important because chloroprocaine, an amide anesthetic, may exacerbate anxiety attacks in patients with severe behavioral problems.[1] A medication history must be taken because beta-agonists can have side effects that affect the manage-

ment of anesthesia in a patient (such as hypokalemia). A history of allergies should be documented. This history should include allergies to sun screen lotions. Some sun screens contain para-aminobenzoic acid (PABA) derivatives. Patients allergic to PABA may be allergic to ester local anesthetics.[3]

A physical examination should also be performed before an anesthetic is given. In an emergency situation the oral airway, lungs, and heart must be examined by the anesthesiologist. Failure to do so can result in increased morbidity or mortality for both the mother and fetuses. The physical examination before the administration of a nonemergency regional anesthetic must include a brief neurologic examination that includes the lower extremities with tests for muscle strength, sensation, and reflexes. This examination may be rapidly performed. Before the anesthesiologist discusses a regional anesthetic with the patient, the distance between the spinous processes must be estimated. The anesthesiologist can determine the potential difficulty at the time of spinal needle or epidural needle placement if the distance between adjacent spinous processes is narrow. If the anesthesiologist anticipates difficulty with regional anesthesia, the patient and obstetrician should be informed. Furthermore, the anesthesiologist should confer with the obstetrician regarding any pertinent laboratory studies that may be necessary before an anesthetic is started.

The anesthesiologist must then assign a classification to the patient based on the American Society of Anesthesiologists' Physical Status Classification:[4]

   I   Normal healthy patient
   II Mild systemic disease

III   Severe systemic disease

IV   Severe systemic disease that is a constant threat to life

V   Moribund patient not expected to survive 24 hours with or without an operation

E   Emergency

The patient's classification should be recorded on the anesthesia record and on the progress note in the patient's chart. A notation concerning the type of anesthetic that the patient, anesthesiologist, and obstetrician agreed on must also be included in the patient's chart. The obstetrician should be informed of the patient's choice of anesthetic. Because of the potential for a significant blood loss during delivery in the patient with multiple births, a large-gauge intravenous catheter should be in place when the patient is in labor.

With respect to preterm labor, several anesthetic issues must be taken into consideration to provide a safe anesthetic for the patient. General considerations include supplemental oxygen for the patient in the labor room. If the patient had oxygen in the labor room and if fetal distress occurs, oxygen should be continued with a portable oxygen tank during transportation to the delivery room. The anesthesiologist must avoid supine hypotension during the transportation of a patient. Epidural catheter dosing must be done slowly to prevent hypotension, and a local anesthetic with a slow onset, such as bupivacaine is recommended. Left uterine displacement is necessary after epidural catheter placement because the patient with a multiple gestation is more susceptible to hypotension than the patient with a single gestation. Beta agonists administered during labor can cause hypoglycemia or pulmonary edema.[13] It would be

prudent to place a pulse oximeter on the patient's finger before giving a fluid bolus of 10 to 15 ml of crystalloid. Prehydration is standard practice before the administration of a regional anesthetic in pregnant patients.

For vaginal delivery, epidural anesthesia offers advantages over spinal anesthesia in that analgesia is provided during both labor and delivery. Spinal anesthesia provides pain relief during the second and third stages of labor. Hypotension associated with a lumbar epidural blockade is essentially not affected by tocolytics. If it is administered properly, a lumbar epidural anesthetic can prevent the sudden maternal urge to bear down. It is important for the anesthesiologist to maintain an adequate sensory level (thoracic dermatome level 10) to allow for the rapid initiation of a cesarean section if needed. For this reason, a continuous epidural infusion should be considered.

A subarachnoid anesthetic offers the advantage of a quicker onset than epidural anesthesia. This is important if a rapid onset of anesthesia is desired. However, the incidence of hypotension may be greater with spinal anesthesia compared with epidural anesthesia. Motor blockade is greater with spinal anesthesia, and consequently the patient may not be able to voluntarily expel the fetus when necessary. Hypotension after the administration of a regional anesthetic may be treated with phenylephrine when a patient has been treated with beta agonists and has a significant increase in her heart rate.[24] Ephedrine is usually given intravenously for the treatment of hypotension in the pregnant patient. Epinephrine is often mixed with a local anesthetic to prolong its duration of action or is used in a test dose for the detection of intravascular epidural needle or catheter placement. Both of these vasopressors can worsen tachycardia in the patient who received beta agonists. Ephedrine could increase the heart rate in a patient who may have tachycardia after beta agonist administration. Phenylephrine given in 50 μg increments does not adversely affect uterine artery blood flow, increases maternal blood pressure, and may decrease the maternal heart rate.

A combined epidural-spinal anesthetic technique is becoming increasingly popular in the practice of obstetric anesthesiology.[9] However, its advantage over the techniques mentioned previously remains to be studied.

For a cesarean section, either a subarachnoid or epidural anesthetic may be given. Spinal bupivacaine has a slower onset of action than either lidocaine or tetracaine and may therefore attenuate the incidence of hypotension. Prehydration must be done with caution in the patient receiving beta agonists because of the potential for pulmonary edema. When a general anesthetic must be given, the anesthesiologist must be aware that beta agonists can cause tachycardia, arrhythmias, and hypokalemia. Beta agonists may inhibit hypoxic pulmonary vasoconstriction.[11] Because of this failure to redistribute pulmonary perfusion effectively, maternal hypoxia may be out of proportion to radiographic findings. Other anesthetic implications exist when a patient receives beta agonists. Beta agonists may cause increases in maternal stroke volume and cardiac output. Because of the increased myocardial oxygen demand that can be caused by beta agonists, some patients may report episodes of chest pain that

usually subside when the beta agonist is discontinued. Beta agonists can also cause uterine atony because of relaxation of uterine smooth muscle.[19] Therefore the obstetric anesthetist must be vigilant and closely monitor the maternal blood loss during delivery. Ideally, the anesthesiologist should wait 30 minutes after beta agonist discontinuation to induce general anesthesia. Halothane should be avoided as an inhalational agent if general anesthesia must be induced, because this volatile anesthetic may cause arrhythmias in patients who have received beta agonists. Beta adrenergic therapy may cause hyperglycemia, and patients with diabetes may require insulin.[5] The anesthesiologist must monitor serum glucose levels intraoperatively at hourly intervals if the patient must have a cesarean section. Beta agonists may also cause a decrease in the maternal systemic vascular resistance. As a result, a conduction anesthetic must be given slowly and the patients blood pressure must be monitored at 1-minute intervals to prevent profound hypotension. Because oxytocin also causes vasodilation one must be careful not to infuse intravenous oxytocin too rapidly if a patient is hypotensive. If a general anesthetic is administered, hyperventilation must be avoided because it can cause uterine artery vasoconstriction and worsen hypokalemia by causing plasma potassium to move intracellularily. Magnesium sulfate can potentiate both depolarizing and nondepolarizing muscle relaxants. As a result, curare should not be given to attenuate succinylcholine fasciculation before the induction of general anesthesia because respiratory depression can occur. Ethanol is rarely used to inhibit labor. However, in instances where ethanol is used to inhibit labor, inebriation, nausea, and vomiting are side effects that may make a patient uncooperative and at a greater risk for aspiration resulting from decreased gastric motility if general anesthesia is induced. On the other hand the patient may not cooperate for the placement of a regional anesthetic. Furthermore, ethanol may decrease the gastric emptying time and decrease maternal serum glucose. Prostaglandin synthetase inhibitors may cause a prolongation of the patient's bleeding time.[6] It would be prudent for the obstetric anesthetist to obtain a bleeding time before a regional anesthetic is given if a patient has recently received one of these agents to treat preterm labor. Calcium entry-blocking agents may cause uterine atony that may be unresponsive to oxytocin and prostaglandin $F_{2\alpha}$.[14] Appropriate blood crossmatching might be considered before delivery if a patient is receiving nifedipine as a tocolytic agent. The anesthesiologist must be aware that patients in preterm labor may deliver precipitously. Therefore when the patient is admitted to the hospital, the obstetrician may request that the epidural catheter be placed before active labor and that the patient be given a local anesthetic when needed.

The anesthetic management of the patient with severe preeclampsia can also be difficult. Severe preeclampsia is present when any of the following symptoms are present in the patient: a systolic blood pressure greater than 160 mm Hg or a diastolic pressure greater than 110 mm Hg, recorded on two occasions 6 hours apart with the patient at bed rest; proteinuria greater than 5 gm/day; oliguria; cerebral disturbances; pulmonary edema; coagulopathy; or epigastric pain.[22] Hypertension can become worse and potentially life-threatening during laryngoscopy and intubation. Decreases in plasma proteins can result in higher plasma levels of drugs that are highly protein bound. Generalized edema (if present) can make intravenous line placement difficult, and if laryngeal edema is present, endotracheal tube placement may be extremely difficult.

Three hemodynamic subsets of severe preeclampsia exist and have been described by Clark et al.[10]: (1) low to normal cardiac output (CO), low pulmonary capillary wedge pressure (PCWP), and high systemic vascular resistance (SVR); (2) high CO, low SVR, and normal PCWP; and (3) low CO, normal or high PCWP, and high SVR. Cotton and Benedetti[12] reported that the use of a pulmonary artery catheter in patients with severe preeclampsia during labor provided a more complete profile of a patient's disease status and provided accurate information on the efficacy of therapeutic modalities used. The following three case reports demonstrate the usefulness of pulmonary artery catheter hemodynamic measurements and the different treatment modalities used in the management of patients with three different hemodynamic subsets of severe preeclampsia.

Case 1

A 19-year-old, 68 kg, Gravida$_2$, Para$_1$, Abortion$_0$ (G$_2$P$_1$Ab$_0$) patient was admitted to the hospital with a blood pressure (BP) of 148/110 mm Hg with +3 proteinuria. Both the patient and her obstetrician requested epidural analgesia for labor and delivery. The patient did not have a coagulopathy. A pulmonary artery catheter was placed. Magnesium sulfate infusion was initiated by the patient's obstetrician. Her baseline hemodynamic values were: PCWP,

1 mm Hg; central venous pressure (CVP), 2 cm H_2O; CO, 4.8 L/min; pulse, 96 beats/min; and SVR, 1788 dynes $-$ sec/cm^{-5}. Intravenous lactated Ringer's solution (1600) was slowly infused until a PCWP of 10 mm Hg was attained and the following values were noted: BP, 138/90 mm Hg; CO, 6.2 L/min; CVP, 11 cm H_2O; and SVR, 1225 dynes $-$ sec/cm^{-5}. An epidural catheter was inserted, and the patient was given 10 ml of 0.25% bupivacaine followed by an infusion of 0.125% at 8 ml/hr, and the patient was delivered of healthy twins without incident or further medication.

Case 2

A 26-year-old, 98 kg, $G_3P_1Ab_1$ patient was admitted to the hospital in labor with a BP of 140/114 mm Hg, +3 proteinuria, pulse of 88 beats/min, and a normal coagulation profile. A pulmonary artery catheter was placed, and intravenous magnesium sulfate was infused before epidural analgesia was initiated. The patient's baseline hemodynamic values were: PCWP, 15 mm Hg; CVP, 10 cm H_2O; CO, 3.1 L/min; and SVR, 2906 dynes $-$ sec/cm^{-5}. Because of the significantly increased SVR, hydralazine was administered intravenously by the patient's obstetrician in increments to a total dose of 10 mg. Twenty minutes after hydralazine administration and prehydration of 10 ml/kg of lactated Ringer's solution, the hemodynamic values were: PCWP, 13 mm Hg; CVP, 9 cm H_2O; CO, 4.9 L/min; pulse, 110 beats/min; and SVR, 1605 dynes $-$ sec/cm^{-5}. An epidural catheter was placed, and the patient was given 10 ml of 0.25% bupivacaine followed by an infusion of 0.125% bupivacaine at 10 ml/hr. The patient's hemodynamic values remained stable, and the patient was delivered of twins without incident.

Case 3

A 20-year-old, 82 kg, $G_1P_0Ab_0$ patient with a twin pregnancy arrived at the hospital in active labor. Her blood pressure was 134/88 mm Hg, and her pulse was 92 beats/min. An epidural catheter was placed, and the patient was given 8 ml of 0.25% bupivacaine followed by an infusion of 0.125% bupivacaine at 8 ml/hr. After 12 hours, the patient became oliguric and tachycardiac. Her blood pressure increased to 150/110 mm Hg. The patient was afebrile. One fetus became bradycardic after the initiation of intravenous magnesium sulfate. The patient's obstetrician chose to do an emergency cesarean section. The epidural catheter was used to administer 0.5% bupivacaine until a bilateral sensory level of T5 was attained. A pulmonary artery catheter was placed when the patient was in the cesarean section room. The following hemodynamic values were noted immediately before delivery: BP, 168/114 mm Hg; PCWP, 28 mm Hg; CVP, 6 cm H_2O; pulse, 124 beats/min; CO, 13.5 L/min; and SVR, 782 dynes $-$ sec/cm^{-5}. The patient was treated with 5 mg of intravenous labetalol at the time of delivery and with labetalol infusion for approximately 16 hours. Her BP decreased to 150/100 mm Hg within 5 minutes of the initiation of labetolol, and her pulse decreased to 94 beats/min. There were no statistically significant changes noted in her other hemodynamic values. Her first twin was resuscitated by the neonatologist present at the time of delivery. The second twin was born with an Apgar score of 8 at 1 minute. The patient was admitted to the intensive care unit for 24 hours postpartum while the labetalol infusion was gradually weaned.

These three cases emphasize the importance of accurately diagnosing the patient's hemodynamic status before instituting fluid and antihypertensive therapy. They also demonstrate that the obstetrician and anesthesiologist must readily communicate and approach the patient as a team. Both the first and third patients were oliguric. Oliguria can be a complication of severe preeclampsia and is defined as a urine output of less than 30 ml/hr for 3 consecutive hours. It has been recommended that a patient with oliguria be given a fluid challenge of 500 ml. If oliguria persists despite a fluid challenge, a pulmonary catheter may be advocated.

Patients with severe preeclampsia and a high systemic vascular resistance and low cardiac output can have reduced plasma volumes. Expansion of the plasma volume alone can result in a decrease in the systemic vascular resistance and a decrease in maternal blood pressure. Joyce, Debnath, and Baker[20] reported that the diastolic blood pressure was proportional to the volume of intravenous fluid needed to restore the central venous pressure to a normal level, but they apparently did not recognize that they were treating only one subset of severe preeclampsia. However, as the previous case reports demonstrated, each hemodynamic subset of severe preeclampsia can have distinctively different intravenous fluid requirements. In patients with low PCWP, low to normal CO, and moderately increased calculated SVR, fluid infusion can increase the CO as the PCWP increases; a decrease in the SVR may also be seen as the PCWP increases. Fifty-six percent of patients with severe preeclampsia are in this category. In patients with normal to high PCWP and high SVR (11%), oliguria can be caused by intense renal artery vasospasm, or de-

creased CO may be caused by generalized arterial vasoconstriction. In these patients, volume loading to a normal PCWP and afterload reduction with hydralazine or preload reduction with nitroglycerine can be beneficial. Lumbar epidural analgesia for labor and delivery has a minimal effect on CO and causes a statistically insufficient decrease in SVR in patients with severe preeclampsia. Therefore epidural anesthesia should not be relied on to effectively decrease the SVR.[16] In patients with normal PCWP, high CO, and low SVR (33%), fluid should be given judiciously and titrated to the PCWP. In such patients, blind volume expansion could cause pulmonary or cerebral edema. In severe preeclampsia, a CVP measurement does not consistently correlate with the PCWP measurement and does not yield as accurate a profile of the patient's hemodynamic status.

The use of sodium nitroprusside in pregnant patients is controversial because of the potential for fetal cyanide toxicity and maternal tachyphylaxis.[21] However, nitroprusside has a rapid onset and short duration of action. It decreases the blood pressure by arterial dilation. Hydralazine, which also exerts its action by arterial vasodilation, has a slower onset of action (15 to 20 minutes) and a half-life of 2 to 8 hours. Because of its low molecular weight, it can pass quickly from the mother to the fetus and cause neonatal hypotension.[28] For this reason, if an epidural analgesic is administered, epidural dosing must be done slowly with a local anesthetic that has a slow onset, such as bupivacaine. Hydralazine can also cause maternal tachycardia.

Nitroglycerine decreases maternal blood pressure by venodilation and by reduction of preload and has been used successfully in patients with severe preeclampsia during general anesthesia for cesarean section. Neonatal hypotension has not been observed with nitroglycerine. However, nitroglycerine dilates arterioles when it is administered in high doses.

Trimethaphan, a ganglionic blocking drug, acts rapidly but has such a short duration of action that it must be given by continuous intravenous infusion. It may be preferable to nitroglycerine in pregnancy because its molecular weight is greater than nitroglycerine and it may not cross the placental barrier as readily as nitroglycerine.[2] Trimethaphan causes vasodilation with reflex tachycardia on occasion. Trimethaphan may cause prolonged apnea when it is administered concurrently with the depolarizing muscle relaxer, succinylcholine. Labetalol attenuates the hypertensive response of the patient with preeclampsia to intubation and has a minimal effect on the uteroplacental blood flow.[23] It has selective alpha- and nonselective beta-adrenergic receptor activity. In pregnant patients who are hypertensive, it has a half-life of 147 minutes and attenuates both the patient's heart rate and blood pressure.

Diazoxide has an unpredictable effect in pregnant patients and is not routinely used. Beta blockers and calcium channel blocking drugs are currently under investigation, and the interaction with regional anesthetics or general anesthetics remains to be reported.

Because of the potential drug interactions that can occur when antihypertensive agents are administered before an anesthetic, the obstetric anesthesiologist should be consulted early if possible. The patient's obstetrician should discuss the planned obstetric management with the anesthesiologist.

Premature rupture of membranes (PROM) is not uncommon in patients with multiple gestations. Controversy exists in the practice of obstetric anesthesiology as to whether a regional anesthetic may be given to patients with premature rupture of membranes who are febrile. Vaddadi et al.[26] reported that no patient with bacteremia from chorioamnionitis who received antibiotics before or after regional blockade developed an epidural abscess. In 1983 Yoder et al.[29] reported that the bacteremia of chorioamnionitis is treatable with appropriate antibiotic selection. Carp and Bailey[8] demonstrated meningitis in bacteremic rats that sustained puncture of the dura. However, no meningitis was reported if the dura was intact. One should be aware that an epidural abscess may arise spontaneously without regional anesthesia in the presence of bacteremia. Blood in the epidural space after the traumatic placement of an epidural needle can become a bacterial culture medium in the epidural space.

If infection is present, antibiotic coverage should be initiated before the institution of regional anesthesia. An epidural anesthetic may then be safely administered. The epidural needle should be placed by an experienced member of the obstetric anesthesiology team to minimize the danger of a dural puncture. If the anesthesiologist doubts the possibility of performing an atraumatic block (for example, because of obesity or lack of obvious landmarks) epidural anesthesia should not be induced. If the patient receives an epidural anesthetic, she should be aware of the signs and symptoms of an epidural abscess: back pain that becomes progressively worse, fever, elevated white cell count, and tenderness and erythema over the needle puncture site. An epidural abscess is an emergency that necessitates an immediate neurosurgical consultation and treatment.

Uterine atony may also occur postpartum in patients with multiple births. A significant blood loss can occur in a short time. As a result, uterine atony can cause maternal death by hemorrhage. If uterine atony occurs during the administration of a general inhalational anesthetic, the inhalational agent should be discontinued and a narcotic should be given intravenously. Fentanyl does not cause a significant decrease in the blood pressure or uterine muscle relaxation. Ritodrine, terbutaline, and isoxsuprine can decrease uterine contractility when they are administered immediately before delivery. Magnesium sulfate may also cause uterine atony. Intravenous calcium chloride may be given if uterine atony is a result of magnesium sulfate administration. Intravenous dantrolene used prophylactically for the prevention of malignant hyperthermia by anesthesiologists may also cause uterine atony.[25] With respect to maternal bleeding, the anesthesiologist must closely monitor the patient's vital signs. The intravascular volume must be replaced with appropriate fluids. The anesthesiologist may be requested by the obstetrician to give intravenous oxytocin. Severe hypotension can occur when oxytocin is given to a patient who has hypovolemia. Tachycardia may also occur. Phenylephrine should be used to treat hypotension and tachycardia caused by oxytocin, because ephedrine could potentially worsen maternal tachycardia. Methylergonovine may be administered intramuscularly in doses of 0.2 or

0.3 mg to decrease bleeding by increasing uterine muscle contraction. It may also be given intravenously if there is profound hypotension. However, the blood pressure must be closely monitored because of the potential for severe hypertension. The anesthesiologist must closely monitor the electrocardiogram when ergot preparations are given because coronary artery spasm can occur. Prostaglandin $F_{2\alpha}$ is often used to treat uterine atony. Bronchospasm, nausea, and vomiting, may occur as side effects.[7] When pharmacologic maneuvers used to stimulate uterine contraction fail, the obstetrician may elect to perform a hypogastric artery ligation or a hysterectomy. With severe bleeding, vigorous fluid volume replacement must be initiated before the induction of general anesthesia to decrease the incidence of maternal hypotension during induction. Ketamine or etomidate used for the induction of anesthesia can preserve maternal blood pressure. Other induction agents may worsen hypotension. Following induction, maintenance anesthesia should be managed with a narcotic-nitrous oxide technique with controlled ventilation and muscle relaxation. With a massive blood loss and severe hypotension, an arterial line, urinary catheter, and central venous line should be inserted. The anesthesiologist should maintain urinary output at 60 ml/hr. If signs of pulmonary edema are suspected after rapid infusion of large volumes of fluids and blood, or if significant decreases in oxygen saturation are noted by pulse oximeter monitoring changes, a pulmonary artery catheter should be placed. Pulse oximetry is useful for measuring hemoglobin saturation. However, if the maternal hemoglobin is significantly low, pulse oximeter readings can be inaccurate, and subsequent periodic arterial blood gas samples should be aspirated from the arterial line both intraoperatively and postpartum at 15-minute intervals until the patient is hemodynamically stable. The hematocrit count, platelet count, and coagulation status must also be periodically monitored by the anesthesiologist during volume resuscitation. The frequency of monitoring depends on the severity of the hemorrhage. Furthermore, periodic arterial serum lactate measurements may reflect the adequacy of tissue perfusion and oxygenation. After volume resuscitation, the patient must be observed closely in the immediate postpartum period in a postanesthesia recovery unit by a nursing staff trained in the management of both the postpartum patient and the critical care patient.

Abruptio placentae may occur in women with multiple pregnancies. The placental separation may be partial or complete. The changes in the patient's hemodynamic profile determine whether a regional anesthetic may be safely administered. The anesthesiologist must be aware that the perinatal mortality rate can be high (40% to 60%) and that acute renal failure or disseminated intravascular coagulopathy (DIC) can occur. When it occurs, vaginal bleeding is usually dark and nonclotting. The anesthesiologist must communicate with the patient's obstetrician and nurse before giving an anesthetic to a patient with abruptio placentae. When the abruptio is confined to the uterine cavity, the uterine mass increases in size and the uterus can become tetanic. During abruptio placentae, the assessment of the patient's blood loss may differ significantly from the actual blood loss. Uterine pain and uterine tetany may not al-

ways be present. The anesthesiologist must confer with the obstetrician regarding the results of ultrasonography. The anesthesiologist must never administer an epidural or spinal anesthetic to a patient with hypovolemia. The obstetric anesthesiologist must also work in cooperation with the obstetrician to ensure that the maternal clotting factors are restored to normal before beginning a cesarean section if DIC is present. When a patient with abruptio placentae is admitted to the hospital, the anesthesiologist should immediately obtain a history from the patient, do a physical examination, and be mentally prepared to induce general anesthesia and rapidly restore the maternal circulating blood volume should the need arise. The anesthesiologist should place two large-bore intravenous lines. An epidural anesthetic may be given for labor and delivery or cesarean section in patients with mild to moderate abruptio placentae if the maternal cardiovascular system is stable and there are no signs of fetal distress. If a patient has an epidural catheter placed for labor analgesia, the decision of whether to use an existing epidural catheter for emergency cesarean section depends on maternal hemodynamic stability. If maternal hemodynamic stability is compromised, a rapid sequence endotracheal intubation must be performed and a general anesthetic must be given. A technique similar to that described for uterine atony should be used.

Most patients do not require blood transfusion until blood loss exceeds 1500 ml. Usually red blood cells are transfused instead of whole blood. Indications for whole blood include the need for simultaneous replacement of blood and oxygen to increase the patient's oxygen carrying capacity. Fresh frozen plasma is administered if the prothrombin time or partial thromboplastin time is 1½ times normal. The usual dose of fresh frozen plasma is 10 to 15 ml/kg. One unit of fresh frozen plasma increases clotting factors by 8%. Platelets must also be monitored in the bleeding patient and replaced as necessary. Platelets should be replaced when the count is less than 50,000. One unit of platelets is derived from one unit of whole blood. Cryoprecipitate should be administered by the anesthesiologist when a significant blood loss has occurred and when the fibrinogen level is less than 100 mg/dl. One may transfuse with O-negative blood (universal donor) but type-specific blood may be preferred. Once 2 or more units of universal donor have been transfused, one should not switch back to type specific blood. The obstetrician and anesthesiologist should determine whether time permits them to use type-specific blood in the bleeding patient.

This chapter demonstrates the challenges faced by the obstetric anesthesiologist in the management of the patient with a multiple gestation. Only with a team effort from each patient's obstetrician, nurse, and anesthesiologist can such patients be managed with minimal maternal and fetal morbidity and mortality.

References

1. Ackerman WE, Phero JC, Juneja MM: Panic disorder following epidural 2-chloroprocaine in pregnant patients, *Am J Psychiatry* 74:940-941, 1989.
2. Ackerman WE et al: Use of the pulmonary artery catheter in the management of the severe preeclamptic patient, *Anesth Rev* 27:37-40, 1990.
3. Aldrete JA, Johnson DA: Allergy to local anesthetics, *JAMA* 207:356-357, 1969.
4. American Society of Anesthesiologists: New classification of physical status, *Anesthesiology* 24:111-113, 1963.
5. Benedetti TJ: Maternal complications of parenteral B-sympathomimetic therapy for premature labor, *Am J Obstet Gynecol* 145:1-6, 1983.
6. Benigni A et al: Effect of low-dose aspirin on fetal and maternal generation of thromboxane by platelets in women at risk for pregnancy-induced hypertension, *N Engl J Med* 321:357-362, 1989.
7. Buttino L, Garite TJ: The use of 15 Methyl F₂ alphaprostaglandin (Prostin 15 M) for the control of postpartum hemorrhage, *Am J Perinatol* 3:241-243, 1986.
8. Carp H, Bailey S: Meningitis after dural puncture in rats, *Anesthesiology* 73:A862, 1990.
9. Carrie LES: Extradural, spinal or combined block for obstetric surgical anesthesia, *Br J Anaesth* 65:225-233, 1990.
10. Clark SL et al: Severe preeclampsia with persistent oliguria: management of hemodynamic subsets, *Am J Obstet Gynecol* 154:491-494, 1986.
11. Conover WB, Benumof JL, Key TC: Ritodrine inhibition of hypoxic pulmonary vasoconstriction, *Am J Obstet Gynecol* 146:652-656, 1983.
12. Cotton DB, Benedetti TJ: Use of the Swan-Ganz catheter in obstetrics and gynecology, *Obstet Gynecol* 56:641-645, 1980.
13. Crawford JS: A prospective study of 200 consecutive twin deliveries, *Anaesthesia* 42:33-43, 1987.
14. Csapo AI et al: Deactivation of the uterus during normal and premature labor by the calcium antagonist nicardipine, *Am J Obstet Gynecol* 142:483-491, 1982.
15. Gieraerts R et al: Increased incidence of itching and herpes simplex in patients given epidural morphine after cesarean section, *Anesth Analg* 66:1321-1324, 1987.
16. Graham C, Goldstein A: Epidural analgesia and cardiac output in severe pre-eclamptics, *Anaesthesia* 35:709-712, 1982.
17. Gronert GA: Malignant hyperthermia, *Anesthesiology* 53:395-423, 1980.
18. Hemmings GT et al: Invasive monitoring and anaesthetic management of a parturient with mitral stenosis, *Can J Anaesth* 34:182-185, 1987.
19. Huddleston JF: *Preterm labor, Clin Obstet Gynecol* 25:123-136, 1982.
20. Joyce TH, Debnath KS, Baker EA: Preeclampsia: relationship of CVP and epidural analgesia, *Anesthesiology* 51:S297, 1979.

21. Naulty J, Cefalo RC, Lewis PE: Fetal toxicity of nitroprusside in the pregnant ewe, *Am J Obstet Gynecol* 139:708-711, 1981.

22. Pritchard JA, MacDonald PC: *Hypertensive disorder in pregnancy.* In Pritchard JA, MacDonald PC, editors: *Williams' obstetrics,* ed 15, New York, 1976, Appleton-Century-Crofts.

23. Ramanathan J, Chauhan D, Sibai BM: The use of labetalol for attenuation of hypertensive response to endotracheal intubation in preeclampsia, *Anesth Analg* 67:5181, 1988.

24. Ramanathan S, Grant GJ: Vasopressor therapy for hypotension due to epidural anesthesia for cesarean section, *Acta Anaesthesiol Scand* 32:559-565, 1988.

25. Storniolo FR et al: *The febrile parturient.* In James FM, Wheeler AS, Dewan DM, editors: *Obstetric anesthesia: the complicated patient,* Philadelphia, 1988, FA Davis.

26. Vaddadi A et al: Epidural anesthesia in women with chorioamnionitis: a retrospective study, *Anesthesiology* 73:A863, 1996.

27. Wong KC et al: Hypokalemia during anesthesia: the effects of d-tubocurarine, gallamine, succinylcholine, thiopental, and halothane with and without respiratory alkalosis, *Anesth Analg* 52:522-528, 1973.

28. Wright JP: Anesthetic considerations in pre-eclampsia-eclampsia, *Anesth Analg* 63:590-601, 1983.

29. Yoder PR et al: A prospective, controlled study of maternal and perinatal outcome after intraamniotic infection at term, *Am J Obstet Gynecol* 145:695-701, 1983.

11 Postpartum Alterations

Stanley A. Gall

The postpartum period, or the puerperium, is commonly thought of as the time immediately after birth. However, conventional thought defines the puerperium as that time from the delivery of the child to 6 weeks after the birth. By the end of the 6 weeks, the reproductive tract and the altered physiologic states of pregnancy (with the exception of ovulation in women who are breast-feeding) have returned to their normal, nonpregnant state.

There are no data to suggest that the involution of the genital and urinary tracts after a multiple gestation is significantly different from that occurring after a singleton pregnancy. Descriptions of the involutional changes may be found in major textbooks of obstetrics. However, postpartum hemorrhage and postpartum endometritis is significantly increased.

Postpartum Hemorrhage

Postpartum hemorrhage is generally defined as a blood loss in excess of 500 ml in the first 24 hours postpartum. The origin of this statement is unclear; it has appeared in textbooks for over 50 years without documentation. Newton[6] measured the amount of hemoglobin lost during the first 24 hours postpartum in 105 women and found the average blood loss to be 550 ml. Pritchard[7] determined that 5% of women who were delivered of their infants vaginally lost more than 1000 ml of blood. He also determined that the estimated blood loss at the time of delivery is only half of the actual loss. DeLeeuw et al.[2] determined that approximately 600 ml of blood is lost during vaginal delivery and within the first 24 hours postpartum. Therefore the average patient whose infants are delivered vaginally experiences a postpartum hemorrhage. The postpartum hemorrhage incidence in multiple gestations is greater than it is for singleton gestations because of the overdistended uterus and the prolonged use of oxytocin.

The predisposing factors and causes of postpartum hemorrhage are listed in Box 11-1.

The primary cause of postpartum hemorrhage in a patient with a multiple gestation is uterine atony. The overdistended uterus is likely to be hypotonic after either vaginal or abdominal delivery. The patient who has been subjected to prolonged oxytocin stimulation is also more prone to postpartum uterine atony. Pritchard et al.[8] determined that the average blood loss after a twin delivery is almost 1000 ml and in some cases much greater.

A postpartum hemorrhage in the patient with a multiple gestation may be

BOX 11-1

Predisposing Factors and Causes of Immediate Postpartum Hemorrhage

TRAUMA TO THE GENITAL TRACT

Large episiotomy that includes extension
Lacerations of the perineum, vagina, or
　cervix
Ruptured uterus

BLEEDING FROM PLACENTAL IMPLANTATION SITE

Hypotonic myometrium—uterine atony
Halogenated general anesthetic agents
Poorly perfused myometrium—hypotension
　Hemorrhage
　Conduction anesthesia

OVERDISTENDED UTERUS
PROLONGED LABOR
RAPID LABOR
OXYTOCIN-INDUCED OR AUGMENTED LABOR
HIGH PARITY (>6)
UTERINA ATONY IN A PREVIOUS PREGNANCY
CHORIOAMNIONITIS
RETAINED PLACENTAL TISSUE

Avulsed cotyledon, succenturiate lobe
Abnormal placentation—accreta, increta,
　or percreta

COAGULATION DEFECT

Intensify all of the above

Modified from Cunningham G editors: Williams obstetrics,
ed 19, Norwalk, Conn., 1993, Appleton & Lange.

more insidious than one in the patient with a singleton gestation. The patient with a multiple gestation may lose large amounts of blood before the maternal pulse and blood pressure undergo alterations. Therefore a patient may lose 1000 ml of blood without significant changes in pulse or blood pressure only to experience severe hemorrhagic shock because the amount of blood lost was grossly underestimated. The clinician was lulled into a sense of false security because of the minor pulse and blood pressure changes.

This concept is even more pronounced in the patient with a multiple gestation and preeclampsia. The incidence of preeclampsia exceeds 25% in patients with multiple gestations. Either the circulating plasma volume fails to expand in these women, or there is actually a constricted plasma volume. These circumstances makes the patient sensitive to or highly intolerant of what may be considered a normal blood loss. Therefore because of the increased risk of postpartum hemorrhage, the clinician must be extremely vigilant for any signs of abnormal blood loss. For instance, it is critical for an experienced person to monitor the patient postpartum. It is not uncommon for the uterine cavity to become distended and harbor 1000 ml of blood while an inexperienced attendant gently massages the enlarged uterus.

The diagnosis of postpartum hemorrhage should be obvious. However, the exact source may not be immediately discernible, and a systematic examination of the vulva, vagina, cervix, and uterus is mandatory. In the vast majority of cases the cause is uterine atony that can readily be determined by pelvic examination. If bright red bleeding persists despite a firmly contracted uterus, lacerations of the cervix or vagina must be suspected.

A similar scenario may occur when a cesarean delivery has occurred. Laceration of the uterus as a result of extension of the uterine incision, either through the uterine artery or a cervical branch of the uterine artery, is heralded by brisk, bright red bleeding. These sources must be carefully identified, since the ureter is likely to be in harm's way. The uterus may be markedly atonic at the time of cesarean delivery, just as it can be at the time of vaginal delivery.

The management of postpartum bleeding in the patient delivered of a multiple gestation must be considered an obstetric emergency. It is critical to activate a plan designed to identify the problem and correct the deficit. This plan should include the following steps:

1. Obtain help immediately. A physician is preferable but any medical attendant is valuable.

2. If you have diagnosed uterine atony, attempt to compress the uterus using the bimanual techniques.

3. Start at least two intravenous access lines with 15-gauge needles or angiocath.

4. Obtain blood for transfusion. Since all patients with multiple gestations should be screened and tested for blood type before labor, blood should be readily available.

5. Add oxytocin to the second intravenous access line. If this does not effectively restore uterine tone, add 250 μg of prostaglandin $F_{2\alpha}$ (carboprost tromethamine) intramuscularly. The prostaglandin may be administered at 15- to 90-minute intervals up to a maximum of 8 doses.

6. Explore the genital tract from the vagina to the cervix to the uterine cavity. If no lacerations are present in the vagina or cervix, curettage of the uterine cavity with a banjo curette may be helpful.

In the vast majority of cases, this procedure allows a correct diagnosis to be

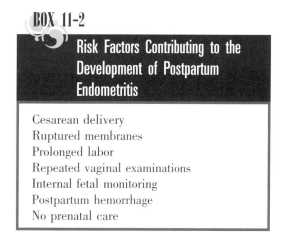

BOX 11-2

Risk Factors Contributing to the Development of Postpartum Endometritis

Cesarean delivery
Ruptured membranes
Prolonged labor
Repeated vaginal examinations
Internal fetal monitoring
Postpartum hemorrhage
No prenatal care

made and the hemorrhage to be brought under control. Fluid and blood resuscitation must be aggressive to maintain adequate circulation volume.

Postpartum Infection

Puerperal uterine infection involves the decidua and adjacent myometrium. The risk factors contributing to the development of postpartum endometritis in a multiple gestation include those shown in Box 11-2.

An elevation of the patient's temperature is usually suggestive of postpartum endometritis. Several commonly used definitions of febrile morbidity include a temperature of 38.0° C (100.4° F) or higher on any 2 of the first 10 days postpartum (exclusive of the first 24 hours), a temperature of 38.0° C (100.4° F) on two separate occasions 6 hours apart and 24 hours after delivery, or a temperature of 101° F (39° C) or higher occurring any time.

These definitions of febrile morbidity are commonly used and represent an effort to be consistent with the Joint Commission on Accreditation of Hospital Organizations (JCAHO) mandate that a pa-

TABLE 11-1

Characteristics of Mothers and Deliveries in Cases of Twin and Singleton Abdominal Delivery

	TWINS (%) N = 122	SINGLETONS (%) N = 761	P
Mothers younger than age 25	31.8	30.7	—
Primipara	62.2	55.5	—
Preterm delivery	69.6	23.0	0.0001
Previous cesarean delivery	7.3	27.5	0.0001
Present operation elective	36.8	40.2	—
Induction of labor	8.2	15.5	0.002
Contractions more than 6 hrs before cesarean section	27.8	44.6	0.001
Senior surgeon	15.7	25.5	0.02
ROM more than 6 hrs before cesarean section	24.0	30.7	—
Blood loss of more than 1000 ml	12.4	10.2	—
Clinical amnionitis	4.9	2.1	—

Modified from Suonio S, Huttunen M: Acta Obstet Gynecol Scand 73:313-315, 1994.

tient with a temperature elevation of 38.0° C (100.4° F) in the postoperative or postpartum period must be seen by a physician. It is a reasonable practice in clinical medicine for a clinician to react to the patient's first significant temperature elevation. The patient should be examined thoroughly, and if no focus of infection is found, the patient should be observed. When the temperature reaches 39.0° C (102.2° F) at any time postpartum or reaches 38.5° C (101.3° F) on two occasions 4 hours apart after the first 24 hours postpartum, the patient should be reevaluated, cultures and blood work should be obtained, and antibiotics should be started.

The risk of infectious morbidity after abdominal delivery is 7 times greater than vaginal delivery. Suonio and Huttunen[10] found the incidence of postpartum endometritis to be nearly 3 times greater after twin deliveries and the rate of abdominal wound infections to be 2 times higher (13.1% versus 4.7% for endometritis;

5.6% versus 3.0% for wound infections). Additionally, significantly more patients with twin deliveries require blood transfusion (10.7% versus 5.3%) (Tables 11-1 and 11-2).

The incidence of endometritis after a vaginal twin delivery was low in this study (2.6%), but it was still 4 times greater than the incidence in vaginal singleton deliveries.[10] The higher rate of endometritis after cesarean delivery is directly related to the increased rate of endometritis found after a vaginal twin delivery. The clinical problems of preterm labor, preterm premature rupture of membranes (PROM), and clinical chorioamnionitis contribute to this greater incidence.

Postpartum endometritis should be suspected when the patient's temperature becomes elevated, as previously described. The patient should be evaluated on the basis of her history, physical examination, pelvic examination, and laboratory test results.

TABLE 11-2

Complications after Twin and Singleton Abdominal Deliveries

	TWINS (%) N = 122	SINGLETONS (%) N = 761	P
Puerperal endometritis	13.1	4.7	0.0001
Abdominal wound infection	5.6	3.0	0.02
Sepsis	0	0.2	—
Wound hematoma	2.1	3.0	—
Thrombotic complication	0.8	0.1	—
Postoperative ileus	0	0.3	—
Blood transfusion	10.7	5.3	0.02

From Suonio S, Huttunen M: Acta Obstet Gynecol Scand 73:313, 1994.

The evaluation of the patient's history should focus on the length of hospitalization, because stays longer than 3 days before surgery are associated with colonization of hospital flora; on the history of preterm PROM and preterm labor, because they predispose the patient to colonization of the chorion and amnion with vaginal bacteria; on the use of antibiotics, because they alter the host microflora; and on a careful review of the operative records from the cesarean delivery.

A general physical examination should be performed to rule out sites of infection other than the operative site. The pelvic examination should include inspection of the perineum and a speculum examination of the vagina. The presence of a foul odor is an indication of either an intrauterine infection or the presence of retained products of conception within the uterus. The uterus should be explored. A ring forceps should be placed on the anterior cervical lip, and downward pressure should be exerted. This straightens the endocervical canal and endometrial junction to allow the insertion of an endometrial suction cu-

rette to collect a biopsy specimen, as well as exploration with ring forceps. Thus any lochial plug, blood clot, or retained placenta or membranes can be removed. A specimen of the endometrial lining to culture may also be obtained with the endometrial suction curette. The specimen should be placed in an anaerobic transport vial for the identification of aerobic, facultative, and anaerobic bacteria.

Specimens of blood and catheterized urine for culture should be obtained. A specimen for culture should be collected from the wound if the clinician suspects that the wound might be infected. A complete blood cell count and a serum creatinine level should be obtained. Leukocytosis of more than 15,000 cells/μl is usually found, but these findings may be difficult to interpret in the face of the physiologic leukocytosis of the early puerperium. The white blood cell count is valuable when observing the patient's response to therapy.

The therapy for postpartum endometritis involves broad spectrum antimicrobial agents that have an aerobic and anaerobic spectrum of activity. Parenteral therapy is indicated at this time and should be continued for a minimum of 72 hours and until the patient is afebrile for at least 24 hours. The use of clindamycin plus aminoglycoside has been a popular choice because these agents cover a wide spectrum of facultative and anaerobic bacteria. This regimen produces cure rates of approximately 90%.

The persistence of a fever after 48 to 72 hours is an indication to reevaluate the patient, the drugs being used, and the certainty of the diagnosis. As a general rule the cause of the infection is found at the operative site, but on occasion an extra-operative source can be located. Complications of endometritis that cause persistent fever despite appropriate antimicrobial therapy include parametrial cellulitis or abscess; infected bladder-flap hematomas; uterine incision dehiscence, especially if a vertical incision has been used; surgical incisional and pelvic abscesses; occluded ureters; and septic thrombophlebitis.

The patient must be reexamined. This determines the presence of an abdominal wound infection. A pelvic examination is helpful but may not be rewarding in the presence of a markedly tender uterus with abdominal tenderness. An ultrasonographic examination of the uterus and a computerized tomography (CT) scan should be done to determine the status of the uterine incision and the presence of masses or abscesses.

As mentioned, the initial course of therapy with appropriate antimicrobial agents achieves a cure rate of 90%. New information by Dinsmoor, Newton, and Gibbs[3] indicates that there is no benefit to prescribing oral antibiotics when the patient is discharged from the hospital if she has received at least 72 hours of antibiotic therapy and has been afebrile for at least 24 hours. This has been one institution's policy for more than 10 years, and no reason has been found to modify the policy.

The availability of newer beta-lactam antibiotics allows the obstetrician to use agents that may be less toxic and less costly than combination agents. Box 11-3 lists agents that offer physicians a wider selection of antimicrobials and that have been shown to be as effective as clindamycin plus aminoglycoside.

The approach taken toward treating the patient who has been delivered of multiple infants should be logical and aggressive. Evaluations should be thorough, and appropriate antimicrobial agents should be used. The vast majority of these patients are cured with a 3-day course of antibiotics. If the patient's fever persists, a thorough reevaluation must be done. The antibiotic may be changed, an abscess or hematoma may be drained, or a retained fragment of placenta may be removed. Use of single antibiotic agents may be benefi-

BOX 11-3

Antibiotic Agents Found to be Effective in Obstetric Infections

PENICILLINS

Mezlocillin
Ticarcillin
Piperacillin
Ampicillin/sulbactam
Ticarcillin/clavulanate
Piperacillin/tazobactam

OTHERS

Imipenem

CEPHALOSPORINS

Ceftizoxime
Cefotaxime
Cefotetan
Cefoxitin
Cefmetazole

cial because of ease of administration and decreased risk of adverse reactions.

Breast-Feeding Multiple Infants

The recommendation to feed full-term infants human milk for 1 year after birth derives from the milk's nutritional benefits, contributions to host defenses, gastrointestinal growth, and psychologic benefits of mother-infant bonding.[4] Preterm delivery presents an additional challenge to breast-feeding because of the physical separation of the mother from the hospitalized neonates and the realization that preterm infants are at risk for certain nutritional deficiencies of protein, sodium, fat, vitamin, calcium, and phosphorus. Nursing should be encouraged, because even partial human-milk feeding enhances host resistance. Multicomponent fortifiers are available to bring human milk up to meet the appropriate requirements for preterm infants.

The medical literature rarely considers breast-feeding issues that mothers of multiple infants face. They must confront a number of complicating issues. The mother has at least two newborns to feed and care for, but twins are more than 5 times as likely to be preterm or small for gestational age as a singleton infant. The maternal-fetal attachment process is often more difficult because of the physical separation of mother and infants.

Prenatal preparation for breast-feeding multiple infants should begin as early as possible. The mother-to-be must be made aware of the possibility of breast-feeding, advised of the possible complicating factors that could interfere with breast-feeding, and encouraged to assess her social support situation.

The advantages of breast-feeding multiple infants is that it ensures numerous mother-infant interactions and the enhancement of infant immunity by passively transferred immunoglobulin and lymphocytes. A relative disadvantage is that of the number of feedings. This drawback can be overcome by substituting expressed breast milk or artificial formula for some of the feedings.

Initiating lactation depends on the circumstances surrounding the birth and the condition of the mother and infants. When the infants are full-term and the mother is in good condition, the initiation of breast-feeding is the same as for singletons. Unrestricted breast-feeding for each infant is advised, because it fits the feeding stage and pattern of each infant. Avoiding night feedings during hospital stays and alternating breast-feeding with bottle feedings are to be avoided (Box 11-4). The simultaneous breast-feeding of two infants is not recommended until the mother demonstrates proper positioning and latch-on with each infant.[5]

If a preterm birth occurs, breast-feeding is often delayed for several weeks. The nurse should reinforce the benefits of breast-feeding and develop an acceptable breast-pumping routine. The pumping routine should begin as soon after delivery as possible. Most mothers prefer simultaneous pumping because of efficiency. Providing breast milk creates a meaningful relationship with the neonate during the time that breast-feeding is not possible. A new intervention (Kangaroo positioning) designed to promote closeness between the preterm infant and the mother has recently been described.[12,13]

As breast-feeding is initiated, feedings need to be coordinated. Any plan works,

BOX 11-4

Factors That May Enhance or Reduce Maternal Milk Supply

ENHANCERS	REDUCERS
Frequent milk expression	Failure to express milk often
Complete emptying at each session	Incomplete breast emptying
Rest and relaxation	Fatigue, anxiety, stress
Infant's improving condition	Worsening in infant's condition
Medication	Medication
Metoclopramide	Bromocriptine
Oxytocin	Antihistamines
Reserpines	Oral contraceptives
Phenothiazines	
Skin-to-skin contact	Maternal illness
Initiation of breast-feeding	Return to work
	Increased commitments in or out of the home

From Schanler RJ, Hurst NM: Semin Perinatol 18:476-484, 1994.

as long as the both neonates latch onto and obtain milk from the breast, each infant feeds often enough, and both breasts are offered if infants express interest. A variety of plans are available for incorporating alternating breasts and infants and days.[5] Whereas demand breast-feeding in the early weeks stimulates lactation, once lactation is established the goal is for mothers to attempt to establish infant routines that save time and coordinate simultaneous feedings.

Summary

Although many of the postpartum conditions are similar for mothers delivering singletons and multiple infants, the incidences of postpartum hemorrhage and endometritis are significantly increased with twin or higher-order multiple pregnancies. The obstetrician must be alert to these conditions. Postpartum hemorrhage should be anticipated and actively managed in a prospective manner. The incidence of postpartum endometritis can be decreased with prophylactic antibiotics. Endometritis occurs despite prophylactic antibiotics, and the obstetrician should be able to diagnose and treat the condition.

Breast-feeding is to be encouraged in women with multiple gestations, but prenatal planning is essential. Excellent communication between the physician and patient and the patient and lactation consultant is needed. With careful planning and continuing support of the patient, multiple neonates can be successfully breast-fed.

References

1. Cunningham G et al, editors: *Williams obstetrics*, ed 19, Norwalk, Conn, 1993, Appleton & Lange.
2. DeLeeuw NK et al: Correlation of red cell loss at delivery with changes in red cell mass, *Am J Obstet Gynecol* 100:1092-1101, 1968.
3. Dinsmoor MJ, Newton ER, Gibbs RS: A randomized, double-blind, placebo-controlled trial of oral antibiotic therapy following intravenous

antibiotic therapy for postpartum endometritis, *Obstet Gynecol* 77:60-62, 1991.

4. Fomon SJ et al: Recommendations for feeding normal infants, *Pediatrics* 1979;63:52-59, 1979.

5. Gromada KK: Breast-feeding more than one: multiples and tandem breast-feeding, *NAACOG Clinical Issues* 3:656-666, 1992.

6. Newton M: Postpartum hemorrhage, *Am J Obstet Gynecol* 94:711-717, 1966.

7. Pritchard J: Changes in blood volume during pregnancy and delivery, *Anesthesiology* 26:393-399, 1965.

8. Pritchard J et al: Blood volume changes in pregnancy and the puerperium. II. Red blood cell loss and changes in apparent blood volume during and following vaginal delivery, cesarean section, and cesarean section plus total hyster-

ectomy, *Am J Obstet Gynecol* 84:1271-1282, 1962.

9. Schanler RJ, Hurst NM: Human milk for the hospitalized preterm infant, *Semin Perinatol* 18:476-484, 1994.

10. Suonio S, Huttunen M: Puerperal endometritis after abdominal twin delivery, *Acta Obstet Gynecol Scand* 73:313-315, 1994.

11. Suonio S et al: Risk factors for fever endometritis and wound infection after abdominal delivery, *Int J Obstet Gynecol* 29:135-142, 1989.

12. Wahlberg V: Alternative care for premature infants: the "kangaroo" method advantages, risks and ethical questions, *Neonatologica* 4:362-367, 1987.

13. Whitelaw A et al: Skin-to-skin contact for very low birthweight infants and their mothers, *Arch Dis Child* 63:1377-1381, 1988.

12 Outcome

Deward H. Voss

The increased morbidity and mortality associated with multiple gestation may not be limited to the antepartum period. Although much of the neonatal morbidity and mortality of multiple gestations is related to prematurity, the long-term growth, development, and survival of the infants and children of these pregnancies are also of concern. Antepartum and peripartum events, as well as factors unique to multiple gestation, may influence the subsequent development. This chapter examines the morbidity and mortality associated with multiple gestation, as well as antenatal and peripartum factors that influence the subsequent long-term outcome.

Perinatal/Neonatal Morbidity and Mortality

When twin pregnancies are compared with singleton gestations, there is a significant increase in perinatal and neonatal mortality and morbidity. This increase is an international problem. National data from Austria, Hungary, New Zealand, Sweden, England and Wales, and the United States[10] show great variation in twinning incidence and perinatal mortality rates. Nonetheless, the risk of perinatal mortal-

ity consistently had an inverse relationship to birth weight and length of gestation.

Although it is higher than the mortality rate associated with singleton gestations, the mortality rate of infants from twin pregnancies, like that of singletons, has decreased in the past 30 years. In 1991 the Linked Birth/Infant Death Data Sets from the National Center for Health Statistics from 1960 and 1983 were used to compare the infant mortality rates of twins and singletons.[21] When data from 1960 were compared with data from 1983, the survival rate had improved for both twins and singletons when birth-weight–specific data were used. Infant mortality among twins in 1983 was still 4 to 5 times that of singletons. Twins did have a survival advantage when their birth weights were in the 1250 to 3000 gm range, even after adjustment for gestational age. The twin mortality risk related to neonatal respiratory disease, maternal causes, neonatal hemorrhage, and short gestation and low birth weight was 6 to 15 times that noted for singletons. The relative risk of sudden infant death syndrome (SIDS) for twin infants was twice that observed in singletons.

The relative risk and population-attributable risk for twins compared with singletons in the United States was reported by Powers and Kiely[30] in 1993. This study was based on the U.S. Linked Birth/Infant Death Data Sets from 1985 to 1986. Stillbirths were not recorded, and triplets or higher-order multiple births were not included for analysis. The data included infants with lethal congenital anomalies, and the relative risks reported were not corrected for these infants. The data set included 7,357,550 singletons (97.91%) and 156,690 twin infants (2.09%). When compared with singletons, twins were noted to have relative risks for all adverse outcomes analyzed. The high relative risk of infant death for all twins (5.43) was thought to be primarily secondary to the elevated relative risk of neonatal death (7.06). Even those twins who survived the neonatal period carried an increased relative risk of postneonatal death within the first year of life (2.75). The relative risks of very low birth-weight (VLBW) and low birth-weight (LBW) infants were elevated in twin gestations. Eighty-nine percent of the infants who did not survive the neonatal period were of VLBW (less than 1500 gm), whereas VLBW infants comprised only 59% of the neonatal deaths among singleton births. The association between VLBW and an increased relative risk of death for twins was strong in each of the time intervals examined.

The importance of birth weight was echoed in a study by Herruzo et al.[19] in which 488 twin pregnancies with neonates of 1000 gm or more were reviewed. In this report, 80% of the neonatal deaths involved newborns weighing less than 2000 gm. The neonatal mortality rate was not significantly different for twins (5.3/1000) and singletons (2.2/1000) when the neonates weighed 2500 gm or more.

Factors Influencing the Perinatal/Neonatal Outcome

The effect of gestational age and birth weight on the subsequent survival and ultimate outcome of an infant from a multiple gestation is apparent. Other factors, such as the route of delivery, birth order, and management of a malpresenting twin, have been studied to identify any compounding variables in the outcome of the multiple gestation. Because these factors are confounding and difficult to control independently, the results of the published studies are conflicting.

The route or method of delivery has been examined repeatedly for its potential influence on the survival and development of children from multiple gestations. Much of the information is conflicting, and many of the studies are hampered by low power because of the small numbers of multiple gestations. However, Rydhstrom, Ingemarrsson, and Ohrlander[34] studied the national data bank in Sweden, the Medical Birth Registry, National Board of Health and Welfare, Stockholm. This study was based on the outcome of 9368 LBW twins delivered between 1973 and 1985. During this time frame the perinatal mortality rate dropped, and the cesarean section rate increased from 7% to 10% to 45% to 50%. There appeared to be three distinct divisions in those 12 years that related to changing trends in obstetric practice. Despite the anticipated correlation between the perinatal mortality rate in the LBW infant and the route of delivery, when the data were analyzed for these three different periods, no causal relationship was found. The authors concluded that factors other than the increased rate in cesarean sections were responsible for the decreased perinatal morbidity observed.

Outcomes of twin pregnancies over an almost identical period were reported in a smaller, retrospective study in the United States by Thompson, Lyons, and Makowski.[41] The study group consisted of 341 pregnancies delivered at the University of Colorado Health Sciences Center from 1973 to 1983. When gestational age and birth weight were eliminated as variables there was no statistically significant difference between Twin A and Twin B in overall outcome, although Twin B was noted to have a higher morbidity in the 35- to 39-week group. The perinatal mortality rate for Twin B was noted to be significantly greater than that for Twin A if both were delivered vaginally. This statistical difference was not seen if Twin A was delivered vaginally and Twin B was delivered abdominally. Notably, the overall perinatal mortality rate for both twins was higher when both were delivered vaginally than if both twins were delivered by cesarean section. This difference was not related to gestational age or a higher rate of morbidity in the operative delivery of Twin B. The authors noted that the numbers reported were small and that a recommendation to deliver all twins by cesarean section could not be supported by the results of their review.

Specific factors that may place the second born at increased risk were studied by Young et al.[42] in 80 twin pairs. Those factors found to be significantly in favor of

Twin A included the 1-minute Apgar score; umbilical venous pH, pO_2, and pCO_2 values, and the level of umbilical arterial pO_2. These differences were persistently in favor of the firstborn twin despite controls for other confounding factors such as route of delivery, interval between delivery of the twins, and possible effects of malpresentation. The authors suggested that the second-born twin may be at increased risk for hypoxia and trauma.

The influence of birth order has also been noted by several other authors. In 1990 Spellacy, Handler, and Ferre[39] reported a retrospective review of infants weighing more than 500 gm, including 1253 twin gestations. As in other studies, the mortality rate for each twin was significantly higher than that for a singleton. The rates of neonatal death for Twin A and Twin B were 33.3/1000 and 33.9/1000, respectively, compared with a rate of 5.6/1000 for singletons. Even more striking, the perinatal death rates for Twin A and Twin B were 48.8/1000 and 64.1/1000, compared with a rate of 10.4/1000 births of singletons. Birth weight did appear to influence this factor as well. When stratified by birth weight, the neonatal mortality rate for Twin A was lower than that for singletons weighing 2500 gm or less, but the rate for Twin B was higher than that for Twin A and for singletons. If the birth weight was more than 2500 gm, the neonatal death rate for both twins was higher than that for singletons; however, at this birth weight the neonatal death rate for Twin A was higher than that for Twin B. Moreover, if the twins had concordant weights, the perinatal mortality rates for Twin A and Twin B were similar. However, when weights differed by more than 10%, there was an increasing difference in perinatal mortalities rates. If a difference of more than 25% was noted, the mortality odds ratio became 1:7.

Also in 1990, the factors associated with neonatal morbidity and mortality in twin gestations in Israel were reported by Fraser, Picard, and Picard.[15] The outcomes of 644 twins with birth weights of 500 gm or more were compared with a control group of 656 singletons. A fourfold risk of antepartum death was noted in twins over singletons; however, this risk was not significant when birth weight was eliminated as a confounding variable. In fact, when other outcome measures were examined, such as rates of hyaline membrane disease (HMD), hypoglycemia, hyperbilirubinemia, anemia, and septicemia, hypoglycemia was the only factor with an increased risk after adjustments for birth weight. Controlling for route of delivery and gestational age were not as effective as controlling for birth weight.

The relationship of birth weight and birth order was also noted by Herruzo et al.[19] Although it was not significantly different, a general trend was noted. Neonatal mortality in the first twin was only 12.1%, versus 24.2% in the second twin. Again, when the outcomes for infants with birth weights less than 2000 gm were examined, Twin B had a poorer outcome. This difference was more pronounced if the birth weight was less than 1500 gm. Among the twins with birth weights of 2000 gm or more, first-born twins again had a higher mortality rate than second-born twins.

The issue of birth order, as well as the effects of gender and intrauterine growth retardation (IUGR), on the neonatal outcome of VLBW twins was examined by Chen, Vohr, and Oh.[11] Forty-four pairs of live-born twins with birth weights of less than 1501 gm were studied. Twins were defined as having IUGR if their birth weights were less than the 10th percentile for their gestational age. A multiple logistic regression analysis was performed with the predictor variables of gestational age, IUGR, and sex; the outcome variables were mortality rate, bronchopulmonary dysplasia, and interventricular hemorrhage. When confounding factors were controlled, the only variables that had a significant effect on outcome were gestational age and IUGR. Gestational age influenced the mortality rates with an increase in the odds ratio of 1:8 (CI = 1.3 to 2.3) for each week that gestational age decreased. Each decreasing week of gestational age also increased the odds ratio for bronchopulmonary dysplasia and intraventricular hemorrhage (2:2 [CI = 1.4 to 3.5] and 4:3 [CI = 1.2 to 1.9] respectively). The presence of IUGR increased the odds ratio of twin neonatal mortality (5:2 [CI = 1.5 to 18.1]). Male gender was associated with an odds ratio for bronchopulmonary dysplasia of 4:3 (CI = 1.1 to 15.8). Other risk factors that did not significantly influence the measured outcome parameters included presentation at birth, mode of delivery, or birth order.

The specific influence of route of delivery on the second-born twin with a non-vertex presentation has been the subject of many recent studies and controversy. In 1988, Laros and Dattel[22] reported the results of a 10-year retrospective review (1976 to 1985) of 206 pairs of twins. A significant difference was seen if sets of twins delivered by cesarean section were compared with sets of twins delivered vaginally. The perinatal mortality rate for twins delivered by cesarean section was 121/1000, compared with a rate of 336/1000 for those delivered vaginally. There were 36 infants with birth weights of less than 750 gm in the vaginal delivery group, compared with only two in the cesarean group, which may have biased this comparison. When twins delivered by cesarean section were compared, only the 5-minute Apgar and the umbilical artery pO_2 were noted to be slightly lower in Twin B. Similarly, statistically significant differences in 1-minute and 5-minute Apgar scores and cord blood gas levels were seen between Twin A and Twin B if the twins were delivered vaginally. In this study no significant correlation was seen if the interval between deliveries, the method of delivery of Twin B, and the second-twin malpresentation were eliminated as confounding variables.

The management of the nonvertex second twin was examined by Gocke et al.[16] in a 1989 study of 682 consecutive twin deliveries. There were 136 sets of vertex-nonvertex twins with birth weights of more than 1500 gm identified. Second twins delivered by a primary attempt at external version, attempted breech extraction, and primary cesarean section were compared. No statistically significant differences were noted in the incidence of neonatal morbidity or mortality among the groups. The influence of the presentation and method of delivery on the outcome of the second twin was also the subject of a study reported by Adam, Alexander, and Baskett.[1] There were 397 sets of twins with birth weights of more than 1000 gm and no lethal anomalies identified in 578 sets of twins delivered from 1980 to 1987. When the fetal weight was greater than 1500 gm, there was no significant difference noted in the perina-

tal death rate, nor was there a significant difference in perinatal mortality when the second twin was delivered by cesarean section instead of vaginally. The only significant perinatal morbidity or mortality was found in infants with weights less than 1500 gm or fewer than 32 weeks' gestation.

The influence of method of delivery and presentation on the outcome of second twins, including infants weighing less than 1500 gm was also the subject of a report by Greig et al.[18] A retrospective study comparing the outcome of 457 sets of twins delivered between 1985 and 1990 was conducted. Second-born infants from these deliveries were stratified by 500-gm weight intervals and divided into the following four groups by presentation and route of delivery: nonvertex/cesarean, nonvertex/vaginal, vertex/cesarean, and vertex/vaginal. No significant differences were noted in 5-minute Apgar scores, venous and arterial pH, number of days of hospitalization, number of infants intubated, length of mechanical ventilation, and incidence of intraventricular hemorrhage among the four groups. Mortality rates were not significantly different among the four groups when birth weight and gestational age were controlled. Similarly, in 1992 Davison et al.[14] compared the outcomes of 54 second twins delivered by breech extraction with weights between 750 and 2000 gm with the outcomes of their siblings and 43 sets of twins delivered by cesarean section for malpresentation. Although the first-born twins delivered vaginally had a significantly shorter length of mechanical ventilation than the breech-extracted siblings, the second-born twins delivered by breech extraction did not differ in any neonatal outcome measure from the second-born twins delivered by cesarean section. These results were unchanged when infants weighing more than 1500 gm were excluded from analysis.

Long-Term Outcome

In addition to increased perinatal and infant mortality, infants from multiple gestations contribute significantly to the number of infants with postneonatal handicaps. The mortality rates and the risk of handicap for infants from singleton, twin, and triplet pregnancies were presented by Luke and Keith.[26] In this study the rates of infant mortality, postneonatal mortality, and handicap were extracted from the National Infant Mortality Surveillance (NIMS) Project, and birth-weight–specific postneonatal handicap rates were taken from the Office of Technology Assessment report Healthy Children in proportion to the 1988 U.S. birth cohort. As in other studies, the risks of an LBW infant or a VLBW infant were markedly elevated in the multiple gestation. The risks of infant mortality were 6.6 and 19.4 for twins and triplets, respectively, when compared with singletons. Infants of twin and triplet gestations who survived the neonatal period had relative risks of severe handicap of 1.7 and 2.9, respectively, when compared with singletons. The overall relative risk of handicap was likewise increased for twins and triplets to 1.4 and 2.0, respectively. The rate of severe handicap in surviving twins was 34/1000 compared with 57.5/1000 and 19.7/1000 for triplets and singletons, respectively.

The potential increased risk of poor performance for the LBW twin was the focus of a report by Akerman and Thomassen[3] in 1992. Thirty-four pairs of twins without evidence of cerebral injury at birth were evaluated at ages 9 months, 18 months, and 4 years for development and behavior. These twin pairs were tested with the Griffiths Mental Development Scale in the following areas: locomotor abilities, personal-social skills, hearing and speech, hand and eye coordination, performance, and practical reasoning. Prematurity was defined as delivery before 37 weeks' gestation, and LBW was determined to be less than 2500 gm. Six infants were noted to have physical handicaps and were among the twins who did have some impairment at 4 years of age. Seven twin pairs were premature, and at ages 9 months and 18 months demonstrated statistically significant lower quotients in all subscales and total test scores than full-term twins. Although the total test scores remained significantly lower for premature twins, there was no significant difference noted between 4-year-old premature twins and full-term twins in the subtests for personal-social skills, hearing and speech, and performance. When LBW twins were compared with twins having birth weights of 2500 gm or more, these differences were smaller than they were when prematurity was studied. At age 4, 22 children (32%) were found to have significant physical and emotional problems. Nineteen of the 22 were either born prematurely or weighed less than 2500 gm at birth.

The long-term outcome of the surviving, VLBW infant was reviewed by Leonard et al.[23] The study population consisted of all infants with birth weights of 1250 gm or less delivered between 1977 and 1987 at the University of California at San Francisco. Ninety-two percent, or 365 infants, were available for evaluation at age 1. Subsequently, 73% of these infants were available for analysis at school age. Neurodevelopmental examination and standard developmental tests were used to assess outcome. Variables studied and included in logistic regression analysis were type of gestation, birth weight, gestational age, intracranial hemorrhage, chronic lung disease, and social risk factor. At age 1, there were no significant differences in the neurologic outcomes of the infants from multiple gestations and the infants from singleton pregnancies. At school age, the outcome of the two groups was again similar. Eight percent of the children from multiple gestations and 8.6% in the singleton group had cerebral palsy or some other functional motor deficit. In the multiple-gestation group, birth order was not associated with or predictive of outcome, and single survivors of multiple gestations did not demonstrate an improved outcome over multiple survivors. Of the independent variables studied, chronic lung disease was the only medical risk factor that showed a significant relationship to subsequent decreased cognitive performance. Those infants who required at least 60 days of supplemental oxygen therapy may have been more chronically ill and may have had significantly lower cognitive function when tested. Additionally, children in both groups were at an increased risk of a poorer outcome at school age if they had been referred to children's protective services. The authors concluded that the developmental outcome in VLBW infants was related to medical and social risk factors but was not significantly worse in infants of multiple gestations.

The influence of fetal nutrition or malnutrition and in utero growth on subsequent growth and development was examined in a cross-sectional study by Chamberlain and Simpson[9] in 1977. In this study, the physical growth of children who were the products of twin gestations, postmature infants, and small-for-dates infants were compared with that of children in a random control group. There were 198 3-year-old twins examined. The twin children were found to be lighter and shorter (p < 0.01), but their body build did not vary significantly from that of the random controls. The children of twin pregnancies had relatively large heads for their bodies. At this same age, the differences noted between postmature infants and the random controls had disappeared. These findings suggest that intrauterine malnutrition, unless it is the result of a prolonged postdate pregnancy, may have some influence on subsequent growth and development.

A study examining some perinatal, environmental, experiential, and developmental characteristics of twins in contrast to singletons was presented by McDiarmid and Silva[27] in 1979. The study was based on a population of 24 twin and 1013 singleton infants with follow-up at age 3 as part of a longitudinal study performed in New Zealand. These children were delivered between April 1, 1972 and March 31, 1973. The occurrence of birth hypoxia was noted in 8% of twins versus 1% of singletons, and twins had decreased birth weights and gestational ages when compared with singletons. The early development of twins was significantly slower (smiling, talking in single words and sentences, self-feeding with a spoon, bladder control), and twins were noted to be significantly shorter and lighter and to have smaller head circumferences. Additionally, twins were noted to have significant delays in verbal comprehension and verbal expression, with a delay in language of approximately 3 months. There was no delay in motor development or in the incidence of abnormal behavior. When twins were matched for the risk factors noted above, almost every measurement lost significance. The only developmental difference that retained statistical significance after matching for perinatal risk factors was an early delay in using single words and sentences. At the age 3, differences in verbal comprehension and expression, as well as in differences in physical development, motor development, and abnormal behavior, were not significant.

Silva, McGee, and Powell[37] provided subsequent follow-up data on this same study population at the ages of 5 and 7. All growth measurements were significantly different; the twins were 4.7 cm shorter, 2.8 kg lighter, and had head circumferences that were an average of 1.4 cm smaller. They also had mean IQ scores that were 7 points lower at age 7. There were no significant differences in verbal comprehension, verbal expression, or reading abilities. Silva and Crosado[36] provided additional follow-up data at ages 9 and 11. At age 9, 21 pairs of the twins were studied, and at age 11 only 13 pairs were available for study. This study failed to demonstrate any significant differences between twins and singletons in verbal comprehension or verbal expression at age 9, and there were no differences in reading or spelling skills at either age. The mean full scale and verbal IQ of the twins studied was significantly lower than that of the singletons, but there was not a significant difference in the performance IQ at either age. The opinion of the authors was that these differences were not of any practical importance. The differences

noted in physical growth in all previous assessment were again noted and could not support any "catch-up" growth by twins.

Differences in the physical growth and mental and neurologic development of twins beyond infancy, childhood, and adolescence has been the subject of several long-term, ongoing studies. A longitudinal study of twins and singletons from birth to age 18 was provided by Akerman and Fischbein[2] in 1991. This Swedish study was performed on 145 twin pairs and a whole cohort of singletons (n = 114,828) born in 1953. The authors provided a brief review of older studies and summarized previous research, noting a "twin handicap" in both physical and mental growth that is more evident in girls than in twin boys. The contradictions in previous study results was acknowledged. Information was gathered from birth registers regarding complications during pregnancy and from ability tests and questionnaires conducted in school. Additionally, complementary data for boys was collected at time of enrollment to military service. The results show that monozygotic twins tended to have lower average scores on the ability test at grade 6 than dizygotic twins; when compared with singletons, both twin boys and girls had lower average scores. Although both verbal and numerical test scores were significantly lower for the twin girls, the twin boys demonstrated a significantly lower average score only on the verbal test scores. The monozygotic twins tended to have lower school grades than did dizygotic twins in grades 6 and 9, but this difference was only statistically significant in the ninth grade. Differences in twins and singletons with regard to school marks was only significant in grade 9 for twin boys. Differences in physical growth for males was extracted from the data obtained at military enrollment. At age 18, a statistically significant difference was noted in height, weight, and muscular strength between twins and singletons; twins were slightly shorter and lighter, and they had slightly less physical strength than the controls.

In this same study, Akerman and Fischbein[2] examined the importance of birth weight and social background for its influence on subsequent mental growth. When birth weight was eliminated as a factor, LBW (defined as less than 2500 gm), was found to be a significant risk factor for handicap in mental growth at both ages 13 and 18. LBW twins, boys more than girls, had significantly lower test scores on all tests at age 13 and lower spatial ability test scores at age 18. As might be expected, social background was found to influence the abilities of both twins and singletons. A stimulating home environment did allow the LBW twin boys to compensate, but this effect was not seen in the LBW girls at ages 13 and 18. The authors concluded that when compared with singletons, monozygotic twins—particularly twin girls—are at a disadvantage in school achievement and ability testing at ages 13, 16, and 18. Additionally, a "twin handicap" was noted in mental and physical growth for 18-year-old male twins compared with singletons.

Similar long-term follow-up was provided by Moilanen and Rantakallio.[28] In this 19-year Finnish study of 289 twins and 11,623 singletons who were alive at 28 days from a 1-year birth cohort were used to match the twins to two sets of controls. Controls were matched either by maternal factors only or by maternal factors and perinatal morbidity. The twin pregnancies were complicated more often

by premature delivery and by infants who were small for gestational age. The twins had a higher rate of perinatal asphyxia, hyperbilirubinemia, and hypoglycemia. Twins suffered from cerebral palsy and mental retardation in 4/314 (1.3%) and 6/314 (1.9%) of the cases, respectively. The comparable rate of cerebral palsy and mental retardation in singletons was 65/11,744 (0.6%) and 159/11,744 (1.3%), respectively. Although the rates of these complications were higher in twins, the difference did not reach statistical significance. The twins' motor development, assessed by their ability to walk, was delayed. This difference was not seen when the controls, matched by perinatal morbidity and maternal factors, were used for this comparison. The twins had delayed language development when compared with singletons, but not when perinatal morbidity was controlled. With regard to long-term development, "several perinatal and environmental factors" were found by logistic regression that influenced the abilities of these individuals as adolescents.[28] The logistic regression analysis was felt to "confirm the hypothesis . . . that some mild difficulties in the development and education of twins are most probably caused by their high perinatal morbidity and not by the twin situation itself."[28]

High-Order Multiple Births

As with twin gestations, the incidence of high-order multiple births has increased dramatically in the last 2 decades because of increasing maternal age and the increased use of agents for ovulation induction (OI) and other methods of assisted reproduction. Fortunately, as the high-order multiple gestation has become a more common challenge for the obstetrician, improvements in neonatal care have provided an improved outcome for these pregnancies. Although twins have received extensive attention in the literature, the relative rarity of triplets and even higher-order multiple gestations has precluded studies of large series. The current outcome and management of triplet and quadruplet pregnancies was reviewed by Ron-El et al.[32] in 1981. Nineteen triplet and 6 quadruplet pregnancies delivered in Tel Aviv, Israel from 1970 through 1978 were included. The mean gestational ages for triplet and quadruplet pregnancies at delivery were 34 and 35 weeks, respectively. The overall perinatal mortality rate in this population was 185/1000; if only those gestations lasting 28 weeks longer or with infants weighing 1000 gm or more were considered, the corrected perinatal mortality rate fell to 137/1000. The outcome was similar between those infants delivered by cesarean section and those delivered vaginally when gestational age was stratified. Most of the neonatal complications were the result of prematurity. The prematurity rate in this study was 68%.

In a 1989 study that took place in Israel,[24] the outcomes of 78 triplet pregnancies with gestational ages of 20 weeks or more was reported. Neonatal outcomes were reported only if the birth weights were less than 1500 gm, because 49% of the infants weighing more than 1500 gm had been lost to follow-up. The most common complication of these pregnancies was premature labor, occurring in 78.2%. None of the fetuses delivered at fewer than 27 weeks' gestation survived. The perinatal mortality rate was 93/1000, and the neonatal mortality rate was 51/1000 live births. If the birth weights were greater than 1000 gm, the neonatal mortality rate was 5/1000 live births. The perinatal mortality rate in each gestational age was not significantly different for those infants delivered by cesarean section or vaginally in pregnancies with 26 weeks' gestation or more. When birth order was examined, the first- and second-born infants did not differ significantly, but the third-born infant had a significantly increased incidence of a low 1-minute Apgar scores and respiratory disorders. This difference in the third-born infant was significant when comparing vaginally delivered third-born infants with those delivered by cesarean section. In this same study, 1-year follow-up data were available for 38 of the 48 surviving infants with birth weights of less than 1500 gm. Only 10.5% of the infants were found to have severe disabilities.

In a 1990 report from Canada, Gonen et al.[17] provided outcome data on 30 high-order multiple gestations delivered from 1978 to 1988. In this series there were 1 quintuplet, 5 quadruplet, and 24 triplet pregnancies. The perinatal mortality rate was 51.5/1000, and the survival-to-discharge rate was 93%. Seventy-nine percent of the triplet gestations were complicated by premature labor, as were all of the higher-order multiple gestations in this study.

The improvements in perinatal morbidity and mortality in triplet pregnancies was the focus of a review by Creinin, Katz, and Laros.[13] This study was limited to a review of 13 sets of triplets delivered from 1981 through 1988 at the University of California at San Francisco. Three additional sets of triplets were delivered before viability and were not included in analysis. As in other studies, 77% of these pregnancies were complicated by premature labor, and the mean gestational age at delivery was 33.9 weeks. An attempt was made to deliver one pregnancy vaginally; however, intrapartum complications after the delivery of the first infant prompted an emergency cesarean section for the delivery of the remaining infants. Only neonates with birth weights of less than 2000 gm had complications. Neonatal complications noted included hyperbilirubinemia (51.3%), hypoglycemia (30.8%), respiratory distress syndrome (RDS) (28.2%), respiratory compromise (23.1%), anemia (17.9%), patent ductus arteriosus (15.4%), and intraventricular hemorrhage (10.3%). Overall, 80% of pregnancies were associated with some morbidity; there were no neonatal mortalities. All morbidity was in infants with average birth weights of less than 2000 gm and fewer than 35 weeks' gestation. In this study, the second- and third-born infants did not have a significantly higher rate of morbidity.

In 1992 Ron-El et al.[33] provided a report on the outcomes of 46 higher-order gestations, specifically 37 triplet, 7 quadruplet, and 2 quintuplet pregnancies. These births occurred from 1974 to 1984 in Tel Aviv, Israel. Similar to the results of other reports, 78% of these pregnancies ended in premature delivery, which was thought to be the main complication of these gestations. Fetal growth retardation was noted in 15.2%, 12.6%, and 17.3% of triplet, quadruplet, and quintuplet gestations, respectively. The perinatal mortality rate of the study group was 14.8% and did not differ significantly when cesarean section was compared with vaginal delivery. The perinatal mortality rate for those gestations shorter than 28 weeks was 9.4%.

Data from Ireland reported by Byrne et al.[8] support similar outcome results in 19 sets of triplets delivered from 1980 to 1990. The prematurity rate was 79%, the mean gestational age at delivery was 34 weeks, and the overall perinatal mortality rate was 35/1000. These authors noted that prematurity was more important than birth weight or birth order in determining fetal morbidity. The perinatal mortality rate was equivalent to that of twin pregnancies over the same period.

Two contemporary reports on the management and outcome of quadruplet or higher-order multiple gestations were published in 1990. Collins and Bleyl[12] analyzed 71 quadruplet pregnancies delivered between 1980 and 1989. The mean gestational age at delivery was 31.4 weeks, and the mean birth weight was 1482 gm. Ten stillbirths were noted, and there were 33 neonatal deaths. The stillbirth rate was 29/1000, and the neonatal and perinatal mortality rates were 123/1000 and 147/1000, respectively. If these mortality rates are corrected for neonatal deaths that occurred before 28 weeks' gestation, the neonatal and perinatal mortality rates were 37/1000 and 47/1000, respectively. In 70 of the 71 pregnancies, premature labor was noted to be a complication, with a range of gestational age at delivery of 20 to 38 weeks. Seventy-three percent and 87% of the patients were delivered of there infants after 30 and 28 weeks, respectively. The number of fetuses regarded as growth retarded by singleton standards dramatically increased at 34 weeks' gestation.

Lipitz et al.[25] reported a study of 11 high-order multiple gestations delivered from 1975 to 1989. These pregnancies consisted of 1 sextuplet, 2 quintuplet, and 8 quadruplet pregnancies. Seventy-four percent of the live-born infants had birth weights of less than 1500 gm, and 41% were small for gestational age (that is, below the 10th percentile). The fetal loss rate was 23%, and when the stillborn fetuses weighing less than 500 gm were excluded, the perinatal mortality rate was 119/1000. The authors did note that a major problem during the management of these pregnancies was the difficulty and uncertainty of antenatal assessment of individual fetal well-being.

Long-Term Outcome of High-Order Multiple Gestations

Few studies are available that provide insight to the long-term outcome of triplet or higher-order multiple pregnancies. In the 1990 report by Gonen et al.,[17] detailed follow-up was provided. One- to 10-year follow-up of the infants from these pregnancies showed somatic growth between the fifth and ninety-fifth percentile for 94% of the infants. Eighty-six percent of the infants did not show any neurologic deficit. Ten infants (12%) had mild hypotonia that was considered functional and expected to resolve. One of these infants did show mild spastic diplegia, and another one who was delivered at 25 weeks' gestation had a moderate neurologic deficit. Fully 76% of the infants were considered to have normal development. The same 10 infants who showed hypotonia demonstrated a mild delay in gross motor development. Mild language delay was noted in 8% of the infants, and mild delay in cognitive development was recorded in 2% of the infants. Seventy-four percent of the infants did not show any chronic or significant medical problems. The most common medical problems noted in the other 26% were reactive airway disease and otitis; the rate of these did not exceed the anticipated incidence among other children of similar age. The infant born at 25 weeks' gestation did have retinopathy of prematurity. In summary, when the three infants with congenital malformations were excluded, only one of the 84 children (1.2%) demonstrated a major handicap or significant medical problem.

In the study by Lipitz et al.[25] of 11 high-order multiple gestations, 2-year follow-up data was provided. Of the surviving infants, 70% demonstrated normal development, and a diagnosis of IUGR did not show any association with a higher risk of developmental delay. Two-year follow-up was available for seven sets of infants, and in only three of those sets were all of the infants neurodevelopmentally normal.

Special Concerns

For decades, infants of multiple gestations, particularly twins, have been considered to have an increased risk for both cerebral palsy and SIDS. The cause of both problems remains elusive, but the relationship of each to multiple gestations should be examined.

Much of the data available regarding cerebral palsy in the infant of a multiple gestation are outdated and of little help. The increased rate of cerebral palsy that has been noted in multiple births may be related to the increased risk of premature birth and IUGR. An increased risk of cerebral palsy has been suggested for the surviving twin when there is antenatal death of a monoamniotic cotwin.[29,35,40]

Interesting data have been reported about the risk twins have for SIDS. In a comprehensive review of the epidemiology of SIDS in Finland from 1969 to 1980, twins were noted to be more common among SIDS infants than infants from the general population.[31] Of the multiple risk factors examined, the most important risk factor was maternal smoking during pregnancy. A more specific review of SIDS in twins was provided by Kahn et al.[20] There were 114 characteristics of these twin pairs examined, and only 11 variables reached statistical significance. When compared with a control group of normal twins, the importance of these characteristics came into question because they were seen at comparable rates in the normal controls. Although a significant number of the victims of SIDS were noted to have had episodes of cyanosis or pallor or repeated episodes of profuse sweating during sleep, these characteristics could not be found in any of the infants in the control group. Additionally, the SIDS infants were noted to have a lower mean heights and weights at birth and were often significantly lighter than the surviving twins.

The possible importance of birth weight in twins and the relationship of twin gestations to SIDS was again noted by Beal.[5] The incidence of SIDS in South Australia from 1970 to 1988 was reported to be 2.0/1000 live births. Of all births, 0.35% were noted to be twins who were growth retarded compared with their cotwins. In this review, each victim of SIDS was noted to be the twin with the lower birth weight if discordant birth weight had been noted. The twin that was growth retarded when compared with its cotwin was noted to have a risk of SIDS of 44/1000, 22 times the risk of the general population. The subsequent incidence of SIDS in the surviving cotwin was noted to be rare, approximately 1%.[6,7] Simultaneous SIDS in twins, or both members of the twin gestation being found dead on the same day, was reported more often than the subsequent SIDS death of a surviving cotwin.

The phenomenon of simultaneous SIDS death in twins has been the focus of controversy and conflicting reports. In 1986 Smialek[38] lent support to the credibility of this phenomenon. He reviewed the literature and provided a history of 9 such cases (8 in the United States). However, in 1989 Bass[4] subsequently examined 13 of the simultaneous twin SIDS cases in the United States. Although the original investigation had led to a diagnosis of SIDS, he proposed that an environmental hazard was present and the probable cause in each case. The author concluded that in most instances the twins' deaths were preventable.

Controversy surrounding a reported increased incidence of either cerebral palsy or SIDS among infants of multiple gestations is understandable. Both conditions are poorly understood and have multiple causes. Both cerebral palsy and SIDS deaths are more common in the offspring of a multiple gestation, but multiple pregnancies often are complicated by prematurity and low birth weight—factors that may be important risk factors in both cerebral palsy and SIDS. Further investigation into the causes of both conditions and the true incidence of each condition in infants from multiple gestations is necessary before a more definitive statement can be made.

Summary

The higher perinatal morbidity and mortality rates of multiple gestations has been long recognized and is an international problem. Although the rate of twin gestations and higher-order multiple gestations has been increasing, the mortality associated with these pregnancies has decreased in the last several decades because of advances in neonatal and obstetric care. Despite these advances, the risk of perinatal morbidity and mortality in a twin gestation is 4 to 5 times that of a singleton gestation and increases with the magnitude of the multiple gestation. There is clearly a direct relationship between the morbidity and mortality of multiple gestations and the significantly higher rate of preterm deliveries, as well as the increased incidence of the small-for-gestational-age infants associated with these pregnancies. Furthermore, recognizing the increased risk of maternal disease or pregnancy complications, such as pregnancy-induced hypertensive disease, gestational diabetes mellitis, and congenital malformations, is important in understanding the increased risk of the poor obstetric outcome associated with multiple gestations. When gestational age, LBW, or VLBW, as well as congenital malformations and pregnancy complications, are eliminated as confounding factors, the data concerning other possible factors that may increase the perinatal morbidity and mortality of multiple gestations are conflicting and confusing. Some studies have suggested that birth order, fetal gender, route of delivery, and management of the malpresenting twin are important factors in perinatal outcome, whereas other authorities have not been able to confirm these findings and have therefore refuted their importance.

Perhaps an even more difficult issue to study is the long-term outcome of multiple gestations. Infants of multiple gestations who survive the neonatal period, particularly those of VLBW, may be at increased risk of death in the first year of life. The increased risk of SIDS and cerebral palsy that has often been associated with multiple gestations has been questioned in recent years, and studies concerning these issues are also conflicting and controversial. Some studies performed to evaluate the growth and development of these infants through childhood and adolescence have shown an increased risk of delay in somatic growth, motor development, language development, behavioral and emotional development, and even intelligence. As with other outcome measures of multiple gestations, the confounding variables, especially environmental influences, are difficult to control and the data regarding long-term outcomes are conflicting. Although some of the studies have demonstrated a statistical difference in children or adolescents from multiple gestations and controls from singleton gestations, the practical or clinical significance of these differences is questionable. The increased risk of difficulties in the long-term outcome of the infant of a multiple gestation is most clearly related to the increased risk of perinatal morbidity and not so clearly a product of the phenomenon of the multiple gestation.

Since the perinatal and subsequent long-term outcome of the multiple gestation pregnancy is most directly related to the length of gestation and appropriate birth weight, efforts to improve the outcome of these pregnancies should focus on the prevention of prematurity and delivery of the LBW or VLBW infants. Patients who are at increased risk of multiple gestation (such as those undergoing assisted reproduction) or those who are found to have a multiple gestation should be warned of the increased risk of a poor outcome; these patients should be attended to more intensely. With an increasing rate of multiple gestations, additional studies to more clearly define the risk of a poor outcome as well as the factors that influence the outcome are needed.

References

1. Adam C, Alexander CA, Baskett TF: Twin delivery: influence of the presentation and method of delivery on the second twin, *Am J Obstet Gynecol* 165:23-27, 1991.
2. Akerman BA, Fischbein S: Twins: are they at risk? A longitudinal study of twins and nontwins from birth to 18 years of age, *Acta Genet Med Gemellol (Roma)* 40:29-40, 1991.
3. Akerman BA, Thomassen PA: The fate of "small twins": a four-year follow-up study of low birthweight and prematurely born twins. *Acta Genet Med Gemellol (Roma)* 41:97-104, 1992.
4. Bass M: The fallacy of the simultaneous sudden infant death syndrome in twins, *Am J Forensic Med Pathol* 10:200-205, 1989.
5. Beal S: Sudden infant death syndrome in twins, *Pediatrics* 84:1038-1044, 1989.
6. Beal S: Siblings of sudden infant death syndrome victims, *Clin Perinatol* 19:839-848, 1992.
7. Beal SM, Blundell HK: Recurrence incidence of sudden infant death syndrome, *Arch Dis Child* 63:924-930, 1988.
8. Byrne BM, Rasmussen MJ, Stronge JM: A review of triplet pregnancy, *Ir Med J* 86:55-57, 1993.
9. Chamberlain RN, Simpson RN: Cross-sectional studies of physical growth in twins, postmature and small-for-dates children, *Acta Paediatr* 66:457-463, 1977.
10. Chaurasia AR: Perinatal mortality in twins, *Acta Genet Med Gemellol (Roma)* 29:237-239, 1980.
11. Chen SJ, Vohr BR, Oh W: Effects of birth order, gender, and intrauterine growth retardation on the outcome of very low birth weight in twins, *J Pediatr* 123:132-136, 1993.
12. Collins MS, Bleyl JA: Seventy-one quadruplet pregnancies: management and outcome, *Am J Obstet Gynecol* 162:1384-1392, 1990.
13. Creinin M, Katz M, Laros R: Triplet pregnancy: changes in morbidity and mortality, *J Perinatol* 11:207-212, 1991.
14. Davison L et al: Breech extraction of low-birth-weight second twins: can cesarean section be justified? *Am J Obstet Gynecol* 166:497-502, 1992.
15. Fraser D, Picard R, Picard E: Factors associated with neonatal problems in twin gestations, *Acta Genet Med Gemellol (Roma)* 40:193-200, 1991.
16. Gocke SE et al: Management of the nonvertex second twin: primary cesarean section, external version, or primary breech extraction, *Am J Obstet Gynecol* 161:111-114, 1989.
17. Gonen R et al: The outcome of triplet, quadruplet, and quintuplet pregnancies managed in a perinatal unit: obstetric, neonatal, and follow-up data, *Am J Obstet Gynecol* 162:454-459, 1990.
18. Greig PC et al: The effect of presentation and mode of delivery on neonatal outcome in the second twin, *Am J Obstet Gynecol* 167:901-906, 1992.
19. Herruzo AJ et al: Perinatal morbidity and mortality in twin pregnancies, *Int J Gynecol Obstet* 36:17-22, 1991.
20. Kahn A et al: Sudden infant death syndrome in a twin: a comparison of sibling histories, *Pediatrics* 78:146-150, 1986.
21. Kleinman JC, Fowler MG, Kessel SS: Comparison of infant mortality among twins and singletons: United States 1960 and 1983, *Am J Epidemiol* 133:133-143, 1991.
22. Laros RK, Dattel BJ: Management of twin pregnancy: the vaginal route is still safe, *Am J Obstet Gynecol* 158:1330-1338, 1988.
23. Leonard C et al: Outcome of very low birth weight infants: multiple gestation versus singletons, *Pediatrics* 93:611-615, 1994.
24. Lipitz S et al: The improving outcome of triplet pregnancies, *Am J Obstet Gynecol* 161:1279-1284, 1989.
25. Lipitz S et al: High-order multifetal gestation: management and outcome, *Obstet Gynecol* 76:215-218, 1990.
26. Luke B, Keith LG: The contribution of singletons, twins, and triplets to low birth weight, infant mortality and handicap in the United States, *J Reprod Med* 37:661-666, 1992.
27. McDiarmid JM, Silva PA: Three-year-old twins and singletons: a comparison of some perinatal, environmental, experiential, and develop-

mental characteristics, *Aust Paediatr J* 15:243-247, 1979.

28. Moilanen I, Rantakallio P: The growth, development and education of Finnish twins: a longitudinal follow-up study in a birth cohort form pregnancy to nineteen years of age, *Growth Dev Aging* 53:145-150, 1989.

29. Nelson KB, Wallenberg JH: Antecedents of cerebral palsy: multivariate analysis of risk, *New Engl J Med* 315:81-86, 1986.

30. Powers WF, Kiely JL: The risks of confronting twins: a national perspective, *Am J Obstet Gynecol* 170:456-461, 1994.

31. Rintahaka PJ, Hirvonen J: The epidemiology of sudden infant death syndrome in Finland in 1969-1980, *Forensic Sci Int* 30:291-333, 1986.

32. Ron-El R et al: Triplet and quadruplet pregnancies and management, *Obstet Gynecol* 57:458-463, 1981.

33. Ron-El R et al: Triplet, quadruplet and quintuplet pregnancies, *Acta Obstet Gynecol Scand* 71:347-350, 1992.

34. Rydhstrom H, Ingemarsson I, Ohrlander S: Lack of correlation between a high caesarean section rate and improved prognosis for low-birthweight twins (less than 2500 g), *Br J Obstet Gynaecol* 97:229-233, 1990.

35. Scheller JM, Nelson KB: Twinning and neurologic morbidity, *Am J Dis Child* 146:1110-1113, 1992.

36. Silva PA, Crosado B: The growth and development of twins compared with singletons at ages 9 and 11, *Aust Paediatr J* 21:265-267, 1985.

37. Silva PA, McGee RO, Powell J: Growth and development of twins compared with singletons at ages five and seven: a follow-up report from the Dunedin multidisciplinary child development study, *Aust Paediatr J* 18:35-36, 1982.

38. Smialek JE: Simultaneous sudden infant death syndrome in twins, *Pediatrics* 77:816-821, 1986.

39. Spellacy WN, Handler A, Ferre CD: A case-control study of 1253 twin pregnancies from a 1982-1987 perinatal data base, *Obstet Gynecol* 75:168-171, 1990.

40. Stanley F: Cerebral palsy in multiple births [Editorial], *Ir Med J* 82:97, 1989.

41. Thompson SA, Lyons TL, Makowski E: Outcomes of twin gestations at the University of Colorado Health Sciences Center, 1973-1983, *J Reprod Med* 32:328-339, 1987.

42. Young BK et al: Differences in twins: the importance of birth order, *Am J Obstet Gynecol* 151:915-921, 1985.

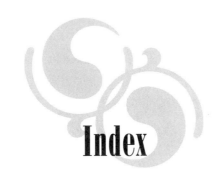

Index